THE CAPE DOCTOR IN
THE NINETEENTH CENTURY
A SOCIAL HISTORY

THE WELLCOME SERIES IN THE HISTORY OF MEDICINE

Forthcoming Title:

Making Health Policy, 1945–2000
Networks in Research and Policy
Edited by Virginia Berridge

The Wellcome Series in the History of Medicine series editors are
V. Nutton, C. J. Lawrence and M. Neve.
Please send all queries regarding the series to Michael Laycock,
The Wellcome Trust Centre for the History of Medicine at UCL,
24 Eversholt Street, London NW1 1AD, UK.

THE CAPE DOCTOR IN
THE NINETEENTH CENTURY
A SOCIAL HISTORY

Edited by
Harriet Deacon, Howard Phillips and
Elizabeth van Heyningen

Rodopi

Amsterdam – New York, NY 2004

First published in 2004
by Editions Rodopi B. V., Amsterdam – New York, NY 2004.

Harriet Deacon, Howard Phillips and
Elizabeth van Heyningen © 2004

Design and Typesetting by Michael Laycock,
The Wellcome Trust Centre for the History of Medicine at UCL.
Printed and bound in The Netherlands by Editions Rodopi B. V.,
Amsterdam – New York, NY 2004.

Index by Indexing Specialists (UK) Ltd.

British Library Cataloguing in Publication Data
A catalogue record for this book is available from the
British Library
ISBN 90-420-1064-9 (Paper)
ISBN 90-420-1074-6 (Bound)

'The Cape Doctor in the Nineteenth Century:
A Social History –
Amsterdam – New York, NY:
Rodopi. – ill.
(Clio Medica 74 / ISSN 0045-7183;
The Wellcome Series in the History of Medicine)

Front cover:
The District Surgeon of Simon's Town inoculating a patient during the bubonic
plague epidemic of 1901 (Source: *Cape Argus Weekly*, 8 May 1901).

© Editions Rodopi B. V., Amsterdam – New York, NY 2004
Printed in The Netherlands

All titles in the Clio Medica series (from 1999 onwards) are available to
download from the CatchWord website: http://www.catchword.co.uk

Contents

List of Illustrations

1

List of Tables

List of Figures

Foreword

The authors of this fascinating and long overdue account of the evolution of medicine and medical practice in the Cape from the British takeover in 1806 through to the establishment of the Union of South Africa in 1910 are to be commended for providing us with a unique window into the origins of contemporary health care in South Africa.

There are any number of impressions and insights to be gained from reading the book. What struck me most upon reading *The Cape Doctor* were the historical parallels from that era that mirror the problems and dilemmas confronting today's medical practice, much along the lines of the trite French idiom, '*Plus ça change, plus c'est la même chose*' ('the more things change, the more they remain the same'). For example, the question of whether doctors should dispense medicines is as much a medico-political flashpoint between doctors, pharmacists (apothecaries) and government regulators now as it was in the 1800s. Then, as now, the establishment was more likely to tolerate dispensing doctors in rural rather than in urban settings.

District surgeoncy is an old tradition, having had its origins in the Dutch East India Company's *chirurgijns* (colonial surgeons) of the 1700s. However, during the subsequent British occupation, district surgeons were usually British immigrants who were perceived as serving the political interests of the government of the day, in the same way that district surgeons came to be regarded during the apartheid years. The book says that they were 'drawn into the [Boer-British political] conflict through their work in examining slaves beaten by their masters', in contravention of British law, and it would seem that many district surgeons identified with the British policy to 'civilise' the Boer.

There are other parallels which emerge from reading *The Cape Doctor*, including the conflict between allopathic physicians and practitioners of 'alternative' or 'complementary' medicine. 'Real' doctors were those that were formally trained in European medical schools. But later – and as happened in the new South Africa – the registration of 'foreign' (then meaning non-British) medical

7

qualifications was severely restricted. The history of medicine in the Cape is inseparably interwoven with the political history of the region, and medical care and practice were profoundly influenced by political change of the time, much as the current health care system was profoundly influenced by the political changes of 1994.

The Cape Doctor is well researched and provides a wealth of data on a large variety of medical-historical topics, *inter alia*, the origins of the Somerset and other early hospitals, medical associations, the *South African Medical Journal*, and Cape medical education. The authors are to be commended on a project well done.

Professor Dan J. Ncayiyana
(Editor, South African Medical Journal, *and*
Deputy Vice-Chancellor, University of Cape Town).

Note on Contributors

Harriet Deacon (PhD Cantab.), Elizabeth van Heyningen (PhD UCT) and Howard Phillips (PhD UCT) are social historians of medicine working in Cape Town, the first two as independent scholars and the latter as an associate professor in the Department of Historical Studies at UCT. Anne Digby (PhD University of East Anglia) is Research Professor in History at Oxford Brookes University. Sally Swartz (PhD UCT) and Felicity Swanson (MA UCT) both worked on the history of colonial psychiatry in the Cape for their higher degrees and are now on the staff at UCT, the former in the Department of Psychology and the latter in the Centre for Popular Memory.

Acknowledgements

Many people and institutions have been involved in the making of this volume. Research funds and facilities have been generously provided by the University of Cape Town, Oxford Brookes University, the Wellcome Trust, the Beit and Oppenheimer Funds in Oxford, the Queen's College in Oxford, and by the Robben Island Museum. We are very grateful for this assistance. Invaluable assistance has been rendered to researchers by the staffs of the Manuscripts and Archives Division of UCT Library, the UCT Medical Library, the African Studies Division of UCT Library, the Cape Archives Depot and the Cape Medical Museum in Cape Town, as well as the Cory and Killie Campbell libraries. Many colleagues have also contributed to the book through incisive commentary and debate when individual chapters were presented at conferences and seminars, particularly at the Medicine and the Colonies conference in Oxford in 1996, in the History of Medicine seminar series at UCT in 1997-1999 and the conference on indigenous medicine hosted by Professor Anne Digby and Helen Sweet at Oxford Brookes University in 1999. Thanks are also due to Professor A.J. Christopher for permission to use maps from his book and to Ann Westoby for drawing all the maps.

The authors

Note on Terminology

Practitioner / Doctor

We have used 'practitioner' to refer to medical practitioners of any sort, including indigenous and alternative healers, but we have used 'doctor' to refer to those practitioners trained specifically in mainstream western medicine.

Black / White

In this book we recognise the importance of understanding racial discrimination as part of the history of the medical profession in South Africa. We have therefore used racial terminology (black / white) to distinguish between those who were accepted by the colonial authorities and by colonial society as 'Europeans' or whites, and those who were not (blacks). This is of course a social rather than a natural distinction.

Khoisan / Khoekhoe / Khoi / San

Some of the indigenous peoples who lived off the land around Cape Town and in the interior, mainly to the west and north, were hunter-gatherers, and others were pastoralists. The Dutch called the former 'Bushmen' and the latter 'Hottentots'. Although later scholars have attempted to get away from the pejorative uses of these words by inventing new terms (San and Khoi or Khoekhoe respectively), which we have used in this book, there has also been a recognition that the distinction between the two is not always sustainable (hence the use of the term Khoisan as well).

Coloured

In the *apartheid* era as well as during the British colonial period in South Africa, lighter-skinned people descended from a mixture of Khoisan, settler, African or East Asian parentage were called 'coloured'. To some extent it has now been accepted as a term of self-definition.

13

Kafir / Caffre / African / Xhosa / Native

Although we accept that those who lived in Africa, and certainly those who lived there before 1652, could all have been termed Africans, in this book we have used the term African specifically to refer to those black indigenous inhabitants of the Cape who were probably not identified as Khoisan, 'Malay' or 'coloured'. For the purposes of this book, most of the African groups mentioned in the text would have been Xhosa-speaking. During the nineteenth century the word 'Kafir' or 'Caffre' was often used to designate either Africans in general (in the specific sense mentioned above) or Xhosa-speaking Africans living in the eastern Cape. Sometimes used in a derogative way during the nineteenth century, by the twentieth century it had become, like 'native', a generally derogatory term. We have thus avoided the use of these terms except in quotations.

Dutch or Cape Dutch Settlers / Afrikaners

The Dutch-speaking white settler community at the Cape came from a range of continental European countries, but predominantly from the Netherlands and Germany. Most immigrated to the Cape before 1806. Although there was considerable intermixing with the local slave and Khoisan population, by the end of the nineteenth century those who saw themselves as 'white' had developed a strong racialised identity as Afrikaners. We have referred to this group as Dutch or Cape Dutch settlers in the early part of the century, and as Afrikaners in the latter part of the century.

Dutch / Cape Dutch / Afrikaans

By the eighteenth century a creole language, sometimes called 'kombuistaal' or 'kitchen language', based on Dutch with an infusion of African and East Asian languages, had begun to develop at the Cape. As a kind of shorthand, we have referred to this creole as 'Dutch' or 'Cape Dutch'. This was formally recognised by the Afrikaner nationalist movement of the mid- to late-nineteenth century as Afrikaans, which term we have used for the later chapters.

Abbreviations

BMA	British Medical Association
CA	Cape Archives Depot, Cape Town
ChB	Bachelor of Surgery
CMC	Colonial Medical Committee (Council from 1891)
CO	Colonial Office
Col. Sec.	Colonial Secretary
CPP	Cape Parliamentary Papers
DEIC	Dutch East India Company
DSAB	Dictionary of South African Biography
DRC	Dutch Reformed Church
DS	District Surgeon
GP	General Practitioner
JAH	Journal of African History
JMASA	Journal of the Medical Association of South Africa
JSAS	Journal of Southern African Studies
LBS	Ladies' Benevolent Society
LMS	London Missionary Society
MB	Bachelor of Medicine
MC	Master of Surgery
MD	Doctor of Medicine
MLA	Member of the (Cape) Legislative Assembly
MOH	Medical Officer of Health
NSH	New Somerset Hospital
OSH	Old Somerset Hospital
PRO	Public Record Office, London
QBSAL	Quarterly Bulletin of the South African Library
RCA	Cape Town (Bouquet Street), Archives of the Roman Catholic Church
RM	Resident Magistrate
RUCL	Rhodes University, Cory Library
SACA	South African Commercial Advertiser
SAMA	South African Medical Association
SAMJ	South African Medical Journal

Abbreviations

SAMR	South African Medical Record
SESA	Standard Encyclopedia of South Africa
SMC	Supreme Medical Committee
St MMBS	St Mary's Mutual Benefit Society
TMJ	Transvaal Medical Journal
UCS	Under Colonial Secretary
UCT	University of Cape Town

1

Introduction:
The Cape Doctor in the Nineteenth Century

Harriet Deacon

The Cape Doctor, named after the profession as well as the wind that sweeps the Cape Peninsula of dangerous miasmas, is a social history of medicine, seeking to place formal western medicine within its political, social and economic context. Besides Shula Marks' study of South African nurses, *Divided Sisterhood,* no previous work has brought such a breadth of material about South Africa's medical past under the framework of social history. This work provides clear evidence of the way in which the Cape medical profession excluded all but a few women and black practitioners, and discriminated along lines of race, class and gender in their practice, but it also moves beyond the classic revisionist tradition (documenting the emergence of a society divided along lines of race and gender) by providing examples of cultural crossover and medical pluralism.

> Without the south-easter (or 'Cape Doctor') they must have fevers etc.; and, though too rough a practitioner for me, he befits the general health.[1]

The 'Cape Doctor' is a nickname for the south-east wind that blows in the hot summers of the western Cape, especially around Cape Town. It was so named by early European settlers because it was thought to have healing properties, cooling the overheated air and blowing away the disease-bearing urban air. It is thus a fitting title for this book, which is the first comprehensive social history of the 'Western' medical profession in the nineteenth-century Cape Colony. *The Cape Doctor*[2] is a social history of medicine, seeking to place formal Western medicine within its political, social and economic context. Besides Shula Marks' study of nurses,[3] no previous work has brought such a breadth of material about South Africa's medical past under the framework of social history.[4] This work provides clear evidence of the way in which the Cape medical profession excluded all but a few women and black practitioners, and discriminated along lines of race, class and gender in their practice. It revises traditional whiggish and linear accounts of professional advancement, but it also moves beyond the classic revisionist tradition (documenting the emergence of a society divided along lines of race and gender) by providing examples of cultural crossover and medical pluralism.

Although its temporal and geographical scope is limited, this work provides one view into a broad historical process within which one can understand present debates about the most appropriate health policies in South Africa today. South Africa's current health system is characterised by huge disparities between urban and rural facilities, between private and public health services and between the high-tech preoccupations which drove the first heart transplant at Groote Schuur hospital in Cape Town in 1967 and the pressing need for primary health care. These disparities can be blamed only partly on the policies of racial discrimination implemented during the *Apartheid* years between 1948 and 1994, for the architects of *Apartheid* drew also on accepted international practice, and built on the foundations laid by the profession and British colonial government during the nineteenth century. South Africa has adopted a form of what Fox has called 'hierarchical regionalism', a set of assumptions behind health care policy uncritically adopted by most developed countries during the twentieth century. This approach centralises the production of medical knowledge, focuses on cure rather than prevention and unwittingly creates a situation in which health costs spiral upwards.[5] Concerns about the high cost of biomedicine and a loss of faith in its superior efficacy in curing or preventing all complaints has resulted in a softening of the official approach to alternative practice, both in South Africa (where traditional healers have always cornered the largest slice of the market) and elsewhere.

The ideologies, practices, and institutional and professional structures behind modern health care have also been deeply influenced by changes in health care provision and practice during the nineteenth century. Belief in the continuous progress of medical science and its applications developed in the late nineteenth-century with new scientific methods and approaches.[6] The roles of institutions, the state and the medical profession itself, were profoundly altered during the course of the nineteenth century which provided the foundations for a centralised, urban-biased, hospital-oriented, largely white male medical profession in the twentieth century. These disparities have helped to cement divisions between doctors, alternative practitioners and other medical professionals like nurses and midwives. In this volume we examine the roots of class, race and gender disparities in a biomedical profession that remains under-representative of its clients even today, as well as the urban focus of doctors and the emergence of hospital practice as an element of professional advancement.

One of the most interesting features of the history of the medical profession at the Cape is its place within a diverse medical market. While the authors do not dispute the fact that biomedical therapies can and do offer some therapeutic advantages over other therapies today, they question the often-stated corollary that alternative therapies, however unscientific, do not, and that biomedicine is, almost by definition, more efficacious.[7] What we wish to suggest in this volume is that the advancement of the biomedical profession at the Cape during the nineteenth century had less to do with therapeutic efficacy or preordained superiority than with political and socio-economic factors. Although there are clear differences between western medicine and forms of traditional healing used in South Africa, until the last quarter of the nineteenth century western medicine had little therapeutic advantage over other therapies. Doctors had secured state support for a monopoly on legal practice as early as 1807, and it was this fact which allowed the profession to expand within both private practice and public institutions in spite of the fact that most South Africans continued to consult traditional healers. By examining the emergence of a powerful, state-sanctioned medical profession in an environment where home remedies and other forms of household medical care have always been the first resort, and where alternative practice is usually the second therapeutic choice, this book can help us to think more creatively about addressing the problems and examining the possibilities of high-tech biomedicine in developing countries today.

This book can contribute to the process of transformation in the medical sector today by helping us to understand a range of issues in South African medical history, including the plurality of the medical market, the consolidation of the medical profession, and discrimination within policy and medical care. The book is an edited volume which attempts to do more than simply provide a collection of related papers: it provides the reader with a series of thematic chapters organised on a roughly chronological and geographical basis. It is a book primarily about doctors, so it cannot do full justice to the histories of other practitioners such as nurses, midwives, diviners, herbalists and homeopaths. The book does however try and understand the western doctor as only one group within a broader medical market. Although most of the doctors were white males, we have included examples of female and black practitioners where possible, and have discussed the ways in which the profession excluded, and competed with, female and black practitioners. Focusing on broad trends which affected doctors, the book does not seek to replace the detailed analyses provided by other works. In order to provide some historical detail, however, we have combined pithy analysis with case studies. Although biographical case studies have been used in previous works, we use biography to enrich our analytical points rather than to provide a heroic history of the great doctors of the nineteenth century. Historical detail about the lives and professional careers of medical practitioners is often also useful in identifying unexpected differences and similarities between past and present, and across geographical borders – issues which are often flattened and hidden by comparative analysis.

The colonial context

To introduce the debates covered in the rest of the book, we now outline the colonial context, discussing the broad trajectory of colonialism at the Cape, the influence of metropolitan models on the medical profession, and comparing the Cape with other British colonies. Then we prepare the ground for the more detailed analyses in subsequent chapters by discussing a few key features of the medical profession at the Cape.

Metropolitan models

There is an interesting dialectic between metropolitan and local influences on Western medicine in colonial contexts. As both David Arnold and Shula Marks have pointed out recently, there are important 'precedents and parallels' between metropolitan and colonial patterns of medical professionalisation and competition for a share of the medical market. These common features were no accident, as the majority of nineteenth-century doctors in Australia, New Zealand and the Cape were born and/or trained in Europe. Colonial doctors, like other settlers and officials, projected many European concerns onto the colonial context. For all its supposed universality, 'scientific' medicine was neither race-, class- nor gender-blind – not in Europe, nor in its colonies.[8] In addition, what European professional organisations and their members did, often served in the colonial context as a definition of best practice – in professional education, legislation, organisation and the management of competition. These metropolitan ideals (perpetuated by medical societies in the colonies) were of course not always as fluid and heterogeneous as metropolitan (or colonial) realities.

European empires influenced Europe as well as being affected by it.[9] Medical practices and priorities thus did not only travel from metropole to colony, but also in the other direction. It has recently been suggested that evidence gathered in the Cape encouraged Robert Knox to postulate his phrenological theories of scientific racism in Scotland, for example.[10] Cape doctors were not however renowned for their contributions to European science or medical procedure in the nineteenth century. William Atherstone's successful experiment with anaesthesia in 1847 was perhaps the most famous Cape medical experiment of the time,[11] but it was one of many similar experiments elsewhere in that decade and did not substantially change the practice of anaesthesia in Europe. Nor did Cape doctors add significantly to the medical pharmacopoeias of Europe during the mid-nineteenth century, the only Cape additions to the British pharmacopoeia being *buchu* and aloe in the eighteenth century. Some Cape doctors did publish in British medical journals, but their international scientific profile was generally low.[12] Cape doctors did not play a key role in the development of European scientific medicine in the nineteenth century. Perhaps the South African medical event of the twentieth century most influential in medical science worldwide was the heart transplant conducted by Dr Chris Barnard in Cape Town in 1967.

The Cape was unusual, although not unique, among European colonies in having more than one metropolitan tradition influencing its medical profession during the nineteenth century. At the beginning of the century, a majority of Cape doctors had been trained in Germany and the Netherlands, but by the end of the century, most had been trained in Scotland and England (see Chapter 4). Cape doctors thus drew on different European professional traditions and models in order to meet their needs at different times. One example of this is the conflict over the legal right of rural doctors to dispense medicines in the first half of the century. Under the legislation of 1807, drawn up jointly by British and German doctors for the Cape governor, Cape Town doctors were prevented from dispensing medicines while rural doctors were permitted to do so. In continental Europe, it was common practice for dispensing to be left to apothecaries, but in Britain, provincial general practitioners were allowed to dispense medicines freely. Cape apothecaries, many of whom were continentally trained in the first half of the century, used European precedent to call for enforcement of the 1807 regulations against dispensing doctors. These doctors, an increasing number of whom were British-trained, invoked British practice and local necessity to justify their dispensing activities and to call for legal change (see Chapter 3).

While the professional concerns of the Cape doctor, and other medical practitioners, were quite close to those of their European counterparts, these concerns were expressed under different circumstances. The local situation affected the timing of protective legislation and the establishment of professional education at the Cape – two key markers of professionalisation. The close relationship between the Cape medical establishment and the colonial state, and the absence of entrenched rival professional bodies, hastened the implementation of protective legislation for the Cape medical profession in the nineteenth century. Cape legislation which assured European-trained doctors of a monopoly over medical practice and registered physicians, surgeons and apothecaries, defining their different roles under the same professional umbrella, was passed as early as 1807, almost half a century before the Medical Act of 1858 in England did the same. Even then, the British legislation did not ban unlicensed medical practice, as Cape law had. Under Cape law, nurses and midwives were registered from 1891, again some years before their British counterparts received legal protection and government ratification of their training.

Colonial comparisons

Medical training, professional organisation, medical legislation and individual doctors themselves were born and reshaped in an imperial context that took in not only the metropole and its individual colonial offshoots, but the whole network of inter-colonial contacts. The Cape doctor had much in common with doctors in Australia, India, New Zealand and Canada in the nineteenth century. Military doctors transferred between the various colonial medical services and army outposts. Civilian doctors also sometimes travelled from colony to colony, working with men who had trained in the same medical schools, under professional bodies closely linked to European colleges and guilds, governed by colonial legislation that had been carved from the same metropolitan models or shared between colonies independently of the metropole.

The south-western Cape had been added to the European colonial empire as early as 1652, and European settlement began in earnest during the early eighteenth century, well before Australia or New Zealand. Yet the Cape profession took longer than the Australasian colonies to develop its professional confidence and colonial identity *vis a vis* the metropolitan profession. The Cape lagged far behind India and Australia in starting its own medical school, and even further behind Canada. It was only early in the twentieth century that the first Cape medical school opened its doors (see Chapter 4). The establishment of colonial medical schools was linked to the presence of a strong local professional lobby. In Upper Canada, rivalry between professional medical organisations, competition with U.S. medical schools and the fear that Canadian doctors would be trained in the U.S.A. encouraged the establishment of Canadian medical schools.[13] The only Cape-based professional organisation of any long-term significance before the 1880s was the Medical Committee, appointed by the government to undertake a limited range of registration and advisory activities related to the 1807 Act and its successors. British professional organisations such as the Royal College of Surgeons, to which many Cape doctors belonged by mid-century, had little interest in or impact on professional organisation in the colony until local branches of the British Medical Association were established in the 1880s.

Over the last decade there has been growing interest in the history of medical legislation in South Africa, an interest linked to the attempt to analyse the emergence of legal racism before apartheid.[14] The framework and content of nineteenth-century medical legislation was copied and adapted by countries in Europe and its sprawling nineteenth-century empire, illustrating the often close connections between spatially distant administrations. One clearcut example is the contagious diseases legislation, adapted from British legislation to protect the health and discipline of the British army at the Cape.[15] Differences in the form or application of medical legislation among colonies and between colonies and the metropole can be very revealing as to local priorities and possibilities. An interesting example is legislation passed in the late-nineteenth century to stem the spread of leprosy, then believed to be a highly contagious disease spreading from black and Chinese people to white colonials and even possibly to countries like America. In the latter country the main focus was on immigration controls for Asians, and on local institutionalisation. In India, paupers alone were institutionalised. Of all the options selected for controlling leprosy, the solution found in the Cape Colony was the most severe: compulsory institutionalisation of all identified sufferers. This solution can be clearly linked in contemporary documents to the (incorrect) belief among Cape officials that leprosy was a black disease and that there was not a large number of sufferers.[16]

Doctors themselves also moved between colonies within the European empires, making comparisons and connections as they moved. This was as true of the Cape under Dutch East India Company (DEIC) rule in the eighteenth century as under British rule in the nineteenth century. One particularly interesting medical traveller was John Fitzgerald, whose professional work in New Zealand and the eastern Cape of South Africa showed remarkable similarities. Elizabeth van Heyningen[17] has traced the career of Fitzgerald from one colony to the other, pointing out how his ideas were shaped by the dual interaction with Maori and African healing traditions. An interesting feature of Fitzgerald's career is his ongoing link to the colonial governor of New Zealand and later the Cape, Sir George Grey. This underlines the connections which should be made both between and within colonial medical history.

Patterns of colonisation at the Cape

Patterns of settlement, demographics, shifting professional status and economic fortunes which can be identified among Western-trained doctors at the Cape were rooted in broader patterns of colonialism in Southern Africa and the rest of the Empire. The area around Cape Town was the first part of South Africa to be colonised by Europeans in 1652. In 1795 an expanding territory stretching from the Buffels River in the north-western Cape to the Fish River in the eastern Cape was an outpost of the DEIC, with one main town, Cape Town, servicing DEIC ships on the East Asian trading routes. There were a few outlying villages, surrounded by wheat, wine and stock farms where settlers employed East Asian and African slaves and indigenous Khoisan in varying degrees of harsh servitude. When the British took over administration of the colony in 1795 (with a brief gap between 1803 and 1806), they continued to push the boundaries of the Cape colony northwards and eastwards into the lands of Griqua, Tswana, Xhosa and other indigenous Africans. With the settlement of British immigrants on the colony's eastern borders in the 1820s and the expansion of the wool trade in that area thereafter, towns like Port Elizabeth and Grahamstown flourished. Until the 1870s, most European settlement was thus concentrated in the narrow coastal belts between the ports of Cape Town and Port Elizabeth, with scattered inland stock-farming and trading making up the balance.

In the interior by mid-century, disaffected Dutch-speaking

settlers had moved northwards to establish the Orange Free State and the South African Republic (the Transvaal), while on the east coast, British settlers had established another colony called Natal. After the 1870s, with the discovery of diamonds (near Kimberley) and later gold (on the Witwatersrand), the economic engine of the colony shifted to the interior, and moved into a higher gear. Mining essentially drove the industrial revolution in Southern Africa in the last quarter of the century, creating conditions in which there was high European immigration, great population mobility within Southern Africa and systematic exploitation of black labour through the migrant labour system. It was also the quest to control gold resources which prompted the South African (Anglo-Boer) War in 1899-1902. Britain's victory ensured the Union of South Africa under British rule in 1910, which united the Cape with Natal, the Orange Free State and the Transvaal.[18]

To illustrate some of these trends, Figure 1.1 (overleaf) shows the growth of the Cape's political boundaries, and Figure 1.2 shows the expansion of European settlement over the course of the nineteenth century.

The Cape medical profession

Patterns of European colonisation in the Cape and elsewhere, coupled with metropolitan models, provided the framework within which western-trained doctors entered the medical market. There are several key features of the nineteenth-century Cape profession and the medical market within which it operated:

- Doctors at the Cape were predominantly white male immigrants who came from Europe. At the beginning of the century, the profession was dominated by Dutch and German men, but after 1820 increased British immigration led to the numerical dominance of British-born and British-trained doctors by mid-century.

- The total number of doctors practising at the Cape was never very high, ranging from about 45 licensed in 1807-8 (in a settler population of just under 30,000) to about 629 in 1904 (in a settler population of around 580,000).[19]

- In the absence of a fully fledged local medical school before 1920, doctors all had to acquire, or at least complete, their medical training outside South Africa in order to be licensed.

Figure 1.1
General political boundaries in South Africa
(A.J. Christopher, Southern Africa, p14)

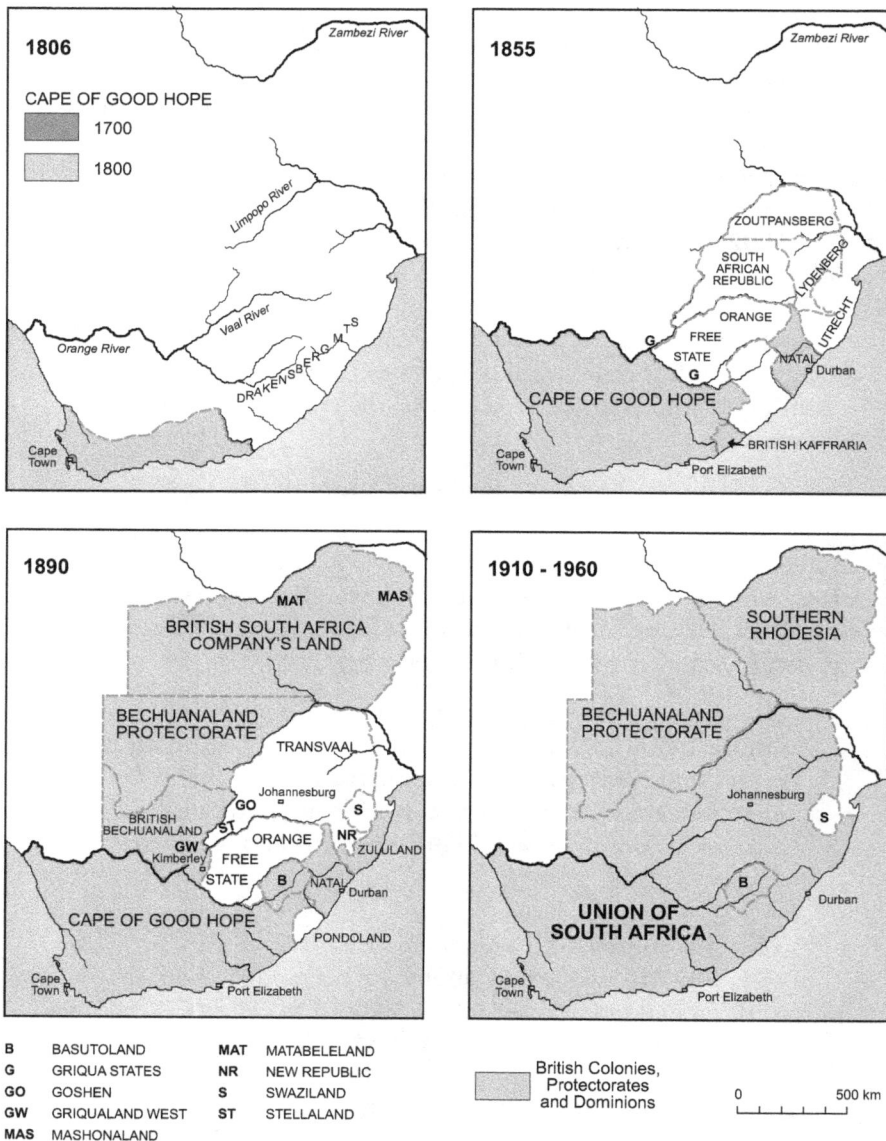

B	BASUTOLAND	MAT	MATABELELAND
G	GRIQUA STATES	NR	NEW REPUBLIC
GO	GOSHEN	S	SWAZILAND
GW	GRIQUALAND WEST	ST	STELLALAND
MAS	MASHONALAND		

British Colonies, Protectorates and Dominions

0   500 km

Figure 1.2
European settlement also showing major black groups in the sub-
continent (A.J. Christopher, Southern Africa, *p247)*

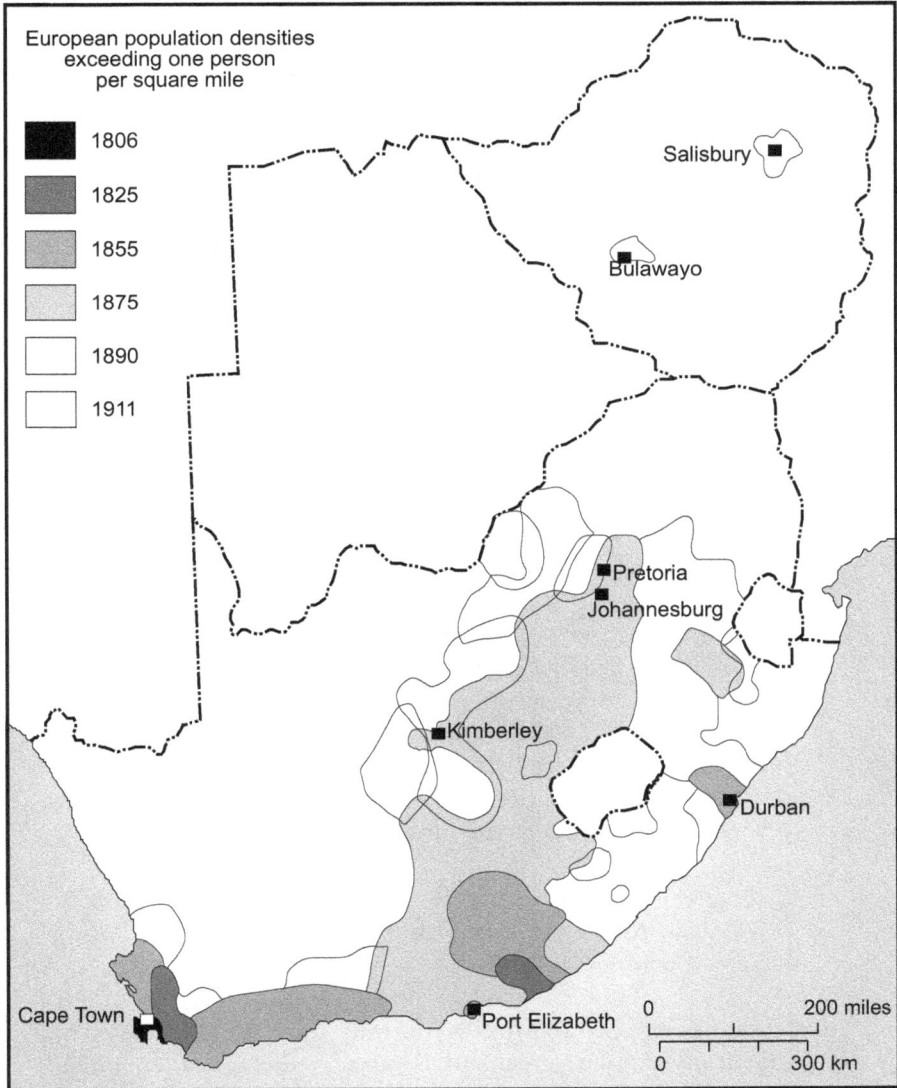

- Doctors congregated where most of their patients were – in the major coastal towns before the 1870s and among the mobile populace seeking gold and diamond wealth thereafter. Doctors thus had to be adaptable (many rural doctors sold medicines or had second occupations) and mobile (as they sought to establish sizeable practices in an increasingly oversupplied medical market).

- Cape Town was the largest town in the colony and as the focus of colonial government it was also a key administrative centre. It was therefore the main locus for doctors' attempts at professionalisation until mid-century and still the key centre for private practice and institutional appointments thereafter.

- Doctors' patients were considerably more heterogeneous in terms of class, gender and race than were the doctors themselves. Although many of these patients would have been white and relatively wealthy, the medical market was not as racially segmented as one might have expected in an increasingly racist colonial society. Some white patients consulted black practitioners, and some black patients consulted white doctors, even where they were not forced into that relationship through institutionalisation.

- Although doctors were nervous about comparisons with tradesmen in the first half of the century, growing economic pressures and more secure social status meant that they were more willing to talk about the economics of medical practice in public fora than were British doctors 'at home' by the end of the century. The difficulties of establishing viable private practices contributed to the mobility of the profession.

- In spite of legislative support for professional regulation as early as 1807, in reality the market for medical services was poorly regulated before the 1890s.

- Western-trained doctors were only one small group of practitioners in a large and diverse medical market which included medical missionaries, indigenous Khoisan (known to early settlers as 'Hottentots' and 'Bushmen') and other African healers, Muslim practitioners (often descendants of slaves), alternative Western healers and midwives.

The nineteenth century was a critical period in the emergence of the modern profession. During the course of the century the social, economic and professional standing of Cape doctors improved significantly, and their profession developed into what would today be a recognisable form of the modern profession. Doctors distanced themselves from other medical practitioners by invoking distinctions of gender, culture, race and class as well as by imposing legal, financial and educational barriers to entering the profession. The foundations of a hospital-based, urbanised, curatively oriented and professionally exclusive medical profession were laid by the end of a century within which the professional ideal had metamorphosed from gentleman doctor into scientist and health-policy professional. By 1900, heroic therapeutics modelled on humoral theories of disease were outmoded and interventions based on germ theories of disease were more common. Most important, however, was the emergence of a state-sanctioned, powerful and united medical profession which claimed high social and economic status and superiority over alternative practitioners. Today's biomedical professionals, who would not recognise themselves in the apprentice-trained doctors of 1800, would have much more in common with the university-trained, biomedically oriented doctors of 1900.

To illustrate the changes within the profession during the nineteenth century, we provide a view of the world as would have been seen by two Cape doctors: one who visited at the beginning of the nineteenth century, when the profession was very small and unsure of itself; and the other who lived and worked there at the end of the century, when a much more mature and self-confident vocation was facing new challenges as a result of the socio-economic upheavals engendered by the mineral revolution.

Soon after the beginning of the nineteenth century, during the Batavian (Dutch) occupation of the Cape from 1803-5, the German doctor Heinrich Lichtenstein (1780-1857) toured the Cape extensively. He was employed as personal physician to the family of General J.W. Janssens, who was then governor of the Cape, and as tutor to his son.[20] Lichtenstein was not entirely impressed with the small, parochial colony, in which European colonists 'gradually deteriorated [and]... declined culturally'.[21] But he was interested in the botanical, zoological and geological richness of the colony, which then extended as far east as the Fish River, as far west as the Hantam

Table 1.1
Doctors and the Cape population

Date	1805[i]	1807-8[ii]	1820[iii]	1865[iv]	1891	1904[v]
Number of doctors	55	45	55	143	336	629
Doctor: Cape settler	1:490	1:666	1:781	1:1,226[vi]	1:1,122	1:922
Doctor: Cape population[vii]			1:1,884	1:3,353	1:4,545	1:3,831

[i] The figures for doctors before 1865 are gleaned from H.J. Deacon's database of doctors, based on licensing records from the Cape Archives for the period 1807-1860. The population figures are based on an estimate of the settler population of the time at around 27,000 – A.J. Christopher, *Southern Africa* (Folkestone: Dawson, 1976), 248. The relatively high number of doctors in relation to the settler population may be as a result of the fact that, in the absence of census data, licensing regulations or comprehensive records of medical practitioners, we have used a database which includes some doctors who may not have been in active practice at this time or who were later excluded from the profession. The high proportion of doctors to settlers helps to illustrate the weak control that the profession exercised over entry into western-style medical practice before 1807.

[ii] For population figures in South Africa see R. Elphick and H. Giliomee, 'The origins and entrenchment of European dominance at the Cape, 1652-c.1840' in R. Elphick and H. Giliomee (eds) *The Shaping of South African Society, 1652-1840* (Cape Town, Maskew Miller Longman, 1989), 524; A.J. Christopher, *op. cit.* (note i), 248.

[iii] The population figures are from R. Elphick and H. Giliomee, *op. cit.* (note ii), 524.

[iv] A. Digby, 'A Medical El Dorado?: Colonial Medical Incomes and Practice at the Cape', *Social History of Medicine*, 7(3) (1995), 474, 477.

[v] *Ibid.*, 474, 477.

[vi] English doctor–patient ratios are around 1:1,400 at this time.

[vii] Unfortunately, because of the nature of colonial records, it is very difficult to get accurate black population figures for the colony.

mountains and as far north as the Nieuweveld Mountains up to the confluence of the Orange and Zeekoe Rivers.[22] In support of Batavian government policy at the Cape, Lichtenstein was interested in using the cowpox vaccine against smallpox developed by Jenner in England in 1796. In 1805 he travelled through the Karoo and the eastern Cape to vaccinate people against smallpox.[23] Lichtenstein's patients ranged from Cape Dutch settlers to their slaves and Khoisan employees, but he advocated a racist public health policy on smallpox, suggesting enforced segregation in 'abandoned farms' for black 'slaves and Hottentots [Khoisan]' and home isolation for white 'Christians'.[24] At this time there were probably around fifty-five doctors of various types (excluding apothecaries) practising in the Cape.[25] Just over half of these doctors were of German origin, the rest mainly Dutch or British. There were no comprehensive regulations restricting entry into medical practice at this time and some of those who styled themselves as doctors had been informally trained or locally apprenticed. Their therapeutic methods had more in common with humoral folk practices than the biomedical science of the late nineteenth century. Although in performing vaccinations Lichtenstein worked with some of these doctors, such as the surgeon Bekker in Tulbach, he also delegated vaccination duties to laymen.[26]

By the end of the century, the Cape medical profession would have presented a very different picture to another medically trained observer, Leander Starr Jameson (1853-1917) who was Prime Minister of the colony in the early twentieth century.[27] The Cape had by this time expanded its borders to approximately the current extent of the Western, Eastern and Northern Cape provinces of South Africa. Like most of his contemporaries within the profession by this time, Jameson was a British-born medical immigrant trained in a British university within a framework which emphasised the scientific nature of medicine and the importance of clinical investigation. He worked as a hospital doctor and private practitioner in Kimberley during the diamond boom of the 1880s, where, faced with the choice between ethical practice and financial reward, he sided with the latter (discussed further in Chapter 8). The mining boom and the South African (Anglo-Boer) War (1899-1902) brought a renewed flood of medical immigrants in the last decades of the century; in 1891 there were 336 licensed doctors on the Cape register and in 1904 there were 629. In the latter year, all but twelve of the doctors were white men.[28] Entry to the profession was regulated by a new law of 1891, which replaced earlier regulations first passed in 1807, and the profession itself was much more tightly organised and focussed through the establishment of professional associations (e.g. local branches of the British Medical Association [BMA]), local medical journals (e.g. the *South African Medical Record* [SAMR]) and by plans for a local medical school.

Cape doctors and colonial society

The social status of the Cape medical profession was enhanced by its ability to restrict entry into its ranks, both with respect to numbers and the social profile of those licensed to practise. Doctors worked hard to establish and protect a public image of themselves, first as professional gentlemen and later also as scientists, specialists or public policy experts.

Compared to Europe, America or even other settler colonies like Australia or Canada, the Cape Colony did not have large numbers of licensed Western-trained doctors during the nineteenth century. But if it is true that they found clients mainly in the settler population then competition between doctors would have been more intense in the Cape than in England, especially at the beginning and end of the century. Doctors in other colonial settlements also experienced more intense competition than in the metropole.[29] Table 1.1 shows how the Cape profession grew, and how this compared to the growth in the general population. At the Cape, only eighty-two doctors were formally licensed during the first fourteen years of licensing after 1807, of whom around fifty-five were still alive or in the country in 1820. Yet the settler population was small too: in 1820, it was only around 43,000. By the time of the first full census in 1865, the ratio of doctors to the settler population was rather more favourable for doctors. If one adds a few thousand black patients to the likely settler patient population, Cape doctor–patient ratios are quite comparable with metropolitan ones at this time. By the end of the century, however, the Cape had an increasingly marked oversupply of medical doctors.[30]

Throughout the nineteenth century, doctors were concentrated in urban areas of the Cape. This meant that urban doctor–patient ratios were generally higher than figures for the whole colony. In 1865, Cape Town and Grahamstown had far higher doctor–settler ratios than the rest of the colony (see Figure 1.3). The urban–rural disproportion at the Cape was consistent with the pattern in England, where in 1841, London had four times as many doctors, relative to population, as the least well-provided county.[31] This was true of other British colonies too: in Melbourne, Australia, in 1871, the doctor–patient ratio was 1:650 compared to a ratio of 1:1,239 in

Figure 1.3

Figure showing the higher density of doctors per settler populations in Cape Town and Grahamstown, compared to the rest of the Cape Colony, from the 1865 census.

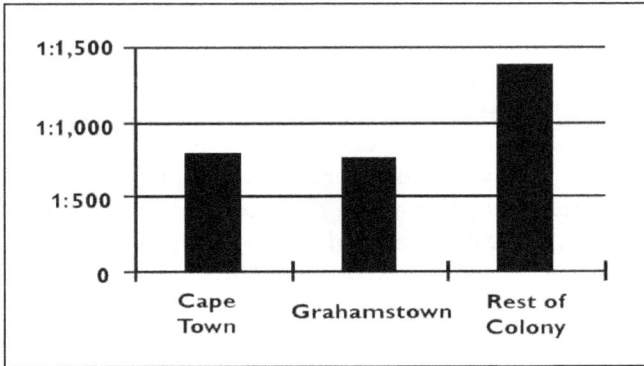

the colony of Victoria as a whole.[32] Pensabene comments that in the colony of Victoria the disparity between doctor–patient ratios in urban and rural areas became even more pronounced between 1871 and 1933, and urban medical markets became overcrowded.[33] In the Cape by the end of the nineteenth century, the problem of oversupply in Cape medical markets[34] would have been even more acute in urban areas.

Youngson has suggested that in the first half of the nineteenth century the English (and to a lesser extent the Scottish) medical profession, 'combined an almost medieval respect for tradition with an excessive admiration for the manners and attainments of an eighteenth-century gentleman'.[35] Professionalisation in Britain, and in colonies like the Cape and Canada,[36] was thus associated with the quest to identify doctors as gentlemen of high social status as well as to acquire the formal trappings of a profession such as legal protection against competitors, professional organisations and specialist training (see Chapter 3).[37] This ideal, although not always realised, became a key influence on the relationship between doctors and colonial society in the early nineteenth century. By the end of the century, more Cape doctors had been trained in clinical techniques at medical schools, and there was a greater emphasis on scientific knowledge as the basis of professional status and expertise. This transition was perhaps somewhat slower and less marked than in America, where Warner suggests that in the 1870s, scientific knowledge became the key to professional identity, whereas before the Civil War practical knowledge, morality and interaction with patients in accordance with shared medical beliefs had defined the essence of professional identity.[38] While scientific knowledge had also become more important to the public image of the profession at the Cape by the end of the nineteenth century, this did not always translate into a change in medical practice or a shift in the image of lower-status doctors.

In their dealings with competitors and clients, Cape doctors were very fortunate in having the support of the colonial government in terms of legislation and professional regulation. This helped the profession to define and protect itself socially and economically by controlling entry to legal medical practice. At the same time, Cape doctors were often called to further the broader aims of colonial expansion and to assist in scattered local struggles in which settlers fought for greater status and control.[39] Doctors were not 'agents of empire' in the sense that they subordinated their personal and professional interests to those of empire, but there were times when medical and imperial or colonial interests meshed very closely, such as during the segregation of parts of Cape Town during the plague scare of 1901.[40] Government-funded public health positions, hospitals and bacteriological laboratories provided some doctors with a platform from which they could launch themselves as public health experts, specialists and scientists.

Like lawyers, many Cape doctors were prominent in village-level society, local politics and in the colonial parliament. The impetus for public visibility was perhaps highest in urban centres (e.g. Cape Town and Grahamstown) and among British medical immigrants who sought Dutch-speaking clients in small country towns. A system of district surgeoncies, established by the Dutch and extended by the British in the 1820s, provided doctors with public office and a small salary, but did not prevent them from practising privately. Holding public positions like these helped doctors to represent themselves as altruistic professional gentlemen. Daniel O'Flinn, for example, an 1820 settler who practised in the largely Dutch-speaking farming Stellenbosch from about 1822 to his death in 1852, and was a district surgeon, served on the Agricultural Society, various other committees and was mayor of the town in 1832.[41] The first Cape parliament in 1854 included a number of doctors, as did the board of the South African Library and various other high-status Cape Town institutions. William Atherstone probably represented the ideal public face of the profession in the second half of the nineteenth century. He was active in promoting medical science and public health matters, advised on the medical legislation of 1891, and prompted the establishment of a Colonial Bacteriological Institute in Grahamstown in the same year. Outside of the medical field he was a prominent local figure, a renowned geologist and a Member of the Cape Parliament in 1881.[42]

Competition and complementarity within the medical market

The Western-trained Cape doctor was not alone in providing medical services to the Cape medical market. Alternative Western medical approaches like homeopathy were not well-represented at the Cape, unlike in Canada,[43] but settler folk medicine was well-established among the Cape Dutch settler community by 1800, and indigenous and slave medical practitioners were the first choice of black residents. Settler folk medicine drew extensively from Khoisan medical techniques and eastern practices brought to the Cape by slaves, feeding into a broad creole medical tradition in the western Cape (discussed in Chapter 2). This creole tradition incorporated European popular medical remedies such as the Halle patent medicines, which were manufactured in Germany and exported to the Cape (these 'Dutch Remedies' continue to be popular among black and white communities in South Africa today). Indigenous African traditions of herbalism and divining (discussed in Chapter 6), were part of the framework in which Africans interpreted and incorporated aspects of Western medicine into patterns of medical care in the northern and eastern Cape. An interesting feature of the heterogeneous Cape medical market during the nineteenth century is that while socio-economic differentiation and segregation of ethnic and racially defined groups increased in society as a whole, white patients continued to consult black practitioners using alternative healing methods, while black patients continued to consult white doctors using western healing methods.

Cape doctors' attitudes towards other practitioners are very revealing of their perceived or desired position within the local medical market. Indigenous practice was probably second only to informal household medicine in terms of its share of the Cape medical market, but licensed doctors generally spurned both indigenous practitioners and their methods. Understanding the spread and resilience of both the indigenous and settler folk sectors of the market still requires extensive research, but it could be that indigenous and settler folk practitioners did not compete in the same market niche as licensed doctors. In this book we suggest that Cape doctors ignored indigenous and folk medical practices partly because

Figure 1.4
Three figures showing the distribution of doctors at the Cape,
1807-1891

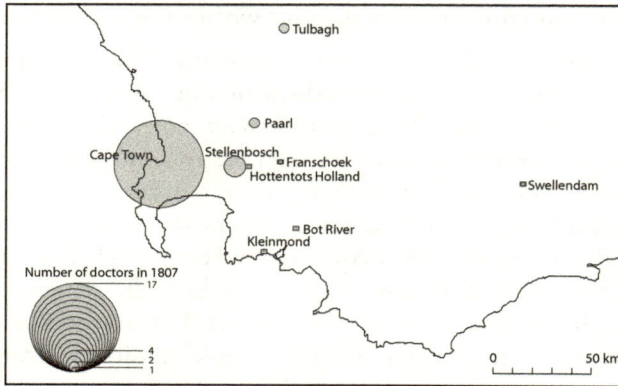

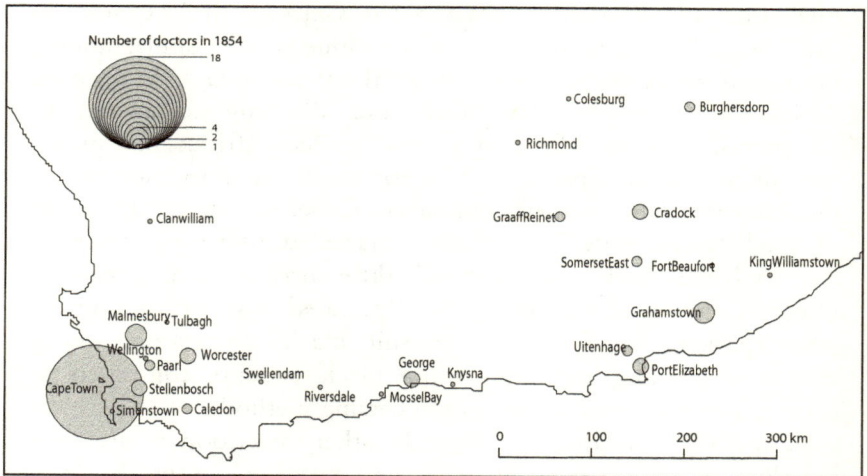

Number of doctors in 1807

Number of doctors in 1854

of ignorance but mainly because doctors felt threatened by acknowledging 'unscientific' practices as medicine, since their own claims to expertise were increasingly, although still hesitatingly, defined in relation to science. Cape doctors gave local midwives more attention than indigenous or folk practitioners. When midwives were mentioned, however, it was seldom with the vociferous antagonism expressed by American or British doctors, and largely to emphasise

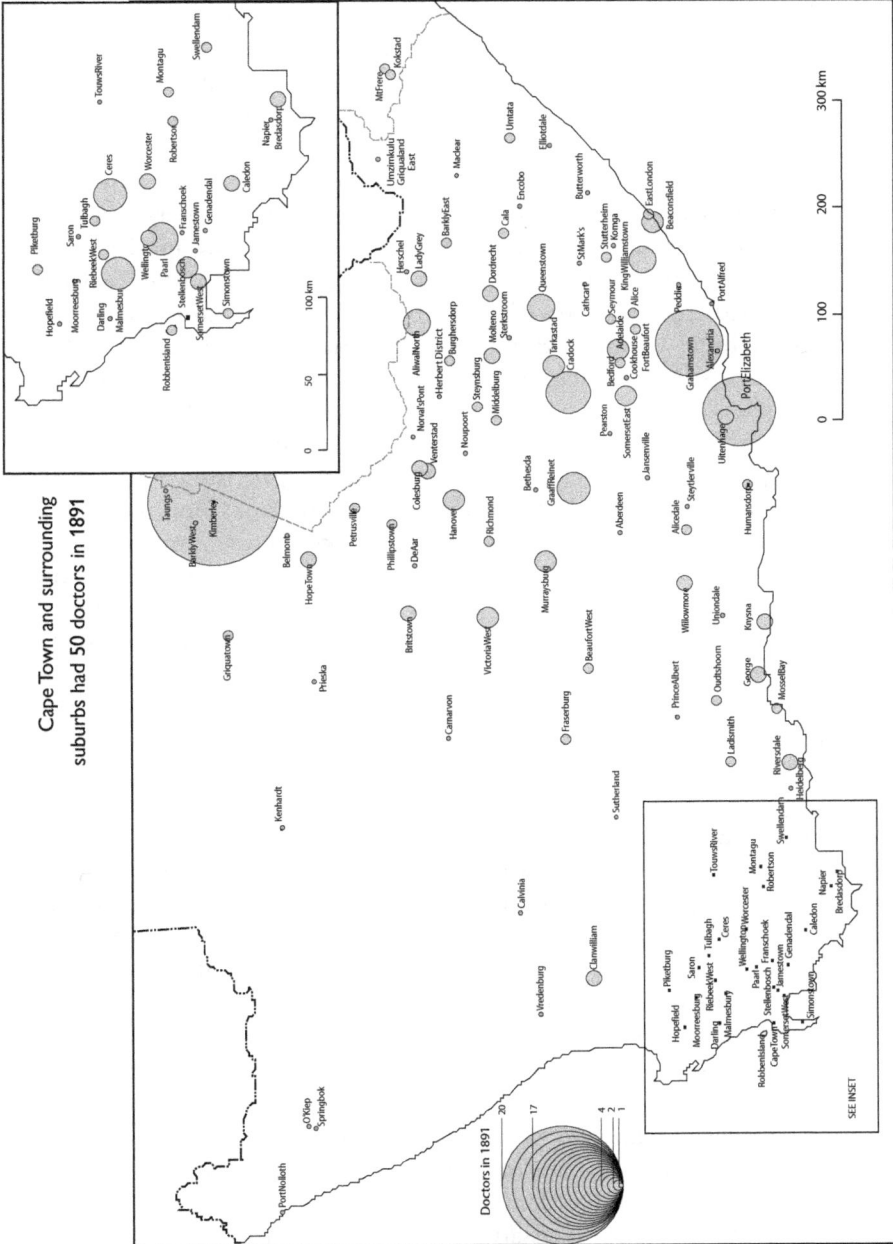

the need for training and the incapacity of untrained midwives. This may have been because of greater complementarity between doctors' and midwives' practice at the Cape than in Britain and America.[44] By the end of the nineteenth century, doctors were more wary of the challenge posed by midwives and formally established their subordinate position *vis a vis* doctors within the 1891 legislation (see Chapter 7).

In the nineteenth century, Cape doctors felt most threatened as professionals not by midwives or traditional practitioners, but by unlicensed practitioners in the Western tradition and by apothecaries and druggists who charged for medical advice and prescribed as well as sold medicines. In the early part of the century, doctors sought to establish their public and professional image as 'gentlemen' who provided medical services rather than 'tradesmen' who sold drugs. They tried to distance themselves publicly from the work of apothecaries and druggists while protecting their economic interests in drug sales and seeking a monopoly over the provision of medical advice. In well-regulated urban environments such as Cape Town and later Grahamstown, this distinction was both more important to doctors and more enforceable by government. The legislation of 1807 specifically prohibited Cape Town apothecaries and druggists from practising medicine, and set out a restricted list of drugs which doctors could sell. The regulatory legislation initially allowed a wider range of practice to both doctors and druggists in country towns, where medical practitioners of any kind were few and far between.

Once district surgeons were appointed to the rural interior of the colony after the 1820s and more druggists settled in these areas, however, competition between the two groups became more intense. District surgeons were allowed to inspect local druggist shops and to sell drugs as part of an incentive package to keep them in country districts, and this became an increasingly important part of their practice. For their part, country druggists did not hold back from practising medicine. Yet official response to the problem of growing competition was slow and ineffectual because of the gap between the interests of urban and rural doctors. In Cape Town the Medical Committee was more concerned to protect the interests of Cape Town apothecary houses, which supplied drugs to a lucrative market consisting of both country retailers and to doctors, than to protect the interests of country doctors. They also made little attempt to improve the regulatory legislation or to implement it more effectively in order to prevent apothecaries in isolated areas from practising medicine (see Chapter 3).[45]

Conclusion

Cape doctors were almost certainly outnumbered by indigenous and folk medical practitioners at the Cape throughout the nineteenth century but they occupied a niche within the medical market which was defined (and protected to some degree) by their legal and social status. This status was modelled on metropolitan ideals, shaped by colonial concerns and negotiated with local stakeholders. The nineteenth century was a key period in the consolidation of the professional, social and economic status of the mainstream Western medical profession in the Cape, as it was elsewhere. During the nineteenth century, Cape doctors fought many of the same battles for professional status and economic survival that doctors were fighting in America, Europe or its other colonies, but with slightly different emphases and outcomes.

Like professionals elsewhere, Cape doctors appealed for the assistance of government to cement their professional credibility and control, and to protect their claims to a share of the medical market. From as early as 1807, licenses for medical practice were issued only to doctors with a traditional European medical training. Perhaps this continued link with European medical schools was one reason why Cape doctors followed metropolitan models of training and practice even more closely than did colonial doctors in Upper Canada and Australia, where local medical education had already begun by 1870. Local circumstances, such as a heterogenous medical market in which Western-trained doctors were a small (though politically powerful) minority, also influenced doctors' professional identity. They sought to define themselves as professional gentlemen as opposed to tradesmen druggists, whose practice was clearly distinct from the 'old-fashioned' and supposedly 'irrational' practices of settler folk healers and indigenous practitioners.

Now that we have introduced the themes which will run through the rest of the volume, we will develop them in the essentially thematic chapters which follow. The second chapter looks at licensed doctors' relationships with other practitioners in the Cape medical market. It seeks to explain the dismissive attitude of the medical profession towards the use of indigenous medicinal plants, which were central to indigenous and folk settler and slave therapeutics. The third chapter explores the first steps towards professionalisation in the first half of the nineteenth century, especially in relation to the medical legislation of 1807, 1823 and 1830 and the development of an urban-rural divide within the profession. The fourth chapter examines the educational background of these doctors, discussing the implications of the relatively late introduction of university medical education at the Cape.

The fifth chapter discusses the effects of employment in the military, in civilian hospitals, charities, friendly societies and district surgeoncies on the early professional and economic status of Cape doctors. The next chapter examines the particular position of doctors working in frontier regions like the eastern Cape, where military doctors and medical missionaries played an important role within the profession. The seventh chapter discusses the emergence of a mature profession in the latter part of the nineteenth century, with particular reference to the establishment of professional authority through public health policy work. Thereafter, the eighth chapter explores the opportunities and limitations experienced by the medical profession in salaried employment within specialist hospitals (asylums) and industries spawned by the mineral discoveries of the 1870s. The ninth chapter examines the economic position of a number of such doctors in the last part of the nineteenth century, discussing both disparities within the profession and between doctors and people in other sorts of employment. The final chapter brings all these strands together to reflect on the importance of historical analysis to modern students of medicine and its place in South African society.

A social history of Western medicine during the nineteenth century can thus help us to understand not only more about the roots of the modern medical profession in South Africa, but also about its relationship with alternative practice, employers, the state and society in general. Through the relatively well-documented history of professional medicine, we can broaden our knowledge about the poorly documented history of indigenous medical practices, creole folk medicine and about some aspects of colonial society, such as the question of colonial identity and professionalisation, which are only now beginning to receive due attention from historians. In this book we hope to integrate these debates, traditionally seen as part of social history, with discussions relating to demographic and economic data so as to understand more fully the position of the medical profession in the nineteenth-century Cape.

Notes

1. L. Duff Gordon, *Letters from the Cape* (London: 1861-2), cited in J. Branford, *A Dictionary of South African English* (Oxford: Oxford University Press, 1978).

2. The term 'doctor' has been used to describe a medical practitioner trained in the mainstream Western medical tradition of the time. The term 'practitioner' has been used more generally to refer to all types of healers: see Note on Terminology.

3. S. Marks, *Divided Sisterhood: Race, Class and Gender in the South African Nursing Profession* (London: Macmillan, 1994).

4. The best existing study of the medical profession in the nineteenth-century Cape, which is written in an earlier historical paradigm and thus provides a limited investigation of the profession's social context, is E. Burrows, *A History of Medicine in South Africa* (Cape Town: Balkema, 1958). Other studies of the nineteenth-century Cape medical profession now read as eulogistic accounts of medical progress and an uncritical examination of the 'birth' of various sectors of the medical profession; P. Laidler and M. Gelfand, *South Africa: Its Medical History* (Cape Town: Struik, 1971); C. Searle, *A History of the Development of Nursing in South Africa 1652-1960* (Cape Town: Struik, 1965).

5. D. Fox, *Health Policies, Health Politics: the British and American Experience 1911-1965* (Princeton: Princeton University Press, 1986), introduction and epilogue.

6. *Ibid.*, 207.

7. B. Good, *Medicine, Rationality and Experience: An Anthropological Perspective* (Cambridge: Cambridge University Press, 1994), 28 suggests that we should compare the cultural constructions of illness in alternative medicine and in biomedical science rather than their claims for efficacy.

8. S. Marks, 'What is Colonial about Colonial Medicine? And What has Happened to Imperialism and Health?', *Social History of Medicine*, x, 2 (1997), 205–219.

9. A.L Stoler and F. Cooper, 'Between Metropole and Colony' in F. Cooper and A.L. Stoler (eds) *Tensions of Empire: Colonial Cultures in a Bourgeois World* (Berkeley: University of California Press, 1997), 1.

10. A. Bank, 'Of "Native Skulls" and "Noble Caucasians": Phrenology in Colonial South Africa', *JSAS*, xx, 3 (September 1996).

11. Burrows, *op. cit.* (note 4), 170–72.

12. S. Swartz, '"Work of Mercy and Necessity": British Rule and Psychiatric Practice in the Cape Colony 1891-1910', *International Journal of Mental Health*, xxviii, 2 (Summer 1999), 72–90.

13. B.R. Tunis, 'Medical Licensing in Lower Canada: The Dispute over Canada's First Medical Degree' and J.F. Kett, 'American and Canadian Medical Institutions, 1800-1870' in S.E. Shortt (ed.) *Medicine in Canadian Society* (Montreal: McGill-Queen's University

Press, 1981), 137–63, 189–205.

14. D. Foster, 'Introduction' in S. Lea and D. Foster (eds) *Perspectives on Mental Handicap in South Africa* (Durban: Butterworths, 1990); H.J. Deacon, 'Racial Segregation and Medical Discourse in Nineteenth-Century Cape Town', *JSAS*, xxii, 2 (1996), 287–308.

15. E. van Heyningen, 'The Social Evil in the Cape Colony 1868-1902: Prostitution and the Contagious Diseases Acts', *JSAS*, x, 2 (1984), 170–97.

16. H.J. Deacon, 'Leprosy and Racism at Robben Island' in E. van Heyningen (ed.), *Studies in the History of Cape Town*, vii (Cape Town: University of Cape Town Press, 1994), 45–83.

17. E. van Heyningen, 'Medicine and Empire: The Transmission of Ideas and Disease between India, Australia, New Zealand and the Cape Colony in the Nineteenth Century', Paper presented at the Ninth Historical Geography Conference, Perth, 1995.

18. See A.J. Christopher, *Southern Africa* (Folkestone: Dawson, 1976) for a historical geography of South Africa.

19. For European populations in South Africa see R. Elphick and H. Giliomee, 'The Origins and Entrenchment of European Dominance at the Cape, 1652-c.1840' in R. Elphick and H. Giliomee (eds), *The Shaping of South African Society, 1652-1840* (Cape Town: Maskew Miller Longman, 1989), 524; Christopher, *op. cit.* (note 18), 248. Unfortunately because of the nature of colonial records and the shifting boundary of the Colony it is very difficult to get accurate and comparable black population figures for the Colony.

20. See for example W.H.C. Lichtenstein, *Travels in Southern Africa*, 2 vols (Cape Town: Van Riebeeck Society, 1928-30).

21. W.H.C. Lichtenstein in O.H. Spohr (ed.), *Foundation of the Cape*, (Cape Town: Balkema, 1973), 15.

22. C. Koeman (ed.), *Tabulae Geographicae: Eighteenth-century Cartography of the Cape Colony* (Amsterdam: Hollandsch-Afrikaansche Uitgewers, 1952), 62.

23. E.M. Sandler, 'Lichtenstein's Vaccination Tour – 1805', Supplement to the *SAMJ*, xlviii (1974).

24. *Ibid.*, 12–13.

25. From H.J. Deacon's database of doctors, based on licensing records from the Cape Archives for the period 1807-1860.

26. Sandler, *op. cit.* (note 23), 7, 9.

27. Burrows, *op. cit.* (note 4), 258–9.

28. A. Digby, 'A Medical El Dorado?: Colonial Medical Incomes and Practice at the Cape', *Social History of Medicine*, vii, 3 (1995), 474.

29. *Ibid.*, 476.

30. *Ibid.*, 474, 477.
31. A. Digby, *Making a Medical Living: Doctors and Patients in the English Medical Market* (Cambridge: Cambridge University Press, 1994), 20.
32. T.S. Pensabene, *The Rise of the Medical Practitioner in Victoria* (Canberra: Australian National University, 1980), 74, 80.
33. *Ibid.*, 75.
34. Digby, *op. cit.* (note 28), 478.
35. A.J. Youngson, *The Scientific Revolution in Victorian Medicine* (London: Croom Helm, 1979), 15.
36. R.D. Gidney and W.P.J. Millar, *Professional Gentlemen: The Professions in Nineteenth Century Ontario* (Toronto: University of Toronto Press, 1994); T.M. Romano, 'Professional Identity and the Nineteenth Century Ontario Medical Profession', *Social History*, xxviii, 55 (May 1995).
37. On professionalisation see E. Friedson, *Profession of Medicine: A Study of the Sociology of Applied Knowledge,* 2nd edn (New York: Harper & Row, 1988), 72.
38. J.H. Warner, *The Therapeutic Perspective: Medical Practice, Knowledge and Identity in America, 1820-1885* (Princeton: Princeton University Press, 1986), 1, 13, 15–16.
39. E. van Heyningen, 'Agents of Empire: The Medical Profession in the Cape Colony, 1880-1910', *Medical History,* xxx (1989), 450–71.
40. C. Saunders, 'The Creation of Ndabeni: Urban Segregation and African Resistance in Cape Town', *Studies in the History of Cape Town,* i (Cape Town: University of Cape Town, 1984); and E. van Heyningen, 'Cape Town and the Plague of 1901', *Studies in the History of Cape Town,* vi (Cape Town: University of Cape Town, 1984).
41. Burrows, *op. cit.* (note 4), 89.
42. *Ibid.*, 173.
43. J. Connor, 'A sort of Felo-de-se: Eclecticism, Related Medical Sects and their Decline in Victorian Ontario', *Bulletin of the History of Medicine*, li (1991), 503–27.
44. H.J. Deacon, 'Midwives and Medical Men in the Cape Colony, 1800-1860', *Journal of African History*, xxxix (1998), 271–92.
45. H.J. Deacon, 'Cape Town and Country Doctors in the Cape Colony during the First Half of the Nineteenth Century', *Social History of Medicine*, x, 1 (1997), 25–52.

2

The Cape Doctor and the Broader Medical Market, 1800-1850

Harriet Deacon

Regularly trained and licensed Cape doctors in the nineteenth century operated within a medical market which accommodated other suppliers of medical care, both competing and complementary.[1] These 'alternative practitioners' included shopkeepers selling patent medicines, apothecaries, chemists and midwives, Muslim folk healers and indigenous Khoisan or African healers. Licensed doctors also provided medical services for a wide variety of clients – white settlers, their slaves, servants, free blacks and indigenes, usually in decreasing order of frequency. Most of these patients probably consulted alternative practitioners as well, often in preference to the Western-trained doctor. Cape doctors distanced themselves very firmly from alternative healers and folk medical traditions in order to establish their niche within the medical market and to secure state support by creating a strong profession.

Introduction

The first indigenous Cape inhabitants to be documented by Europeans were Khoisan living in the Western Cape coastal area from Cape Town to Saldanha Bay. Early travellers were interested in these 'Hottentots', 'Bushmen' and 'Strandlopers' as independent societies and wrote about their medical practices and customs and about indigenous flora and fauna. Cape settlers were also interested in Khoisan knowledge about local herbs and remedies, some of which settlers adopted and adapted for medicinal use (e.g. *buchu*). Slaves, imported from east Asia as forced labour for the growing settlement, brought with them a range of other folk medical knowledges (such as *snake stones* which were used to absorb the poison from snake bites). Much of the folk medicine of slave origin was associated in settler and visitor accounts with poisons and poisoning.

45

A creolised folk medicine began to emerge which drew from European, Eastern and indigenous sources. As the colony spread away from the small DEIC hospital at Cape Town, which was staffed with European barber-surgeons, this folk medical tradition strengthened and changed, incorporating new plants and materials found outside the unique floral kingdom of the western Cape. Although it was shared to some degree by slaves and servants, the folk medicine tradition became a part of the Trekboer quest for independence from DEIC and British colonial control emanating from Cape Town. Imported European patent medicines became an intrinsic part of the Cape Dutch folk medicine tradition (and later also indigenous medical traditions), which necessitated dependence on country retailers who were supplied by Cape Town merchants or apothecary houses. Although relatively isolated and independent, Trekboers were thus also inescapably linked to colonial and international markets in medicinal supplies, as well as coffee, gunpowder and sugar. In addition, when Western-trained doctors were available, Cape Dutch settlers did not baulk at requesting medical help. Like the Afrikaans language, which also had creole roots, this eclectic Cape Dutch folk medicine was, rather ironically, drawn into the broader movement to create a white Afrikaner ethnic identity in the late nineteenth century.[2]

Although settlers, slaves and indigenous Khoisan shared some elements of their medical knowledge with each other, for most of the nineteenth century, licensed doctors did not publicly seek to acquire or apply this folk knowledge about medicinal indigenous plant use. Some botanists and botanist-doctors collected and published information about indigenous medicinal plants during the eighteenth and nineteenth centuries, but few licensed practitioners engaged publicly with these scientific accounts. Botany was regarded as a 'puerile hobby horse' and doctors preferred to use established European plant remedies. It was only after the late nineteenth century, with the emergence of a new discourse of pharmacological analysis and extraction, that professional medical interest in indigenous plant remedies became more acceptable, although not of high status. Even then, this was not a very widespread interest within the profession.

Figure 2.1
Map of South Africa showing towns mentioned in the text

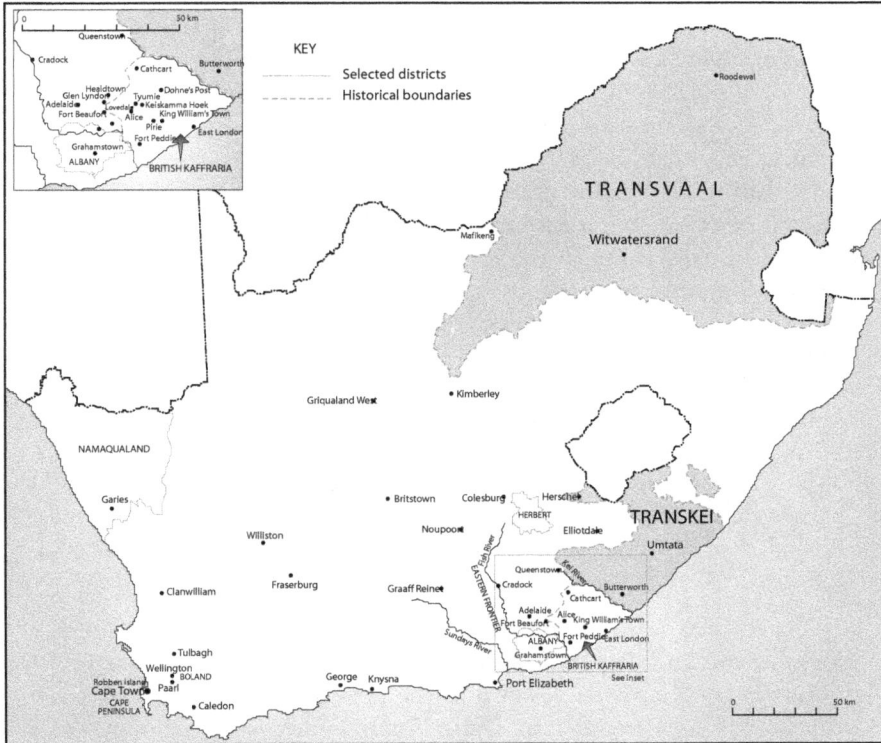

The Cape medical market

The co-existence of different healing traditions was not unique to the culturally heterogenous Cape, nor were the legal and social pressures on patients to consult certain healers and not others.[3] While it is important to recognise the divisions within the Cape medical market, it would be wrong to suggest that this resulted in a firmly segregated medical market or the disappearance of whole realms of medical practice. However much some contemporaries might have wished it to be so, the various healing traditions at the Cape did not exist in isolation from each other. They influenced one another to varying degrees and patients would often turn to a whole range of traditions for healing a difficult complaint. In both irregular as in regular practice, the cultural-racial divide continued to be crossed in spite of the increasingly segregated history of colonial South Africa.

47

Different cultural, economic or political conditions sometimes encouraged patients to select medical practitioners in terms of certain gender, ethnic, educational or organisational characteristics. Particular types of practitioners were thought to have skills in curing certain diseases: Western-trained doctors in surgery (particularly of the eye), Muslim healers in poisoning cases or exorcisms and traditional healers in scrofula.[4] The association between doctors, urban environments and new diseases sometimes turned communities against Western medicine. A missionary wife wrote in 1839 during a measles epidemic in the eastern Cape that local Africans believed the disease to originate in schools. Although many Africans initially came to the missionaries for a cure for the disease, she said that after realising 'they can get through without [Western] medi[cine,] [g]reat numbers [of Africans began to] take medicine of their own'.[5] A similar response occurred in the rural Afrikaner community of the western Cape, where one farmer's wife commented in the same year:

> I see that more people are dying [of measles] around the Doctors than on the distant farms, therefore the Doctors cannot help us, if God does not give his sanction. I have used nothing but home remedies.[6]

There was also a power imbalance among practitioners. Government and legal support for formally trained and licensed doctors at the Cape, fee levels and the growing status of doctors as professionals – especially in Cape Town – helped to cement the official status of the Cape doctor over his rivals. All unlicensed practitioners were legally banned from practising for payment after 1807.[7] While witchcraft, witch-finding and ordeals were universally banned, other colonies did not always follow the Cape's lead in restricting licensing to Western-trained practitioners. Natal, for example, recognised and licensed traditional herbal doctors from 1891.[8] Whatever the legal provisions for banning alternative medical practice, however, at the Cape as elsewhere in colonial Africa, little attention was devoted towards prosecuting unlicensed practitioners who did not compete directly with European-trained and licensed doctors. But, although alternative practice was made illegal in law after 1807, and it was only in 1985[9] that alternative healers were placed on a similar footing to regular practitioners in the eyes of the law, alternative practice has survived and even thrived in both urban and rural South Africa.

Various terms are currently used to describe alternative practitioners: alternative, folk, traditional, informal, popular or holistic practitioners, or witch-doctors, faith-healers, irregulars, quacks, and so on. One objection to these terms is that they are often used to distinguish practitioners by race and class: 'traditional' is usually used to refer to black practitioners, 'folk' to white practitioners with poorer clients and 'alternative' or 'holistic' to those attending wealthier clients. While ethnic and class divisions may be important elements in analysing the social and economic dimensions of the medical market, when embedded in the terms of analysis they may obscure important similarities between the practitioner groups or regional and historical differences within them.

Indigenous medical practices, of course, were not and are not discrete and unchanging systems of medicine. Traditional African healers do not all share the same unchanging therapeutic system today, nor did they do so in the past, nor were they necessarily practising differently from Cape Dutch folk healers during the nineteenth century. Their practices probably varied between regions and certainly changed over time. The Khoisan, for example, rapidly incorporated European imports, such as tobacco, into their medicinal remedies. In turn, Cape Dutch settlers incorporated and altered remedies used by indigenes in their medical practice. Yet much of the historical information we have about alternative practitioners comes packaged in racial or class-specific terms, and extensive research is required to group them in more illuminating ways. It is also difficult to move beyond the current consensus that Western medicine has proved to be a more effective tool against many forms of disease than alternative medical practices. This view has to be challenged if one is to look beyond the characterisation of indigenous medical practices simply as 'belief systems' with no scientific validity.[10] While it is true that Khoisan medical practices were, for example, closely linked to broader belief systems, this is no less true of biomedicine today.

In this chapter we shall not try to solve these problems, but shall draw out some of the connections between the various alternative and licensed practitioners by looking at organisation, contact and therapy among various medical groups described in the contemporary literature. Our focus will be on the ways in which the theoretical background, training, origins and professional development of the Cape doctor influenced his interaction with alternative practitioners in the Cape medical market.

Harriet Deacon

The licenced Cape doctor

The Western medical model

Early Cape doctors were operating within a system of medical knowledge that had drawn heavily on classical Greek and Arabic humoral theory, as well as innovations in the Renaissance and the Enlightenment, such as the discovery of blood circulation and the invention of the obstetric forceps. The Classical writers had interpreted disease as arising out of an imbalance of the four humours: blood, bile, black bile and phlegm. The humours were linked to the four seasons and the four elements, binding man, nature and the universe tightly together.[11] 'Airs, waters and places' influenced disease patterns by changing the humoral balance. After the early modern period and the discovery of new parts of the world, environmental influence on human health and culture was considered even more important than before, an idea which was taken up and extended in the seventeenth and eighteenth centuries by writers like Sydenham, Montesquieu, Buffon and others.[12] Curing a disease involved restoring the balance between the humours inside the body by making the patient bleed, vomit, excrete wastes, become hotter or colder, and so on.

The early-nineteenth century doctor did not use such modern techniques such as anaesthesia (which was first used in the 1840s), antisepsis (which was introduced in the 1860s) or the scientific theory of germs as disease agents (which was consolidated in the 1880s). Germ theory challenged some of the tenets of humoral theory and introduced a biomedical understanding of disease. Much ink has recently been expended in blurring the distinction between scientific biomedical medicine and its more holistic and environmental predecessors. Here, it will suffice to make the point that humoral theories of disease as employed by formally trained doctors were often more compatible with folk theories of disease before the 1880s than were the biomedical models afterwards.[13]

In the early-nineteenth century formally trained and licensed Cape doctors thus used a system of medical knowledge which had much in common with folk theories of disease. It was relatively unproblematic for them to incorporate into their practice remedies from folk medicine which relied on humoral theory, as had been done in the previous centuries. Their training and practice still relied on much botanical knowledge. This did not make Cape doctors lie any closer to folk or indigenous practitioners than their modern

50

counterparts do, however. During the nineteenth century, as Cape doctors sought professional status and a niche in the competitive medical market, they generally tried to distance themselves more firmly from alternative practitioners, both in social and clinical terms. They had little therapeutic advantage over most alternative practitioners, except possibly in surgery, and had to compete with them for clients. There were circumstances in which a more collaborative attitude was fostered, for example between urban doctors and midwives,[14] but seldom did Cape doctors seek similar collaboration with indigenous or folk healers.

Licensing regulations

Formal licensing for medical practice at the Cape was introduced in 1807 under regulations which were scarcely altered until 1891. A central aspect of the licensing regulations was their insistence on European medical training. Two proclamations in 1807 established a Medical Committee, consisting of Western-trained doctors based in Cape Town. These men[15] were empowered to license Western-trained doctors for medical practice and the sale of medicines at the Cape. Applicants for the licences had to produce proof of apprenticeship and/or tickets of attendance at medical lectures at a European university, hospital or private medical school. They also needed to show some professional British certificate, such as the Licenciate of the Society of Apothecaries (LSA), Membership of the Royal College of Surgeons or Physicians (MRCS or MRCP), or a guild membership from a continental town. Apothecaries initially had to be apprenticed in Europe, but in 1829 this rule was relaxed after an acrimonious debate over standards.[16]

The emphasis on European training was matched by the dominance of immigrant Europeans within the Cape profession. In general, the Cape licensing system favoured those born in Europe who immigrated to the Cape after completing their training, because for Cape-born men, foreign training was expensive and difficult to arrange without good contacts abroad. This meant that most of the Cape-born doctors who studied abroad were sons of reasonably wealthy medical families, and it was not surprising that many of them settled in Cape Town, the most prestigious and lucrative place to practise.[17] Immigrant doctors predominated, however. During the period of Dutch colonial rule at the Cape, which finally ended in 1806, a number of Dutch and German doctors had settled there. Most of these men were surgeons working for the DEIC at the hospital in Cape Town. They had usually come as ship surgeons –

many had been trained on the job. Others arrived as soldiers or sailors and worked their way up the hospital hierarchy. Burgher surgeons, who were not numerous, had usually either trained as surgeons or had not been formally trained in Europe. Some of these men were licensed in the early nineteenth century, others moved out of Cape Town to practise in the less well-regulated countryside and others continued their businesses illegally.

There were few British doctors at first, but by the end of the century they outnumbered those of Continental origin. Some of the British residents of Cape Town complained that 'in consequence of the regulations... adopted [in 1807]... there is not one English practitioner of medicine in the Colony, and the only English Apothecary's shop [that of Joseph Mackrill] is ordered to be shut up.'[18] The first British medical immigrants were military and navy doctors. Most came after the end of the Napoleonic Wars in 1815, which created an increasingly competitive medical market in Britain.[19] A government-aided settlement programme in the eastern Cape in 1820 brought more British doctors. Whereas before 1820 only about a fifth of the doctors licensed were British (excluding military doctors), this increased to ninety per cent in the 1820s and did not drop below fifty per cent thereafter.[20] The influx of British doctors soon led to their predominance; by 1880 most Cape doctors were British-born general practitioners (GPs)[21] who had trained in London or Edinburgh.[22]

Medical licensing at the Cape thus both underlined and encouraged the dominance of European rather than local medical cultures, knowledges and training. Licensing conferred authority and status on Cape doctors rather than any real protection against competitors, except possibly in Cape Town. There will be further discussion about the importance of Cape Town for medical professionalisation in the next chapter.[23] In the first wave of licensing the Medical Committee was quite lenient, giving licences to the older and more successful of the doctors already practising in Cape Town without adequate formal training. To protect the Cape Town market and encourage doctors to move to rural areas they also issued restricted licences to those who lacked the requisite qualifications but were willing to practise in the less well-populated hinterland – the 'country'. The licensing rules were more strictly applied during the 1820s, however. In theory, anyone practising without a licence could be fined, but very few people were brought to book under the regulations.

Under the 1807 regulations an applicant could be licensed as a physician, surgeon, apothecary or as a chemist and druggist. Some were also licensed as accoucheurs or man-midwives. The licensing regulations supported and strengthened a distinction within the Cape profession between doctors (surgeons and physicians) and druggists (apothecaries, chemists and druggists), in terms of status, fees and practise. Under the regulations, doctors were distinguished from druggists because the former had the right to prescribe drugs and perform surgery, and the latter could only make and sell drugs. In practice, both apothecaries and druggists seem to have made up and sold drugs as well as doing some prescribing and practising. Cape doctors often prepared and sold their own medicine. This mixture of roles was not illegal in the areas outside Cape Town until 1830, but it seems to have continued well after that in practice, especially outside Cape Town.[24]

The Cape regulations sharpened the distinction between doctors and druggists by reducing the distinction between physicians and surgeons on the one hand and widening the divide between surgeons and apothecaries on the other hand. Physicians and surgeons were not significantly differentiated at the Cape in terms of social status or legal ambit of practise, although in Europe, physicians, who had to have a MD degree, had traditionally concentrated on the theoretical side of medicine and on internal ailments while surgeons, who usually had only an apprenticeship and guild or college membership, were more practically oriented. During the nineteenth century, this distinction was retained more strongly in Britain than in continental Europe (see Chapter 3). If Cape applicants had an MD degree they were usually given a dual licence, as surgeon and physician. In Cape Town both surgeons and physicians were permitted to practise medicine (including surgery) and to prescribe drugs. Apothecaries and chemists were allowed only to make up drugs and sell them.[25] Whatever the differences between Cape law and practice, making medicines was considered a particularly low-status occupation associated with druggists. This may have discouraged Cape doctors from engaging with any seriousness in the collection of indigenous plant remedies and their preparation.

Henry A.J.B. Hammerschmidt: unlicensed practitioner

An interesting example of the indirect power of licensing, and of ways in which the quest for professional status affected doctors' relationships with the indigenous medicines of the Cape, is provided by the brief medical career of an Austrian-born doctor in Stellenbosch, then a small village near Cape Town. Hammerschmidt was an immigrant who applied for a licence to practise as a physician, surgeon and apothecary at the Cape in 1858 on the grounds that he had trained at the University of Vienna and worked as a military doctor in the Hungarian war of 1848-9.[26] The MC refused him a licence because he could not provide adequate documentation of his training – he claimed that some of his testimonials had been lost.[27] Hammerschmidt appealed unsuccessfully against the decision, asking for a provisional licence 'to practise the profession which I had and ever shall have at heart, and for which alone I was ever bred, or born.'[28] Recent research suggests that he had never in fact obtained his MD, although he was enrolled as a medical student in Vienna in 1850-51.[29]

Undeterred by the lack of a licence, Hammerschmidt soon began practising in Stellenbosch,[30] where he probably took over the practice of Dr Schröder, who had been admitted to the Robben Island mental asylum.[31] He seems to have had a large clientele, recording 1,266 cases between October 1858 and June 1860. He practised illegally as a doctor and probably also as an apothecary[32] without being prosecuted by the authorities, partly because the local magistrate seems to have been reluctant to prosecute, and partly because Ordinance 12 of 1836, which provided for better control over unlicensed practitioners, had never been made into law.[33] In spite of this, Hammerschmidt went bankrupt in 1861, complaining that outstanding accounts for medical services rendered, totalling £247/3,[34] were 'irrecoverable [and] the principal cause of his insolvency'.[35] One reason why Hammerschmidt was unable to recover these debts was probably because, unlike licensed doctors, he could not appeal to the Medical Committee or the courts to enforce payment.

Perhaps because Hammerschmidt was situated at the fringes of the Cape medical profession by virtue of his lack of appropriate training and licensing, he tried particularly hard to emulate the medical professional ideal. The inventory of his property in 1861 suggests that he was an avid reader, owning around 100 books and some medical pictures, a large collection for the time. He also had a small collection of bottled 'curiosities', possibly specimens of natural history or medical interest.[36] He published a pamphlet in 1860 about the state of medical health in Stellenbosch, which was deliberately aimed at establishing his scientific credentials in the eyes of the profession and the public, and thereby refuting the 'reiterated provocations and odious insinuations' that he was not a qualified medical man.[37] His attitude makes the pamphlet an important (even somewhat exaggerated) statement of what Hammerschmidt (and probably other local doctors) considered to be the legitimate interests and activities of a licensed doctor. After describing the people, climate and natural environment of Stellenbosch, he listed all the diseases suffered by the patients he had attended, extolling the scientific virtues of statistics, and then supplied notes on his treatment of the various classes of disease. He also included reports on the smallpox and measles epidemics in Stellenbosch.[38]

For the purposes of this chapter it is especially interesting to note that, although Hammerschmidt gives the popular and scientific names of 179 plants found in the Stellenbosch area and elsewhere, he does not show much interest in their healing properties. He notes in the list of plants that *geele bloemetjes thee* [yellow flower tea] ... [was] added to spec. pector. by some apthecaries', that the 'snake root – *garuleum bipinnatum* ... [was] much alike in medicinal properties to *polygala senega*', that the '*platdoorn* [flat thorn] ... [resembled] sassaparilla in its properties' and that '*varkensoren* [the pigs' ears plant]... [was an] antiepileptic, and the leaves [could be used] for corns'.[39] But these comments on medicinal use are exceptional in a list which includes *buchu, geneesblaaren* [healing leaves], *kankerblaaren* [cancer leaves] and other well-known medicinal herbs widely used not only by Khoisan but also by local settlers. Hammerschmidt's chapter on therapeutics is clearly aimed at a professional medical audience; it is peppered with professional abbreviations and Latin terms, refers to medical practices abroad and details the use of acupuncture ('quite the rage' in Europe) and chloroform in his practice. Although indigenous remedies for snake bites abounded, he treated a snakebite victim with chloroform, saliva and solid nitrate of silver,[40] and whereas he had mentioned the use of the *platdoorn* for treating corns, he himself used only 'a plaister composed of *gummi ammoniac* and wax, with a small admixture of verdigris'.[41] This suggests that while Hammerschmidt was aware of local plant remedies for common conditions, he did not feel that the use of these remedies was appropriate in the practice of a licensed doctor.

Cape Doctors and Alternative Practice

The licensed doctor thus entered the Cape medical market armed with a European cultural and medical background and the legal sanction of the colonial government, and influenced, especially in the urban environment, by the desire to move away from the tradesman status of a druggist. This affected his attitude towards other healers who were touting their wares in the Cape medical market. Although medical travellers of the eighteenth century had shown some interest in indigenous and slave therapies, this research was increasingly relegated to the sphere of natural history rather than medical science during the nineteenth century. Although they generally scorned the remedies of settlers, the Khoisan, slaves and other alternative practitioners, much less attention was paid to these groups. Doctors railed against the inroads of travelling drug salesmen and country apothecaries, and tried to control the practice of midwives. This, along with other evidence, may indicate that there was greater competition between doctors and druggists than between doctors and midwives, and even less competition between doctors and slave or indigenous practitioners. The differences in the attitudes of doctors towards other practitioners and medical traditions also reveal much about the kind of public image the profession was trying to carve out for itself.

The use of indigenous medicinal plants

Although it is difficult to suggest a definitive chronology to this without further research, it is probable that it was in the early and middle years of the nineteenth century that Cape doctors were most disinterested in the use of indigenous remedies. The Dutch-speaking DEIC and burgher surgeons of the eighteenth century, often self-taught or apprenticed in the Cape Town hospital, were usually linked more strongly to settler medical traditions than those of the mainstream metropolitan profession. They would perhaps have been more willing to experiment with indigenous remedies, especially given the erratic supply of imported medicines to the hinterland.[42] After 1806, immigrant English-speaking doctors, formally trained in mainstream metropolitan traditions and self-consciously seeking professional status and advancement, were both more isolated from the Cape creole medical traditions and less willing to accept their validity. The British government also showed little concerted interest in exploiting indigenous Cape plants.[43] It was only after the late nineteenth century, with the emergence of a new discourse of pharmacological analysis, that professional medical interest in indigenous plant remedies could be accepted as scientific. Even so, such interest has remained a low-status curiosity within the medical profession even today, belonging more with botany and pharmacology, rather than becoming an accepted sub-specialism within the profession.

There were a variety of reasons why Europeans at the Cape

collected information about indigenous plant remedies. During the seventeenth and eighteenth centuries, settlers and DEIC employees had an interest in rapidly acquiring medical knowledge at the Cape, both for local use and for possible export.[44] Most information about local medicinal plants initially came from the Peninsular 'Hottentots' or Khoi living near the first European settlement at Cape Town. Cape Dutch settlers drew on indigenous knowledge to develop a creolised folk medicine at the Cape. Following the growing European interest in naming and classifying flora and fauna from around the world, travellers investigated the Cape floral kingdom ever more closely. Various writers documented folk and indigenous remedies, notably Peter Kolb (1713) and Dr Karl Thunberg in the eighteenth century and Dr Ludwig Pappe (1847, 1850) and Andrew Smith (1888),[45] a missionary at Lovedale (not the famous explorer of the same name), in the nineteenth.[46] By the mid-nineteenth century, therefore, there was a considerable body of popular and published information about local medicinal plants available to Cape doctors, if they looked for it. But the Cape medical profession as a whole did not seem willing or able to engage in any systematic investigation and use of indigenous plants during the nineteenth century.

In Kolb's account of the Cape in the early eighteenth century, he described the Khoisan as using aloe juice, wild sage, wild figs and fig leaves, *buchu*, garlic and fennel as medicines.[47] *Buchu* was used in powder form in the hair to cure head-itch and headache.[48] As a result of observing Khoisan practise, *buchu* became a common ingredient in Cape Dutch folk medicine.[49] Unusually for a plant indigenous to the Cape, it was also taken up in European medical traditions from where it filtered through to the practise of some Cape doctors. It is probable that some Cape doctors incorporated a few indigenous plants into their medical practice, such as *buchu*, aloe and the *platdoorn* (Arctopus echinatus).[50] But the full extent of indigenous plant use among Cape doctors is unclear. In his account of European diseases at the Cape, Kolb describes three indigenous remedies (besides *buchu*) in use among settlers. Of these the only successful remedy involved the use of aloe juice for stomach complaints, a common Khoisan remedy. Kolb said that this was used by 'the Europeans at the Cape' in general, not specifically by their doctors.[51] Yet Kolb describes a few doctors' (unsuccessful) experimentation with local plants, an oculist using the juices of 'certain of the Cape-Herbs and Flowers' for sore eyes,[52] and a German surgeon using the powdered bark of the *kreupelhout* (literally, crippled wood) tree for dysentery.[53] Other eighteenth-century travellers, Ten Rhyne,

Thunberg and Sparrman, had medical training and were interested in recording the use of indigenous plants. While Sparrman complained about the ignorance of some local doctors about indigenous plants,[54] Thunberg assured a Dutch official that 'the Cape doctors often use indigenous remedies'.[55]

In the early nineteenth century some Cape doctors, such as Joseph Mackrill, James Barry and William G. Atherstone, conducted their own experiments on settler and indigenous plant remedies.[56] Others experimented with remedies which had not yet become part of the creole folk tradition, such as when, in the 1830s, a Cape Town surgeon, Samuel Bailey, reportedly used 'a *Caffre* [Xhosa] medicine... made of herbs from the Caffre country [the eastern Cape]' which 'he put... great faith in.'[57] But this kind of experimentation was not very widespread. When district surgeons were asked to send in accounts of indigenous plants and their medicinal use to the government in 1829, very few responded.[58] The results of this kind of scattered experimentation were not seen as mainstream medical knowledge, nor were they systematically shared among the profession. By the latter part of the nineteenth century Cape doctors were making more concerted efforts to examine the usefulness of indigenous plants as medicines, mainly through pharmacological investigation of remedies identified in indigenous and settler healing practices.[59]

Throughout the eighteenth and nineteenth centuries, a time when one would expect great interest in the potential financial benefits of the export industry, only two medicinal Cape plants were exported on a large scale from its unique and varied floral kingdom to Europe: aloe and *buchu*. Not surprisingly, only these two Cape plants were incorporated into the published British pharmacopoeia (which Cape doctors used, sometimes alongside the Amsterdam one).[60] Cape aloe also got into the German pharmacopoeia.[61] The poor success of Cape medicinal plants as exports may have been due partly to local doctors' lack of interest in indigenous medicinal plants as objects of medical knowledge. It is also true however that there were difficulties in preparing the Cape remedies commercially, both in Cape Town and abroad, because boiling them often destroyed the active agents in the plants.[62] The lack of ready-made products in turn would have retarded the use of these remedies by local doctors who lacked access to the plants or the requisite knowledge to prepare them, and also prevented their appearance in the European pharmacopoeias, on which Cape doctors and apothecaries depended so heavily.

Some of the reason for Cape doctors' inadequate engagement

with indigenous plants and their medicinal use during the nineteenth century may have been a result of their European training. Knowledge of plants and their medicinal utility was an important part of this training, but most of the plants they would have been taught about were European and the Western Cape floral kingdom is botanically unique. Some European medicinal plants grew well at the Cape and obviated the need to seek local replacements. There was also a ready source of foreign medicines coming by ship from east Asia and Holland. In 1847 the botanist-doctor Ludwig Pappe, a rare enthusiast for indigenous medicinal plants, published a list of local plants and their uses in the *Cape Town Medical Gazette*. He noted that the wild chamomile, which grew on the Cape Flats in great quantities and was used widely by 'farmers and the coloured people' in more remote areas for digestive complaints, had not yet been adopted by Cape apothecaries who still imported chamomile from Europe.[63] He made a similar comment in the case of castor oil from the *olieboom* [literally, oil tree].[64] This seems to indicate that Cape apothecaries, like doctors, were largely ignorant of many local species of medicinal plants, although Pappe did ascribe some knowledge and use of the *bitterwortel* [literally, bitter root] to apothecaries.[65]

The medicine trade

In the late eighteenth century, the traveller Sparrman had suggested that Cape doctors were interested only in the commercial possibilities of indigenous medicinal plants for export,[66] not in their local application or botanical importance. He was visited in Cape Town by a doctor who requested to see his herbal collection but did not know the uses of any local plants. Sparrman explained that:

> the worthy physician's income depended more upon merchandise, than upon Apollo and the Muses... to the great prejudice of the sick in particular as well as to that of natural knowledge and the art of medicine in general.[67]

During the nineteenth century, Cape Town doctors sought to raise themselves above the status of tradesman, at least in the way they presented themselves to the public. That apothecaries showed a greater interest in indigenous remedies than doctors by the mid-nineteenth century, according to Pappe, was perhaps a symptom of the growing intra-professional distinction between doctors and druggists in Cape Town. Higher-status doctors associated investigations of indigenous plants with drug manufacture and sale, trading activities unsuitable for the gentleman practitioner. Botanical science was not a key element of this identity. Pappe complained that Cape doctors, who had an ideal opportunity to observe how country people used indigenous herbs as home remedies, 'consider[ed] the study of Botany a puerile hobby horse' and denigrated it to conceal their ignorance of natural history.[68]

Country doctors remained heavily involved in selling medicines throughout the nineteenth century. These medicines were largely imported, however. According to a list in 1953, the Dutch (Hollandse or Hallische) medicines which were purchased by settlers contained no indigenous plant extracts except *buchu*.[69] In fact, country doctors may have considered the authorisation of medicinal plant use a possible threat to their patent medicine sales. A doctor based at Swellendam in 1805 reportedly depended on the sale of Hallische medicines, emetics and purgatives which he peddled around the countryside to secure an adequate income: 'no man in this country can subsist on a proper or regular practice, if every colonist preferred to be their own physician and only called another in cases of extreme necessity.'[70] A Cape Town chemist remarked in 1842, that 'Dr Gill's [a country doctor] and other orders have completely cleared our stocks of Dutch medicines.'[71] While many Cape doctors sold patent medicines of various sorts, they were very sensitive to allegations that by doing so they were practising as 'quacks'. One doctor successfully sued the *Zuid-Afrikaan* newspaper for implying that he was 'a quack, a man-murderer'.[72] As in Britain, where the *British Medical Journal* denigrated patent medicines made from secret recipes but carried advertisements for them, Cape doctors had to sacrifice their principles for the much-needed income.

The association between indigenous plant use and Cape Dutch and Khoisan folk medicine may also have lowered its status in the eyes of Cape doctors. Robert Ross and others have emphasised the close cultural and economic contact between frontier settlers and the Khoisan during the eighteenth and nineteenth centuries.[73] As one German-trained doctor living in Graaff Reinet, J.F. Haszner, believed, Cape Dutch settlers used herbs, plants and roots as charms against disease or misfortune as well as medical remedies.[74] This magical use of plants was also observed among the Khoisan, and was seen by doctors as a sign that their medicine was based on superstition rather than science, like that of European quacks, from whom doctors, as professionals, wished to distance themselves.

Cape doctors did not therefore engage in any extensive and systematic investigation of indigenous plant use, and increasingly distanced themselves from the 'superstitious' side of settler, slave and Khoisan medicine. Licensed doctors could do nothing about the widespread use of home remedies (in particular among frontier settlers), although they could try and control the sale of medicines for this purpose. These consisted predominantly of patent medicines manufactured in Europe.

Khoisan medical traditions

Viljoen argues that until the smallpox epidemic of 1713 the Khoisan generally avoided Western medicine, but they were more willing to try it thereafter because of the new disease environment and the loss of political and economic independence from settler society.[75] Early settlers (including some doctors) and travellers (some of whom were medically trained) were, by contrast, very eager to learn about indigenous medical remedies from the Khoisan, and were irritated by Khoisan 'secrecy'. Yet professional medical interest in indigenous and slave healing traditions was coloured by the value-laden distinction between folk and scientific medicine in Europe. Some European visitors and many western-trained doctors were thus dismissive of indigenous and slave healing traditions and of the creole folk medicine that grew out of contact between Cape Dutch settlers, slaves and Khoisan. Credit was given to these alternative therapies mainly where Western medicine was thought to be weak: in treating poisoning rather than in surgery or internal medicine. Settler interest in indigenous and slave healing traditions was much more general, and many different remedies were shared between the various groups,[76] particularly in the area of midwifery. By the nineteenth century, when this creole folk medicine was well-established, Khoisan and Muslim[77] practitioners seem to have occupied a niche market among Cape settlers, being consulted mainly in midwifery, bewitchment and poisoning cases.

Eighteenth-century accounts of the Cape grudgingly admitted that the Khoisan had some medical skill, which visitors and settlers were keen to acquire. Early travellers compared them to low-status European quacks, however, and emphasised their primitiveness. The traveller Nieuhof commented after his visit in 1654:

> Those Hottentot doctors *seem to have some knowledge*, at least of how to sew up a wound, but the scars remain as if it were cauterised. They carry their charms and medicines with them *as do our quacks*.... In the use of [herbs and roots] lies their art, and they also have some knowledge of their effects.[78] [emphasis added]

Illustration 2.1
Kolb: Khoisan medicine

Two early eighteenth-century engravings from Peter Kolb's *The Present State of the Cape of Good Hope*, showing surgery and midwifery as practised by the Khoisan, whom he called 'Hottentot'. The childbirth picture shows female babies abandoned in the tree and on the ground, as Kolb alleged this was a common Khoisan practice. Kolb, unlike many early and most later European commentators, was however generally complimentary of Khoisan medical skills. The engravings depict the use of ground ox horn, 'lancet' and poultices by specialist doctors and the expert birthing assistance provided by Khoisan women.

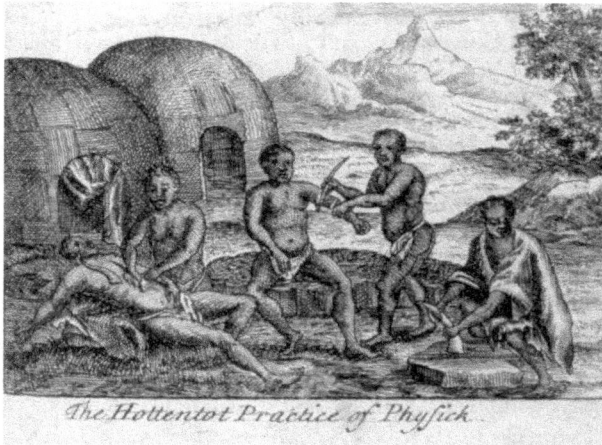

The Hottentot Practice of Physick.

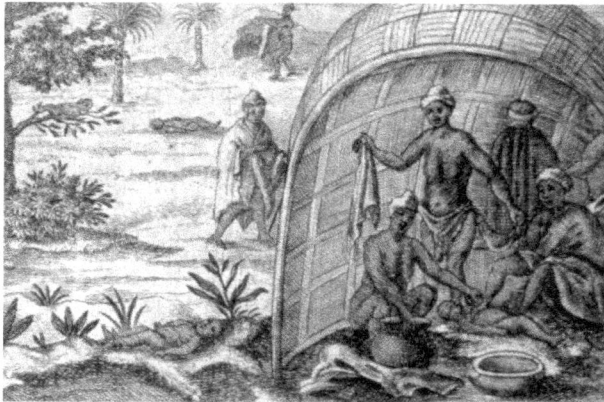

One of the fullest and most positive accounts of Khoisan medical practice during the eighteenth century comes from Kolb. He commented after his visit to the Cape in 1705:

> In every Kraal there is a Physician, in the large ones there are two, who are well skill'd in the Botany, Surgery and Medicine of the Hottentots, and are chosen out of the Sages of each Kraal and appointed to watch over the health of the Inhabitants. This they perform without Fee or Reward. The Honour of the Employment is judg'd a Recompence for all the Trouble of it.[79] But the Candidates for it must be no youngsters. They have great Skill in the Vertues [sic] of their Herbs; and cup, and handle a Lancet well.[80]

Kolb noted that there were also several 'Old Women' in the Kraal who used roots and herbs and were mortally hated by the doctors.[81] Thus far, his account resembles any description of European surgeons who learned through apprenticeship and sought to emphasise their professional detachment by underplaying the importance of payment. But Kolb also suggested that the Khoisan doctor was secretive and dealt in the arcane world of magic, like the European empiric or the unscientific medieval doctor:

> The Doctors suffer none to see 'em gather and prepare their Remedies... [and] keep the Preparations very secret. And if a Patient dies under their Hands, they always assert. that their Remedies had been render'd ineffectual by Witchcraft; and they are always believed.[82]

The reference to magic and witchcraft was to become a common method of differentiating European doctors (and their belief systems based on 'science') from the supposedly more 'primitive' African doctors. Like later writers,[83] both Kolb and Ten Rijne complained that Khoisan doctors were secretive about their methods.[84] Many early European attempts to garner medical information from the Khoisan were disappointed; these doctors' reluctance to give freely of their local knowledge was represented as an unprofessional, unscientific trait. The frequency with which travellers complained about indigenous healers' secrecy could indicate the degree of their interest in finding out Khoisan remedies.

Although few of the eighteenth-century accounts dismissed indigenous doctors' medical skills out of hand, there was much debate in the travel literature about the range of their ability. Khoisan doctors were not thought to be of great skill in setting bones; this was possibly where it was felt that European surgeons were most capable. Hofman[85] said that Khoisan doctors bound broken arms and legs with split pieces of wood. After it had been smeared (probably with fat), the bandaging was continued until the part was healed or rotting. Kolb claimed that 'Of Setting a fractur'd Limb they [Khoisan doctors] know Little or Nothing',[86] although he acknowledged that they could 'bleed, cup, make an Amputation, restore a Dislocation, and perform all the Manual Operations in their Practice with the most surprising Dexterity [using only] a common Knife, a Horn and the Bird's Bone'.[87] In a nineteenth-century account, Campbell described bonesetting among the Damaraland Namaqua, which involved setting bones with a wooden splint, rubbing fat on painful parts, motions over the place, incisions and dropping of wood.[88] He said that 'Bushmen' set a limb by sewing a piece of skin tightly around it.[89] Other groups fared little better. Another nineteenth century traveller described a Bondelswartz doctor setting an elbow joint at an angle to allow for eating as they knew it would be stiff afterwards.[90] The critique of Khoisan skill in setting bones may thus have been part of a broader scepticism about non-Western doctors' skills in this regard. While the traveller Valentijn had some faith in the Balinese and Chinese doctors, for example, he did not think that they were good at setting broken limbs.[91]

Internal medicine was another issue about which European commentators were sensitive. In Europe, internal medicine was a high-status activity: in theory if not in practice, the preserve of the most highly trained physicians. It is thus not surprising that many commentators emphasised the poverty of Khoisan practice in this regard. In one early eighteenth-century account it was alleged that to cure a 'Hottentot's' illness, whatever the cause, their doctors used nothing but sheep- or ox-fat, with which the sufferer's whole body was smeared.[92] Fat was also the most important internal medicine, although here it was taken with certain roots which were pounded and mixed with water. Unlike many of his contemporaries, Kolb suggested that the Khoisan doctors used a number of salves and poultices and internal remedies, although he conceded that there were not as many as in the European *materia medica*. He mentioned remedies for stomach pains comprising aloe leaf juice taken in a little warm broth (cupping was employed if this failed) and headache[93] (shaving some of the hair and powdering the scalp with *buchu*).

One area in which indigenous practitioners, as well as slaves, were thought to be particularly skillful was the treatment of poisoning cases. During the eighteenth century, Khoisan were increasingly brought into conflict with the Cape Dutch settlers who pushed further and further into their territory. One of the ways in which the Khoisan fought back against the settler commandos, and killed settler sheep for food, was by using poisoned arrows traditionally used for game hunting. Khoisan were thus associated in settler accounts with poisoning and the treatment of poison wounds.[94] Poison antidotes were important to settlers who faced natural dangers from new kinds of venomous snakes at the Cape.

The Khoisan used *buchu* leaves to dress a snakebite wound. Another approach was to place snake venom and saliva on the scratched stomach of a poisoned person.[95] Campbell described San ('Bushman') use of scorpion stings and poison against snakebite and the use by 'natives' (probably Khoisan) near Pella of a living frog or a kidney or scarlet bean as an absorbent plaster on a snakebite wound.[96] Barrow described 'several vegetable antidotes' the Khoisan employed against snakebite, noting that they were especially fearful of the *cobra capella*.[97] Moodie described the use of leaves and root of *mellitus* for snakebite. He said the *slangen wortel* (snake root - *catula capensis* and *anthemoides*) was used by 'Hottentot' (Khoi) shepherds.[98] In the late 1820s the District Surgeon of Worcester sent to the government a specimen of the *Slangenbosch* (snake bush) whose root had medicinal properties used for snakebite, other poisonous bites and 'Bushman' arrows. The 'Bushmen' kept the root handy in the form of cakes, while settler farmers used the bruised root soaked in spirits – it was highly prized by them.[99] De Jong noted in 1802 that the Cape Dutch also commonly used a bean, usually a *grooteboon* (big bean) or a *gouverneursboon* (governor's bean), cut open and placed flat on the wound to suck up the snake poison.[100] Cape Dutch settlers also used snakestones.[101] These had been introduced to the Cape by slaves from east Asia, where they were prepared by the 'Brachmans' in a secret process. It was an artificial stone, shaped like a bean with whitish matter in the middle, the rest sky-blue. The stone allegedly soaked up the poison and was then cleaned in milk.[102]

Another reported cure for snakebite was the drinking of snake poison. In 1786 Sparrman wrote that the up-country Khoisan considered snake poison a medicine and preservative against the dangers of snakebite. He pointed out the similarity between this belief and the European (folk) understanding that only the blood-and-venom combination was dangerous,[103] thus drawing the dividing line between folk and scientific knowledge rather than European and African knowledge. In the 1830s another traveller commented on this remedy among the Namaqua Khoi of the north-western Cape coast, whose poison doctors swallowed snake venom so that when someone was bitten they could offer the person water from their cap and thus assist their cure.[104] Moodie noted that Khoi doctors who drank snake poison were called '*gift-drinkers*' (poison drinkers).[105] He mentioned that Cape Dutch settlers also believed this to be efficacious against snakebite,[106] an indication of knowledge transfer between Khoisan and settlers, or the maintenance of older European traditions which Sparrman had described.

Slave and Muslim healing traditions

Settlers also evidenced a great fear of being poisoned by household slaves or, after emancipation, by Muslim domestic servants. Muslims in particular (many of whom came to the Cape as slaves from east Asia) were thought to possess much skill in poisoning and black magic. Although Muslim slaves were considered by settlers to be 'the cleverest and most civilised' among the slaves, they were also thought to be 'vindictive and jealous' when aroused:

> It is also very generally believed among the Dutch, and the lower classes of the English in the colony, that they can administer poison in such a manner as to destroy the health, without occasioning death for many months, or even years.[107]

Muslims were also thought to cast magical charms. Settlers in Cape Town associated Muslims in general with magic and poisoning.[108] This was also true of the rural areas. Moodie records the case of a Cape Dutch farmer who wrapped his head in a piece of flannel and wore a steel ring to cure his rheumatism. He had consulted a 'Malay' (i.e. Muslim) slave who gave him a charm on a piece of paper which he wore on his head under the flannel – 'inscribed with strange characters, probably a sentence from the Koran' – and some powder to rub on his jaws and the inside of his mouth. The farmer believed the charm did him good, not the powder, 'for an English doctor or anybody might have given me a powder, but it would not have helped me'.[109]

If poisoning or black magic was suspected, settlers thus often sought out a Muslim doctor or diviner for a cure. In 1883 a Woodstock resident called a 'Malay doctor' to attend to her servant girl who had 'gone mad or was in a fit'. 'Brutus', the doctor, chanted and sang in the 'vernacular' to ward off the presence of the Devil who, he said, had been in the room the previous night.[110] The association between Muslims and bewitchment became a common element in the delusions of psychiatric patients at the Cape. One man who was sent to the Robben Island asylum in 1886 complained that he could not fish because the 'Malay men' hid under the water and took the fish off his line.[111] Another patient refused to apologise for beating his wife and children because he said 'a Malay had bewitched him'.[112] The idea of being 'Malay tricked' was also a feature of delusional content among Valkenberg Mental Asylum patients (see Chapter 8 for more on the asylum).[113]

The slave healer September

Settler fears of being poisoned or bewitched by Muslims or slaves had a long history. The story of the slave-healer September[114] in the late eighteenth century reveals not only the importance of magical elements in slave healing, but also the harsh response of the authorities to the threat posed by slave resistance, especially where this was linked to bewitchment. In 1760, September was a 50-year-old slave living on the farm of Plattekloof, at the western extremity of the Tygerberg, just north of Cape Town. He worked as a shepherd, but seems to have had considerable latitude, regularly visiting Cape Town. He was a Bugis, having been born in the south of the Indonesian island of Sulawesi, and had been enslaved and sold to the Cape (when and how we do not know).

Particularly among his fellow Bugis, September had a considerable reputation as a healer. His practice, insofar as it can be reconstructed, had two components. The first was his ability to render first aid. On one occasion, he coped with a gun-shot wound 'by spitting [on it] in the Buginese manner', and then binding it up with a handkerchief. The second was his knowledge of the formulas by which other Bugis could 'bewitch their master or mistress, or also... cure one or the other ailment.' These *azimat* were written in the Bugis script, which September admitted being able to copy. He denied being able to read it, or to compose non-formulaic text, but this seems unlikely, and is contradicted by other witnesses. He made the disclaimers in an (unsuccessful) attempt to save his life.

September had to attempt this subterfuge because he had been protecting a group of slaves who had murdered Michael Smuts, a DEIC official, and his wife, in their house on the slopes of Table Mountain in Cape Town. They had then fled north to the dunes along the shores of Table Bay, where they had met September, who had fed them, treated them and set them on their way towards the Xhosa-speaking communities of the eastern Cape. Crossing the Cape Flats (the plains to the north-east of Cape Town), they were intercepted by a commando, and the survivors were forced to reveal

Illustration 2.2
Old Somerset Hospital account

An 1834 bill from the Old Somerset Hospital, which shows how owners like Mr Zastron were billed for the medical care of their slaves. Ironically for the owner wishing to protect his human 'asset', this bill was issued just before all slaves were emancipated by government decree in December 1834. At £15/19/6, representing a year's wages for many working-class people, few would have been able to afford this bill in any case.

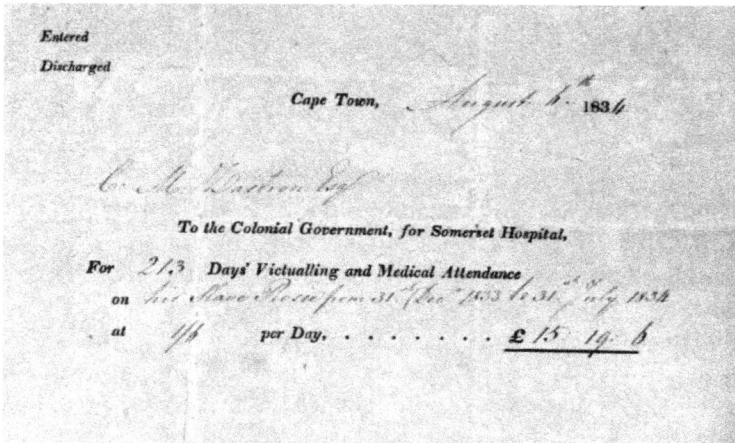

from whom they had received assistance. September was arrested, and in his possession a letter was found from a fellow Bugis slave, Upas, who lived in Stellenbosch. In this letter Upas wrote that he had been sick for two months, and asked September to send him a cure. For the Cape Dutch authorities, who were in a state of panic brought on by the Smuts murders, this evidence of slave literacy, and of forms of communication to which they had no access, and over which they had no control, was sufficient to suggest most dangerous opportunities for plotting, even though Upas's letter contained no suggestion to that effect (their mistranslation of the letter suggested otherwise, however). As a result, the Dutch executed September in one of the more brutal ways at their disposal.

There were probably many other circumstances besides snakebite, bewitchment or poisoning in which settlers found Muslim healers more useful than Western-trained doctors, and much more research needs to be done on this topic. In the eighteenth century one traveller suggested that Javanese slave doctors using medicinal herbs sometimes had a wider practice among settlers than did their Western counterparts.[115] The issue of midwifery will be discussed further below. Suffice to say here that by the nineteenth century, licensed doctors' attitudes towards Muslim healers were not particularly favourable. The Police Surgeon of Cape Town, William Ross, complained in 1874 that a Muslim healer – whom Ross insisted on calling a 'mason' rather than a doctor – had administered 'pungent', possibly sedative, drugs to a man suffering from delirium tremens and forced him to inhale charcoal fumes. In an official memo to the Resident Magistrate, Ross suggested that this was a case of deliberate malpractice:

> I do not know whether Azur calls himself a doctor, but he is an ignorant Malay mason, and allows himself to be consulted as a Native Physician; and when sent for to display his abilities, does not seem to have had any scruples towards giving an exhibition. In conclusion, I am of opinion that a great deal of this rude doctoring goes amongst the coloured classes; and that a successful and prolonged attempt to deprive a man of air can scarcely be regarded as an accident.[116]

Travelling druggists and patent medicines

Country doctors in particular depended on the sale of medicines to augment their incomes and gain clients. They complained vociferously about the sale of medicines by unlicensed practitioners and the practice of medicine by apothecaries and druggists. These people were the main threat to their rural practice.[117] The experience of one angry country doctor can illustrate this point. Charles Orpen, an Irish-born, medically trained church minister living in Colesberg, complained about the 'indiscriminate sale of medicines by unlicensed persons' (probably shopkeepers) in the 1840s.[118] In his biography, Orpen's son described the case of an old farmer called Jan Wessels living in the area who was sought out for medical care because he was supposed to have a good knowledge of medicine and a large supply of it. He treated a local farmer, Jan Zwart, who stayed with Wessels for a week seeking to be cured of his rheumatic fever, but without success. Zwart was then visited by Orpen, who prescribed a medicine that was made up by a Colesberg chemist and administered with good results. Orpen's son explained:

[Wessels had] a ship captain's medicine chest of the biggest sort, which he had got hold of by some extraordinary chance. The ordinary medicine chest of a Boer's house was a well-known little japanned tin box with 'Huis Apatheek' [sic – Home Apothecary] printed upon it. Wessels' big box gave him medical prestige.... [Orpen] looked through the [medicine chest's contents] and said the names given on the prescriptions were ones of about a century past, some being good but none quite suitable [for treating Zwart].[119]

Patent medicines were widely used at the Cape by Cape Dutch settlers. Most popular were the *Hallische* (from Halle, Germany) or *Hollandse* (Dutch) medicines which contained a book of directions for use that was seldom followed by the settlers, who used their own recipes and additives.[120] In 1834 the Halle Orphanage established a depot for the sale of their medicines at the Cape, a step which a Cape Dutch magazine, the *Zuid Afrikaansche Tijdschrift*, applauded.[121] The Trekboers of the nineteenth century took such medicine chests in their waggons and Louis Trichardt devoted a whole page of his diary to the Halle medicines.[122] The medicines in the traditional *Huis Apotheek* contained substances like 'Hoffman's druppels' (for headaches), eucalyptus oil, rue (both for colds), thyme (for dropsy) and beechwood leaves (for rheumatism).[123]

Homeopaths and other alternative practitioners

Unlike places like Canada, where homeopaths and other alternative practitioners attained, if briefly, the same legal and official status as regular doctors,[124] no homeopath could get a licence at the Cape unless he was also medically trained. There were people who practised homeopathy, but they were too few to pose any real challenge to the Cape doctor.[125] Mrs Langham Dale, the wife of the Superintendent-General for Education in the 1860s, used homeopathic medicine to cure headaches (her husband bought a box of the medicine for £4).[126] In 1888, two men were brought before the Magistrate of Kimberley charged with practising as physicians, surgeons and accoucheurs without a licence. They appealed against their conviction before the Supreme Court, saying that they administered homeopathic rather than allopathic medicines. While the Judge said there was some disagreement in both the legal and the medical profession about the desirability of free trade in services, they had to follow the law. He said under the Medical Ordinance

70

Illustration 2.3
Advertisement for blood-cleansing herbs

This advertisement for blood-cleansing herbs – a steal at only 1 Rd
or 1/6d per packet – offered relief from piles, dizziness, bile, acid,
and for women in 'unusual circumstances', i.e. pregnancy. It was
obtainable at one of the most famous chemist shops in Cape Town,
the 'Angel' *Apotheek*, which the apothecary Juritz took over from Dr
Liesching, and where the 'genuine' Hallische medicines were also
obtainable at 'reasonable' prices.

Bloedzuiverende Kruiden.
TE KOOP
IN DE ENGEL APOTHEEK
VAN
C. F. JURITZ,
No. 29, LOOPSTRAAT, KAAPSTAD.

Met een flesch oude Wyn, op een warme
plaats, dagelyks eenige keer wel omge-
schud, te laten trekken, vervolgens door
Flenny te drukken, 's Morgens en 's
Avonds een kelkje vol te nemen. Dit is
een der beste Bloedverdunnende en Bloedzuiverende Middels, zeer sterk in ge-
bruik tegen Aanbeijen, Duizeligheid in
het hoofd, ook tegen Gal en Slym;—als-
mede tegen Zuur en andere kwalen, by
Vrouwen in andere omstandigheden.—
Alleen te bekomen by
CARL FRIEDRICH JURITZ,
"ENGEL APOTHEEK,"
No. 29, LOOPSTRAAT, KAAPSTAD,
Voormaals de Apotheek van Dr. LIESCHING, alwaar
het Depôt van de opregte Hallesche Medicynen is
opgerigt, en alleen de opregte Hallesche Medicynen
te bekomen zyn tegen billyke pryzen.

Het pakje Bloedz. Kruiden kost 1 Rds.

homeopathic practitioners, like indigenous practitioners, were liable
for fines if they sought payment for their services or medicines but
were unlicensed.[127]

Midwives

While there seems to have been little concern among licensed European-trained doctors that Khoisan, slave or homeopathic practitioners would challenge their status or economic prospects, some midwives may have competed with doctors hoping to expand into man-midwifery. Midwives certainly competed acrimoniously and unsuccessfully with doctors in Britain and America for control over attendance at normal childbirths, although in continental Europe they routinely attended normal births and called doctors in complicated cases. [128] For most of the nineteenth century at the Cape, doctors were interested in practising general midwifery, but public conflict and open competition between midwives and doctors was relatively rare. What bad publicity midwives got from doctors and their supporters was focussed on black midwives, who were tarred with the same racist brush as black women in general at the Cape during this period.

Midwives had been appointed by the DEIC to serve the needs of their employees and slaves during the eighteenth century. Under British rule, however, this system of accreditation fell away. A few continentally-trained doctors were eager to institute a system of local training and licensing of midwives in Cape Town after 1810, possibly to gain professional control over midwifery and to encourage midwives to make referrals in difficult cases. The midwifery training system, which seems to have wound down by 1850, favoured white midwives in its licensing, and provided little professional advantage for midwives in general. Midwives did not organise into professional lobbying groups, nor could they change the legal training requirements. They remained a loose, varied group of practitioners who occupied a low social and economic status in colonial society and were subject to the professional validation of the higher-status doctors. [129]

The Midwife Johanna Blank

While we do not know much about Johanna Blank's midwifery practice itself, [130] we can gather some information about her social circumstances. Most midwives were relatively poor, and many were black. A number of Cape midwives had slave origins but this did not necessarily consign them to social and economic obscurity. Johanna Catherina van die Kaap, although born into slavery, was relatively wealthy for a midwife. Born at the Cape, she was initially owned by C.G. Höhne, during which time she had several children, one at least by her future husband, Jan Anthonie Blank, a first-generation immigrant from Holland. She married him in 1792 and they lived in Cape Town where Jan died in 1818 and Johanna seven years later, aged 87. Although it is not clear what sort of training she had undergone, she could not write her own name. Her practice would probably have included both rich and poor clients – she acted as midwife to the slave Spacie van die Kaap in 1797, and was listed as a licensed midwife in the 1820 and 1825 Cape Town almanacs.

Johanna may have acquired her wealth through her husband's earnings rather than her midwifery practice (they were married in community of property), but she must have gained some personal or financial satisfaction from her work because she continued to practise after her marriage and after her husband's death. The Blanks freed their house slave, Dora, and also probably Johanna's four children, one of whom travelled to Holland. On Johanna's death in 1825 she left 2,000 guilders (about £1,000 at the time) to her daughter. Her estate included two houses on 102 Zieke Dwarsstraat, containing expensive gilded mirrors and some paintings. This relative wealth, compared to most of her colleagues, and her marriage to a Cape Dutch settler, helped Johanna to 'pass' for white in the early nineteenth-century Cape.

Unlicensed midwives were not prevented from practising, and licensed midwives were subject to growing competition from doctors by the 1830s, especially in urban areas where most of the licensed accoucheurs practised. In Cape Town the large status differential between midwives and doctors and growing willingness among immigrant women to consult male midwives in normal births prevented white midwives from gaining a significant advantage over doctors. British immigrants to the Cape, who were concentrated in urban areas, were quicker to consult male midwives than were Cape Dutch families who predominated in country districts. The latter tended to favour female attendants, many of whom were black farmworkers. In the 1860s, a British doctor who attended a Cape Dutch woman's confinement in Fraserburg found 'an old native woman was there as midwife'. The patient's husband stayed in the room because it was so unusual for the Cape Dutch to have a man attending a childbirth.[131] Yet in these country areas doctors were initially more focussed on wrestling with druggists and traders over the drug trade than on capturing the market in normal deliveries from midwives.[132] This reduced the intensity of competition between midwives and doctors in country areas.

Medical remedies to aid childbirth were exchanged between

settlers, slaves and Khoisan, a process probably encouraged by extensive slave and Khoisan attendance at settler births.[133] Early travellers commented on the use of a mixture of *dagga* and milk by the Khoisan to hasten labour, which was altered after the introduction of tobacco to a mixture of tobacco and milk, and in turn adopted by the Cape Dutch. The Cape Dutch also used a mixture of tobacco and water or brandy, which was the most common solvent in settler remedies.[134] A British soldier travelling near George in 1853 noted that the settlers there used a mixture of brandy and the local herb *gaab,* which grew only in Cradock, to assist women in childbirth.[135] Similarly, there are various recorded uses of *pelargonium anceps* (which Pappe calls *peristera anceps*)[136] or *roode rabassum* which was 'a great favourite with the Malays' during the nineteenth century and was still used by the Nama (Khoi in the north-western Cape) in the 1920s.[137] Pappe says it was used by the 'Malays' (Muslims) to promote childbirth, and Laidler records its use as an abortifacient or to hasten labour by the Nama as well as Muslims and Afrikaners. The latter used it for anaemia, weaknesses and fevers, as its redness was thought to strengthen the blood. The association between Khoisan and Muslim women and abortion in the medical as well as the broader settler literature is a sign not only of their marginality within the settlers' moral world, but also their key role in assisting settler women in childbirth and abortions.

Conclusions

Reading the official and public papers relating to the Cape medical profession during the nineteenth century, one could be led to believe that these doctors were operating in small provincial towns in England rather than in an African country with a number of strong alternative medical traditions very different from those in Europe. The practitioners who featured most significantly in doctors' public discourse were those who sold patent medicines, unlicensed practitioners in the Western medical tradition and midwives. Although the legal sanctions existed to hinder indigenous and other alternative practitioners, Cape doctors saw this as a low priority in the early and mid-nineteenth century and showed little interest in investigating African or east Asian medicine. This pattern suggests that there were significant differences in the scope and practise of these two groups of medical practitioners in the Cape medical market. While Muslim and Khoisan healers did attend settler clients, their expertise was thought to reside mainly in areas such as poisoning or exorcism which were not well covered by mainstream

Western medicine or by an already creolised folk medicine. As we will see, Cape doctors did have black clients too, but many of these people were seeking particular remedies for which Western medicine was well known, or were recipients of government or employer-sponsored medical care in hospitals, prisons or settler homes.

While there was no doubt a gap between doctors' public statements and private practice (how large this gap might be we do not yet know), the public face of the Cape doctor is an important indicator of the role the medical profession sought to delineate for itself in the colonial context. Nineteenth-century Cape doctors showed little public interest in indigenous plants and their use partly because they wanted to carve out a new professional identity for themselves, based on formal training in Europe, linked to European models of professional organisation and practice and specifically distinct from any association with the work of informal practitioners and druggists. Country doctors had to continue selling drugs, but these patent medicines were largely of European origin and manufacture. This activity, while necessary for their economic survival, lowered their professional status and was one of the main reasons why country doctors at the Cape, like provincial GPs in Britain, continued to be regarded as lesser members of the medical profession throughout the century. The distinction in professional status and practice between town and country doctors will be elaborated in the next chapter.

Notes

1. The subject of indigenous healing in South Africa has until recently has been sadly neglected in academia, with the exception of the work of anthropologists, e.g. H. Ngubane *Body and Mind in Zulu Medicine* (London: New York Academic Press, 1977) and botanists – the classic work here is J.M. Watt and M.G. Breyer-Brandwijk, *The Medicinal and Poisonous Plants of Southern Africa* (Edinburgh: Livingstone, 1932). The topic is currently receiving more attention from historians, for example C.A. Harrison, 'The King of Native Customs: S.P.D. Madiehe and the Ambiguities of African Traditional Healers' Associations, 1928-1948' (unpublished B.A. thesis, University of the Witwatersrand, 1993); C. Burns, 'Louisa Mvemve: A Woman's Advice to the Public on the Cure of Various Diseases', *Kronos: Journal of Cape History*, xxiii (1996). A research project on medical pluralism at the Cape is currently being conducted by Prof. Anne Digby of Oxford Brookes University in England, with the assistance of Helen Sweet. Less historical attention has however been

paid to imported forms of alternative healing in South Africa such as slave medicine, homeopathy and patent medicines – see for example E. Lastovica, 'Sequah, a Quack in Nineteenth Century Cape Town', *Cabo*, vi, 2 (1987), 10–18.

2. In the same way that Afrikaans was linked in nationalist discourse to Dutch rather than Malay or Khoisan languages, settler medicine was increasingly located in farmers' closeness to the earth rather than their proximity to indigenous healers. Thanks to a student of the University of Natal (Durban) History Department for pointing out the language comparison here.

3. On nineteenth-century Britain see for example, P.S. Brown, 'The Providers of Medical Treatment in Mid-Nineteenth Century Bristol', *Medical History*, xxiv (1980), 297–314. Africa provides numerous examples of multiple healing traditions both before and after European colonialism: see for example, S. Feierman and J. Janzen (eds), *The Social Basis of Health and Healing in Africa* (Berkeley: University of California Press, 1992). In colonial Haiti, slave healers treated slaves, free people of colour and white settlers during the eighteenth century (Karol K. Weaver, History Dept., Penn State University, personal communication 20 April 1998).

4. In an interesting piece of research, K.L. Leonard ('African Traditional Healers: Incentives and Skill in Health Care Delivery', paper presented to the ASA Annual Conference, San Francisco, November 1996) argues that the main factor influencing the choice of traditional or Western healers by patients in modern Africa is not culture or cost, but the combination of treatment requirements (medical effort, patient effort and medical skill) necessary for specific diseases.

5. Letter from Mrs John Ross to her sister, 7 June 1839, U. Long, *An Index to Authors of Unofficial, Privately-Owned Manuscripts Relating to the History of South Africa 1812-1920* (London: n.p., 1947), 238.

6. Letter from Mrs Hugo to B.J. de la Bat, 7 June 1839, CA, Van der Merwe Collection, A 454.

7. In 1807 the regulations detailed the penalty for practising without a licence as 1000 Rixdollars (Rds) and banishment for a second offence (Proclamation by Governor Caledon, 18 August 1807, Section 1 Proclamations 1806-1820, CA, CO 5881). In 1823, the penalty for a second offence was changed to prohibition from further practice in the colony (Government Proclamation, 26 September 1823, Proclamations for 1823, CA, CO 5824), and in 1830 the fine was fixed at £50 (Ordinance 82, 23 December 1830, Proclamations for 1828-31, CA, CO 5829). While the regulations

could prevent unlicensed practitioners from recovering their fees, and could impose a fine, if the unlicensed practitioner could not afford the fine he could not be imprisoned. On this, see Robarts v. Jelly in M.W. Searle (ed.) *Cases decided in the Supreme Court, 1857-1860*, iii (Cape Town: Juta, 1888), 407–8 and Queen v. Maynier in H. Juta, *Reports of Cases in the Supreme Court*, vi (Cape Town: Juta, 1890), 125.

8. M. Last and G.L. Chavunduka (eds), *The Professionalisation of African Medicine* (Manchester: Manchester University Press, 1986), 18–19, fn.19. In the Transvaal, the *Uitvoerende Raad* (Executive Council of Government) refused to limit the free sale of medicines and open access to medical practice in the 1850s, A.N. Pelzer, *Geskiedenis van die Suid-Afrikaanse Republiek*, 3 vols. (Cape Town: Balkema, 1950), i, 36.

9. E. Pretorius, 'Alternative (Complementary?) Medicine in South Africa', *South African Sociological Journal*, xxiv, 1 (1993), 13–17: 15.

10. B. Good, *Medicine, Rationality and Experience: An Anthropological Perspective* (Cambridge: Cambridge University Press, 1994), 28, notes that 'Questions of the efficacy of clinical medicine are often quite distinct from the truth claims of biomedical science'. He suggests that we should compare the cultural constructions of illness in alternative medicine and in biomedical science rather than their claims for efficacy.

11. V. Nutton, 'Humoralism' in W.F. Bynum and R. Porter (eds), *Companion Encyclopedia of the History of Medicine* (London: Routlege, 1993), i, 281–91: 288.

12. C.J. Glacken, *Traces on the Rhodian Shore: Nature and Culture in Western Thought from Ancient Times to the End of the Eighteenth Century* (Berkeley: University of California Press, 1967), 429, 502, 566, 620–2. See also M. Harrison, *Public Health in British India* (Cambridge: Cambridge University Press, 1994), 38.

13. An interesting analysis along similar lines is made by D.V. Hart in 'Bisayan Filipino and Malayan Humoral Pathologies: Folk Medicine and Ethnohistory in South East Asia', Data Paper 76, SE Asia Program, Dept. of Asian Studies, Cornell University, Ithaca, New York, November 1969.

14. H.J. Deacon, 'Midwives and Medical Men in the Cape Colony, 1800-1860', *Journal of African History*, xxxix (1998), 271–92.

15. They, like all the doctors practising at the Cape, at least until the latter part of the nineteenth century, were all men.

16. The request for local training gained support because the son of a high-profile doctor had undergone an apprenticeship in Cape Town

and wished to be licensed for practice in the Colony.

17. More information on early licensing can be found in the classic work on South African medical history, E.H. Burrows, *A History of Medicine in South Africa* (Cape Town: Balkema, 1958), Chapter 6.
18. Memorial of 'subscribers, merchants, traders and others of Cape Town', 16 September 1807, CA, CO 3864, doc.423. In 1810, Mackrill, living at 10 Burg Street, was the only English civilian doctor listed in the *Cape Almanac* as a surgeon in Cape Town. There were of course British military doctors at the Cape in 1807 who probably practiced privately.
19. A. Digby, *Making a Medical Living: Doctors and Patients in the English Medical Market for Medicine* (Cambridge: Cambridge University Press, 1994), 226.
20. These figures were extracted from a database of all medical practitioners in the Cape Colony from 1800-1860, compiled from various sources by the author.
21. A GP in Britain was most commonly a doctor with qualifications in medicine and surgery – surgeon or surgeon-apothecary – who was a Member of one of the various Colleges of Surgeons (MRCS) and Licentiate of the Society of Apothecaries (LSA). Some would have had a midwifery qualification as well.
22. E.B. van Heyningen, 'Agents of Empire: the Medical Profession in the Cape Colony, 1880-1910', *Medical History*, xxx (1989), 452.
23. See also H.J. Deacon, 'Cape Town and Country Doctors in the Cape Colony during the First Half of the Nineteenth Century', *Social History of Medicine*, x, 1 (1997), 25–52.
24. *Ibid.*, 43.
25. The roles of apothecary and druggist were not clearly differentiated in Cape law, but the licensed apothecary usually had a formal certificate like the LSA as well as proof of apprenticeship, and the druggist usually only had the latter.
26. For a biography, see F. and W. Malherbe, *H.A.J.B. Hammerschmidt: Medical Practitioner in Stellenbosch 1858-1860* (Stellenbosch: Stellenbosch Museum, 1999).
27. Memorial of J.B. Hammerschmidt, 6 February 1858, Memorials 1831, CA, CO 4102, doc.H20.
28. Memorial of J.B. Hammerschmidt, 19 February 1858, Memorials 1831, CA, CO 4102, doc.H27.
29. Malherbe, *op. cit.* (note 26), 41.
30. Memorial of E. Schröder, 1 December 1859, Memorials 1859, CA, CO 4111, doc.S131.
31. Malherbe, *op. cit.* (note 26), 23.

32. The Liquidation and Distribution Account of Johan Baptist Henry Anton Hammerschmidt of Stellenbosch, 1861, CA, MOIB 2/943 (159), lists his possessions as including '*1 doos met instrumenten*' (one box with instruments) and a dispensing room containing shelves with medicine bottles on them, pots with ointment, a funnel, glass bottles, measuring glasses, scales, packaged herbs, mortar and pestle, corks and vials, packets of herbs and salts.
33. Malherbe, *op. cit.* (note 26), 25.
34. *Ibid.*, 42.
35. The Liquidation and Distribution Account of Johan Baptist Henry Anton Hammerschmidt of Stellenbosch, 1861, CA, MOIB 2/943 (159), Insolvent Schedule D: Bad debts; 110 accounts for medical attendance to different parties in the year 1858 (value 53/0/0d); 221 accounts for 1859 (130/5/6d) and 92 accounts for 1860 (63/17/6d). All patients residing in Stellenbosch.
36. *Ibid.*, Inventory of goods and effects.
37. J.B. Hammerschmidt, '…and Medical Statistics on Health and Disease during the time from October 1858 to October 1860' (Cape Town: 1860), i–ii. Reprinted in Malherbe, *op. cit.* (note 26).
38. *Ibid.*
39. *Ibid.*, 34, 36, 37.
40. *Ibid.*, 66.
41. *Ibid.*, 61.
42. Pedro Sousa Dias (Faculty of Pharmacology, University of Lisbon, personal communication 14 July 1997) also links interest in indigenous remedies in colonial Brazil and Angola to difficulties in the supply of European medicines and to a shortage of European doctors. Karol Weaver suggests that Western doctors in colonial Haiti turned to slave healers for medicinal herbal knowledge partly because medicines imported from France were 'outdated' (History Dept., Penn State University, personal communication 20 April 1998).
43. Pedro Sousa Dias (Faculty of Pharmacology, University of Lisbon, personal communication 14 July 1997) suggests that the level of interest shown by imperial governments in exploiting colonial medicinal resources also played a key role in the investigation of indigenous remedies by colonial doctors in South America.
44. In colonial Spanish America the Spanish showed even greater interest in collecting information about indigenous herbal remedies because it was believed that local plants would cure locally endemic diseases (this idea sometimes discouraged the adoption of colonial plants in Europe where it was believed they would be less effective). In the

1570s, a special expedition was launched to collect information about Aztec herbal knowledge (Prof. J. Canizares, Assistant Professor of History, Illinois State University, personal communication 16 July 1997).

45. A. Smith, *A Contribution to South African Materian Medica Chiefly from Plants in Use Among the Natives* (Lovedale: Lovedale Press, 1888). Most of his informants were missionaries and local Africans.

46. See J.M. Watt, 'The History of Pharmacology in South Africa', *Journal of the Medical Association of South Africa*, i (22 October 1927), 528–34.

47. P. Kolb, *The Present State of the Cape of Good Hope* 2 vols (London: W. Innys, 1731), ii, 309.

48. *Ibid.*, ii, 250.

49. See travellers' accounts in this chapter, and also 'Folk Remedies', n.d. UCT Department of Manuscripts and Archives, BC 295.

50. P.W. Laidler and M. Gelfand, *South Africa: Its Medical History* (Cape Town: Struik, 1971), 165, 209. See also T. James, 'Sieketroost: Dr James Barry's Contribution to Materia Medica', *SAMJ*, il (15 July 1972), 1013–16.

51. Kolb, *op. cit.* (note 47), ii, 359.

52. *Ibid.*, ii. 355.

53. *Ibid.*, ii, 351.

54. A. Sparrman, *A Voyage to the Cape of Good Hope* (London: G.G.J. & J. Robinson, 1786), 47.

55. E. Bergh, 'Memorie Over de Kaap de Goede Hoop' (1801) in Theal's *Important Historical Documents*, iii (Cape Town: n.p., 1911), 68.

56. C.H. Price, 'Diary of Dr Mackrill', *Africana Notes and News*, xiii (8) (December 1959), 315; James, *op. cit.* (note 50); N. Mathie, *Man of Many Facets: Atherstone, Dr W.G.* (Grahamstown: Grocott & Sherry, 1997-8), ii, 472–4.

57. A.M.L.R., 'An American Girl at the Cape in 1834', *Quarterly Bulletin of the SA Library*, xxiii, 3 (March 1969), 87.

58. One of these was the Worcester District Surgeon's report on *slangenbosch*, see below.

59. See for example, Report on a BMA meeting, 'Notes on the Pharmacology of some South African Drugs', *SAMJ*, vii (October 1899), 123–8; J. Maberley, 'South African Pharmacology', *Transvaal Medical Journal*, i, 4 (1 November 1905), 99–104.

60. BMA, *op. cit.* (note 59), 125. The aloe was later removed because of poor results abroad.

61. Maberley, *op. cit.* (note 59), 100.

62. James, *op. cit.* (note 50), 1014 and BMA, *op. cit.* (note 59), 125.
63. L. Pappe, 'A List of South African Indigenous Plants Used as Remedies by the Colonists', *Cape Town Medical Gazette*, i, 4 (Oct 1847), 83–4.
64. *Ibid.*, 87.
65. *Ibid.*, 86.
66. H. Hoving, 'Thunberg en die Kaapse inwoners' (unpublished MA thesis, University of Stellenbosch, 1939), 336.
67. Sparrman, *op. cit.* (note 54), 47.
68. Pappe, *op. cit.* (note 63), 58.
69. 'Hollandse Medisijne', *SAMJ*, xxvii, 25, (20 June 1953), 532–3. This was probably somewhat different from the nineteenth century range, as it excluded one known ingredient called *Hoffman's Druppels*, but all the major ingredients were imported, as they had been during the nineteenth century.
70. De Mist's Journal of 1803 in E.C.G. Molsbergen (ed.), *Reizen in Zuid-Afrika in de Hollandse Tijd*, iv ('s-Gravenhage: Marinus Nijhoff, 1916-1932), 227.
71. C.H. Price, 'J.T. Pocock – Pioneer – Pharmacist, Part II', *South African Pharmaceutical Journal*, xxvii, 6 (February 1961), 20.
72. Horstock vs. Boniface, Breda and Neethling in W. Menzies, *Cases Decided in the Supreme Court of the Cape of Good Hope* (Cape Town: Juta, 1903), 467–9.
73. R. Ross, 'The Anthropology of the Germanic-Speaking Peoples of Southern Africa', paper presented at the Conference on History and Anthropology, University of Manchester, 1980, 11.
74. J.F. Haszner, 'Medical Handbook' translated and transcribed by L.C. van Oordt, J.F. Haszner Collection, SA Library, MSB 240, v.
75. R. Viljoen, 'Disease and Society: VOC Cape Town, Its People and the Smallpox Epidemics of 1713, 1755 and 1767', *Kleio*, xxvii (1995), 18, 22.
76. More research needs to be done on the political and economic implications of 'sharing' and commodifying medical remedies. For a fine study of narcotic abuse and the politics of early colonialism, see D. Gordon, 'From Rituals of Rapture to Dependence: The Political Economy of Khoikhoi Narcotic Consumption, c.1487-1870', *South African Historical Journal*, xxxv (November 1996), 62–88.
77. Both before and after slave emancipation in 1838, many ex-slaves were Muslims.
78. J. Heniger, *Hendrik Adriaan van Reede tot Drakenstein (1636-1691) and Hortus Malabaricus: A Contribution to the History of Dutch Colonial Botany* (Rotterdam: Balkema, 1986), 9 – my emphasis.

79. Le Valliant says they are fed a meal of fat first, cited in P.W. Laidler, 'Manners, Medicine and Magic of the Cape Hottentots', unpublished transcript., UCT Manuscripts Collection, BCS 401, 149.
80. Kolb, *op. cit.* (note 47), i, 87.
81. *Ibid.*, 88.
82. *Ibid.*
83. J.W.D. Moodie, *Ten Years in South Africa* (London: Richard Bentley, 1835), i, 233.
84. H.S.N. Menko, *Contributions of the Netherlands to the Development of South African Medicine (1652-1902)* (Amsterdam: De Bussy, 1954), 57.
85. C.F. Hofman, *Korte Beschreijving van de Caab de Goede Hoop* (University of Natal facsimile reproduction, 1967 [n.d. on original]), n.p.
86. Kolb, *op. cit.* (note 47), ii, 305.
87. *Ibid.*, ii, 302–3.
88. J. Campbell, *Travels in South Africa Undertaken at the Request of the Missionary Society* (London: Black and Parry, 1815), 308.
89. Campbell, *op. cit.* (note 88), 316 ff.
90. J. Backhouse, *Extracts from the Journal of James Backhouse* (London: 1840), 44.
91. S. Kalff, 'Batavische Doctoren uit de 17e eeuw', *Staatkundig, Economisch en Letterkundig Tijdschrift*, xxxii (1910), 1290–1.
92. Hofman, *op. cit.* (note 85), n.p.
93. Kolb, *op. cit.* (note 47), ii, 305–6.
94. For a commentary on this see D. Bunn, 'Of Poison and Painting "The Brown Serpent of the Rocks": Bushman Arrow Toxins in the Dutch and British Imagination, 1735-1850', paper presented at the Appropriations conference, Centre for African Studies, University of Cape Town, September 1993.
95. Kolb, *op. cit.* (note 47), ii, 305.
96. Campbell, *op. cit.* (note 88), 316–25.
97. J. Barrow, *Travels into the Interior of Southern Africa* ii (London: T. Cadell & Davies, 1806), 90.
98. Moodie, *op. cit.* (note 83), i, 234.
99. P. McMagh, *The Three Lieschings: Their Times and Contribution to Cape Medicine* (Cape Town: The Society for the History of Pharmacy in South Africa, 1992), 31.
100. C. de Jong, *Reizen Naar de Kaap de Goede Hoop* (Haarlem: Francois Bohm, 1802), 197.
101. Barrow, *op. cit.* (note 97), i, 90.

102. Kolb, *op, cit.* (note 47), ii, 167. See also V. de Kock, *Those in Bondage* (Pretoria: Allen & Unwin, 1963), 134–5.
103. Sparrman, *op. cit.* (note 54), 177.
104. J.E. Alexander, *Expedition of Discovery into the Interior of Africa* (London: Colburn, 1838), 83.
105. Moodie, *op. cit.* (note 83), i, 235. See also 'South African Snake-Bites', *Chambers's Journal,* 29 March 1890, 208.
106. Moodie, *op. cit.* (note 83), i, 236.
107. *Ibid.* i, 197.
108. J.V. Bickford-Smith, *Ethnic Pride and Racial Prejudice* (Cambridge: Cambridge University Press, 1995), 71–4.
109. Moodie, *op. cit.* (note 83), ii, 33–4.
110. *The Lantern,* 25 August 1883.
111. Case of Jan alias Kwaai, n.d., Health Branch, Criminal Lunatics 1893-1899, CA, CO 8050.
112. Case of Bekker, 25 November 1895, Attorney General's Papers, Lunatics 1894-1895, CA, AG 1932.
113. H.J. Deacon, 'A History of the Medical Institutions on Robben Island, 1846-1910' (unpublished Ph.D. thesis, University of Cambridge, 1994), 187.
114. This biographical sketch is drawn with permission from S. Koolhof and R. Ross, 'Upas, September and the Bugis at the Cape of Good Hope: The Context of a Slave's Letter', *SARI: A Journal of Malay Studies,* forthcoming. V. de Kock also mentions the medical practice of a slave called September, in the 1760s; *op. cit.* (note 102), 132.
115. *Ibid.,* 132.
116. Police Surgeon to Resident Magistrate of Cape Town, 1 July 1874, CA, 1/CT 11/43.
117. Deacon, *op. cit.* (note 23), 42.
118. Memorial of C. Orpen, 1 August 1849, and Medical Committee to Secretary to Government, 15 August 1849, CA, CO 4048, Memorials N-P, 1849, doc.55.
119. J.M. Orpen, *Reminiscences of Life in South Africa from 1846 to the Present Day* (Cape Town: Struik, 1964), 27.
120. P.W. Grobbelaar, C.W. Hudson and H. van der Merwe (eds), *Die Afrikaner en sy Kultuur, deel VI: Boerewysheid* (Cape Town: Tafelberg, 1977), 126. *Hallische* is a term referring to the orphanage at Halle, Germany, where they were packed; it was later corrupted to '*Hollandse*' medicines.
121. W.H.J. Punt, *Louis Trichardt se Laaste Skof* (Pretoria: Van Schaik, 1953), 160.
122. Grobbelaar *et al.* (eds), *op. cit.* (note 120), 126 and Punt, *op. cit.*

(note 121), 160.

123. Menko, *op. cit.* (note 84), 125.
124. J. Connor, 'A Sort of Felo-de-se: Eclecticism, Related Medical Sects and their Decline in Victorian Ontario', *Bulletin of the History of Medicine*, lxv (1991), 503–27.
125. On homeopathic remedies and practitioners see also J. Brown, 'Some Reminiscences of Practice in the Cape Half a Century Ago', *SAMR*, xiv (1916), 216–18, 248–50, 321–3, 384–6.
126. J. Murray (ed.) *Mrs Dale's Diary 1857-72* (Cape Town: Balkema, 1966).
127. Queen vs. Sampson and Bacon in Juta (ed.), *op. cit.* (note 7), vi, 279.
128. M.J. van Lieburg and H. Marland, 'Midwife Regulation, Education, and Practice in the Netherlands During the Nineteenth Century', *Medical History*, xxxiii (1989), 301, 305, 316.
129. Deacon, *op. cit.* (note 14), 290–91.
130. This study is drawn from Deacon, *op. cit.* (note 14), 280–1.
131. Brown, *op. cit.* (note 125), 249.
132. Deacon, *op. cit.* (note 14), 286.
133. On this see also R. Viljoen, 'Diseases and Doctoring: Khoikhoi, Diseases and Medicine at the Cape of Good Hope', paper presented at the SSHM Summer Conference, Medicine and the Colonies, July 1996, 27.
134. Kolb, *op. cit.* (note 47), i, 140 and ii, 337.
135. Graham, Lieut. Lumley (Infantry), 'Cape Journal', iii (January 1853-September 1853), Rhodes House, Oxford, Mss Afr.8, 161–6.
136. Pappe, *op. cit.* (note 63), 59.
137. Laidler, *op. cit.* (note 79), 163.

3

Medical Gentlemen and the Process of Professionalisation before 1860

Harriet Deacon

In the early-nineteenth century, the professionalisation of medicine at the Cape began in earnest. Although there were key legislative and professional developments in this period, the notion, outlined in Burrows' seminal work on South African medical history, that it was a 'golden' age of medical reform underplays the extent of intra-professional differentiation and draws attention away from the politics of professional regulation at the Cape. The period was a time of inter- and intra-professional conflict as doctors, druggists and shopkeepers competed to sell drugs and medical advice and it spawned a profession that was deeply divided. In spite of early, general and monopolistic legislation passed in 1807, the process of medical profes-sionalisation at the Cape was very uneven, cementing an intra-professional distinction between doctors in Cape Town and doctors or druggists in the rest of the colony. The special status of Cape Town provided the bedrock for an urban-rural divide in professional regulation and services still present in South Africa today.

Introduction

Friedson[1] argues that the central defining characteristic of the medical profession is that exclusive autonomy has been deliberately granted to them to define who is a 'trained' medical practitioner, what characterises health and illness and the right to treat illness (sometimes this is a legal monopoly right). This technical autonomy is generally, although not necessarily, accompanied by some autonomy over the social and economic context of their work. Other characteristics such as autonomous professional organisations, systems of education based on specialist knowledge, and full-time employment are means towards technical autonomy rather than ends

85

in themselves and in any case are often ideals rather than reality. The definition of a profession is not universally applicable, however, but historically constructed.[2] During the nineteenth century, the relatively small differences between regular doctors' methods and those of their rivals and patients made social differentiation particularly important in constructing the medical profession.

Most recent work on Cape medical history has tended to concentrate on medical professionalisation during the period of industrial development after 1880.[3] Then, doctors were more numerous and attained more of the traditional trappings of a profession: a national professional organisation after 1883, greater say in professional education in the Cape after 1904 and greater authority in a wider range of services in the public sector as their role in public health expanded after the 1880s. But it was in the early nineteenth century, and perhaps before, that the professionalisation process at the Cape really began. Although there were key legislative and professional developments in this period, the notion that it was a 'golden' age of medical reform[4] underplays the extent of intra-professional differentiation and draws attention away from the politics of professional regulation at the Cape. The period was a time of inter- and intra-professional conflict as doctors, druggists and shopkeepers competed to sell drugs and medical advice and it spawned a profession that was deeply divided. In spite of early, general and monopolistic legislation passed in 1807,[5] the process of medical professionalisation at the Cape was very uneven, cementing an intra-professional distinction between doctors in Cape Town and doctors or druggists in the rest of the colony. The special status of Cape Town provided the bedrock for an urban-rural divide in professional regulation and services still present in South Africa today.[6]

In working towards an understanding of the nineteenth-century colonial medical profession in the Cape we need to explore its historical roots in Europe. In Britain and elsewhere there was a gradual increase in the number and status of what were called 'professional gentlemen' during the eighteenth century, whose authority rested on specialist knowledge rather than land or titles. This increase was closely linked to the growth of trade and urbanisation which boosted the service sector of the economy.[7] Gidney and Millar have suggested that in nineteenth-century Britain and Ontario, 'the title "profession" was an indication of the social ranking of particular occupations'.[8] Professionalisation was associated with the acquisition of gentlemanly status; doctors sought to become 'professional gentlemen', although not all of them succeeded. The ideal professional gentlemen were 'respectable' men – exclusively men – who possessed both a liberal education and a recognised specialist training in the church, law or medicine. Their liberal education in the classics and codes of ethics drawn from traditions of gentlemanly behaviour gave them a social status as 'gentlemen', although many were not born into the gentry. This social status gave them the moral authority to represent their career as an altruistic vocation rather than a self-interested money-making venture, and their income as a gratuity rather than a living.[9] John Harley Warner has suggested that even in antebellum America, doctors' professional identity was predicated partly on 'moral character' or social respectability, although social status did not determine whether a man was a doctor or not.[10]

Professionalisation at the Cape

During the eighteenth century, there was little formal control over medical practice at the Cape. The Dutch East India Company (DEIC) appointed surgeons to work in its ships and at its hospitals, but these appointees often lacked formal medical training, even as apprentices. There was even less regulatory control over the accreditation and practice of burgher surgeons who served the settler population at the Cape – these men were often ex-DEIC appointees or immigrant doctors with widely varying educational backgrounds. The lack of formal regulation led to considerable differences in training and social status among Cape doctors trained in the Western medical tradition, and blurred the distinctions between these doctors and alternative medical practitioners. Alternative medical practitioners (including indigenous practitioners) faced no significant legal limitations on their practice during this period. Partly because of the looser regulatory structure before 1807 and partly because of the cheaper and more flexible nature of medical apprenticeship as a mode of training compared to European university instruction, female and black medical practitioners had greater opportunities and more official recognition at the Cape during the seventeenth and eighteenth centuries than in the nineteenth century.

In 1807, regulations were promulgated which provided for the licensing of regular practitioners and the prohibition of unlicensed practice. Thereafter, a growing number of licensed medical practitioners were involved in formal (legal) medical practice. While the 1807 regulations were not strictly applied, and indeed did not provide significant regulatory controls over medical practice outside of Cape Town, they formed a platform for licensed doctors and apothecaries to begin the process of professionalisation. This chapter will examine the ways in which licensed doctors sought the status of professional gentlemen in the Cape between about 1800 and 1860. Doctors and apothecaries were appointed to medical committees which acted in an advisory capacity to the colonial government, they established medical societies and a professional journal before 1850 and claimed a place within the upper ranks of the growing colonial middle class at the Cape. Professional advancement was easier to achieve in the wealthy urban centre of Cape Town (and later in Grahamstown) than in the country areas where competition between apothecaries and doctors was a growing problem.

Cape midwives were an exception to this pattern of inter-professional conflict and intra-professional organisation and lobbying, although they were affected by the urban-rural differences in the medical market and came under state regulation in 1810.[11] As a group, licensed midwives were more racially heterogenous than doctors, including not only white women of Dutch, German and British extraction, but also free blacks (mainly freed slaves) and slaves. In contrast, for the whole of the nineteenth century and much of the twentieth, the vast majority of licensed doctors and apothecaries were European and South African-born men trained in the mainstream Western medical tradition. By 1810, regulations for the licensing of female midwives were in force. These regulations were, like the 1807 provisions, most closely observed in the highly regulated medical market of Cape Town. Yet even in Cape Town, many practising midwives, mainly black women of slave ancestry, were not formally registered. Nevertheless, the 1810 regulations underlined male control over the medical profession: Midwives had to be examined and licensed by doctors in order to practise legally. Licensed midwives (and later nurses) had a lower social status and were less well organised as a profession than were doctors. This status distinction widened during the course of the nineteenth century and was further entrenched by the subordinate position of nurses and midwives *vis-a-vis* doctors in the 1891 legislation.

Certain conditions helped doctors to shape and codify their professional identity in the early nineteenth-century Cape Colony. In Europe these conditions included growing state intervention in public health, scientific advances and urbanisation.[12] The rise of a middle class, the expansion of secondary education, the increasing involvement of the state in medical affairs as well as legislation on

88

professional structure and medical education enabled the reform of education and organisation in Britain.[13] The Cape medical profession was able to take advantage of these trends both through European influence and similar local conditions. Cape doctors, who had to have been trained in Europe to be licensed after 1807, had benefited from scientific advances and educational reforms there and sought to reproduce some forms of professional organisation in the colony. Military doctors seeking greater status abroad and civilian doctors, who became part of a colonial middle class in Cape Town, were eager to exploit opportunities for professionalisation at the Cape. With the full support of autocratic governors and in the absence of pre-existing professional medical bodies, legislative reform was rapid. Professional licensing and regulation was undertaken by a government-appointed Medical Committee from 1807.

After they retook the Cape in 1806, British governors ruled supreme until a colonial parliament was formed in 1854. Autocratic and elitist, the governors were willing and able to push through legal, commercial and administrative reforms of the old Dutch system. A professional class was of particular importance to imperial administrators wishing to recreate in new colonies the structure of British society in the absence of an aristocracy or landed gentry, both as a symbol of British civilisation and as a tool of colonial 'progress'. As Gidney and Millar argue for Upper Canada, professional gentlemen were to 'provid[e] it with its political leadership, its central social values, its ruling ideas, its erudition'.[14] In the Cape, these professional gentlemen, especially in Cape Town and Grahamstown, were an important part of a middle-class campaign for representative government which was granted in 1854; they helped to define the new society as respectable and worthy of self-government. This may have been one reason why doctors had a higher social status in nineteenth-century Australia, Canada and the Cape than in Britain.[15]

Negotiating boundaries

Defining the 'professional gentleman' required a negotiation of the shifting boundaries between male and female roles, those of gentlemen and tradesmen, 'regular' professionals and 'quacks' and also, within the profession itself, between physicians, surgeons and apothecaries. Even within the ranks of regularly trained doctors in Britain, there were some – like the lowly surgeon-apothecary – who could not qualify as 'professional gentlemen'. In the colonial context, where there were relatively few members of the British upper classes, the definition of the 'gentleman' had to incorporate a wider range of social roles and status than in Britain. There were fewer professionals in general and more low-status doctors at the Cape, which tended to encourage the blurring of distinctions of status and role within the profession. A British visitor to the Cape in 1818, Sarah Norman Eaton, described how little social distinction was made between physicians and surgeons:

> After [the church] service, we called on Miss Muddle at Dr, or rather Mr. Bailey's (he being only a surgeon, though it is customary here to give him that title, as well as others in the same line).[16]

This was similar in some respects to the situation in continental Europe, where the divide between physician and surgeon had narrowed by the beginning of the nineteenth century.[17] Although in the 1830s civilian doctors in Cape Town titled physicians 'Dr' and surgeons 'Mr' among themselves,[18] they were reluctant to make these distinctions in the public arena. They protested against the 'invidious distinction' made between physicians and surgeons in the 1823 regulations.[19] This was a reference to the fact that physicians were referred to as having to produce a university diploma for licensing while surgeons, like apothecaries and druggists, had to produce 'such Certificates as is usually required for these Arts'.[20]

The boundaries between doctors and other practitioners (druggists and irregulars) were drawn and redrawn according to local circumstances. In the colonies those able, often for the first time, to represent themselves as 'professional gentlemen' were anxious to create new distinctions as well as new alliances within the profession. Where there were new competitors, such as black midwives and politically powerful alternative practitioners, new forms of social and legal differentiation were sought. These boundaries were defined in terms of social status as well as technical duties and expertise.

Battles over drug sales

The intensity of complaints by Cape doctors against other practitioners was related to the expansion of 'regular' practice into new areas during periods of greater competition; doctors' strategies for dealing with the problem were diverse.[21] After 1790 competition between surgeon-apothecaries and dispensing druggists within the British profession had encouraged the former to seek competitive advantage and greater social status through advances in medical education, greater professional unity and closer co-operation with the state on urban health reforms.[22] At the Cape, fierce competition between doctors, drug-merchants and druggists in Cape Town at the beginning of the nineteenth century was the impetus for the Cape's first professional legislation in 1807, which sought medical controls over the drug trade and a legal monopoly over prescribing and dispensing for the 'regular' profession (this has been discussed in Chapter 2). The regulations of 1807 forbade doctors from selling any medicine outside of a narrow range of items and it forbade apothecaries and others from selling medical advice. This did not, however, apply outside Cape Town. The regulations thus distinguished Cape Town doctors as 'gentlemen' from low-status 'tradesmen', as well as protecting doctors to some extent against competition from within and outside the profession. The distinction between Cape doctors and druggists was later reinforced by the licensing rules, which insisted on European training for physicians and surgeons until the early twentieth century but accepted local apprenticeships for druggists in 1829, as has been discussed in Chapter 2.[23] The insistence on European training for doctors helped to maintain their higher social status *vis-a-vis* druggists and to restrict numbers.

James Barry, a Scottish-born doctor of uncertain gender (see Chapter 4), acted as adviser to the colonial government in place of the Supreme Medical Committee from 1821-25 in his capacity as Colonial Medical Inspector.[24] His complaints about the sale of uninspected drugs in Cape Town, doctors keeping druggist's shops, shopkeepers selling medicines and apothecaries practising medicine resulted in the promulgation of tighter regulations on drug sales in the regulations of 1823. This provoked vociferous protests from shopkeepers.[25] Barry also opposed local apprenticeships for apothecaries. He felt that while the status of medicine had improved at the Cape under British rule, 'the Cape [was] not a School for Medicine' and it was 'absolutely impossible for any Person to procure a Medical Education at the Cape'.[26] His refusal to license Carl Friedrich ('Charles'), the son of Friedrich L. Liesching, as an apothecary after a local apprenticeship (see Chapter 5 for more about the Lieschings) caused great controversy within the profession. To avoid further friction and embarrassment, the Colonial Office moved quickly to replace Barry as Colonial Medical Inspector with a re-assembled Medical Committee in 1825. As a further indication of Barry's loss of influence after 1825, the reconstituted Committee included Friedrich Liesching's other son Carl Ludwig ('Louis')[27] and by 1829 government had overturned Barry's insistence on European training for apothecaries.[28]

The symbolic positioning of doctors as gentlemen rather than tradesmen, dispensing advice rather than medicines, was important for the profession's image, but the practicalities of the medical market outside larger towns like Cape Town (and Grahamstown by the 1840s) forced doctors to trade in medicines and often also in other goods. Medical practice was so difficult in country villages that the colonial government often found itself appointing underqualified men as district surgeons, a continuation of the early nineteenth-century practice of licensing unqualified men as 'country doctors'. Even those who were given official sanction and a small stipend in this post sometimes sought extra income. William Gill (1797-1863), for example, who practised in Somerset East (and was district surgeon there), also dabbled lucratively in merino sheep-farming.[29] More often, however, doctors competed directly with apothecaries and patent medicine salesmen. Country doctors also sometimes found themselves defending their livelihoods against missionaries who used medical practice or dispensing as a way into the hearts and minds of the unconverted, either by virtue of formal medical training, a hasty missionary medical course or possession of medical books and supplies.

The Cape Town medical elite

Although the 1807 and 1823 legislation provided for the regulation of the whole medical profession from physicians to druggists under one body, and followed the standard distinction between physician, surgeon and apothecary in licensing, it made a much more significant distinction within the profession. This was between Cape Town practitioners and those elsewhere. In the first half of the nineteenth century, these differences in legislation as well as settlement patterns, economic and organisational opportunities created a two-tier medical profession in the Cape, with the most powerful sector based in Cape Town. In England, where London hospitals emerged as the major teaching centres, rivalling Edinburgh by the early nineteenth century,[30] and had always been the base for the Royal Colleges, the profession was divided by mid-century into 'consultant' surgeons and physicians (mainly in London), as opposed to general practitioners (who predominated outside London). In Upper Canada, Toronto doctors dominated the Medical Board and medical schools, while country practitioners had different lobbying power and different requirements in securing professional legislation.[31] The medical elite of Upper Canada were the men who edited the medical journals, who served on the Medical Council, were elected as members of parliament and considered to be the 'leading schoolmen' (intellectual pillars of society).[32] In the Cape, even more than in Upper Canada or England, all these kinds of opportunities, as well as legislative and economic advantages, were concentrated in the few major towns. The professionalisation process was thus largely driven and directed by Cape Town doctors, who most ardently and successfully pursued the ideal of the 'professional gentleman'.

By differentiating medical professionals' duties in Cape Town but not elsewhere, the medical legislation of 1807 and 1823 recognised the varying requirements of practitioners in what were two very distinct medical markets. By the end of the eighteenth century Cape Town was the only major urban centre; a small but bustling port town which sustained a variety of competing practitioners. Smaller country towns in the arable regions of the Western Cape could support only a few doctors or apothecaries until mid-century. By then, the Eastern Cape towns of Port Elizabeth and Grahamstown, populated by British settlers and accompanying doctors in the 1820s, had begun to form a second locus of economic stability and organisation for the Cape profession. More isolated stock-farming regions to the interior of the colony were served mainly by itinerant doctors and traders selling patent medicines. Doctors in the sparsely populated country districts often had to ensure their economic survival by selling drugs and farming. Even though clients often combined churchgoing or local auction attendance with seeking medical advice, country practitioners had to travel more widely in order to make their living. This, coupled with poor transport infrastructures and the greater distance between country doctors, made professional organisation and intra-professional differentiation harder to achieve. The enduring isolation and relative poverty of the rural interior has meant that the difference between the rural and urban medical markets remains significant even in the late twentieth century.

During the DEIC period, doctors at the DEIC hospital in Cape Town had been able to conduct their private practices from a secure and authoritative base, serving not only clients from visiting ships but also clients from other areas of the colony who came to Cape Town to sell their produce or get married. By 1806 Cape Town, the oldest and largest colonial town, supported a sophisticated and wealthy white population and a constant stream of visitors who provided an willing clientele for medical men. Regularly trained medical immigrants were attracted to the town where a steady income from private practice allowed the more successful to move away from a reliance on medicine sales. In Cape Town doctors were able to support local secondary education, social clubs, philanthropic societies and scientific associations, while country practitioners had the local agricultural society or school board alone. Professional organisation was also more easily possible in Cape Town, where doctors were most numerous. Fraught with internal dissent, the Cape Town medical elite was particularly interested in attaining greater professional unity, both through fee regulation and a code of ethics which emphasised 'gentlemanly' conduct among themselves. To this end, they formed a Medical Society in 1827 which tried to contain quarrels between doctors as well as disseminate medical knowledge from abroad. Most of their lobbying and professional concerns thus remained local, either diverging from or perceived as competing with those of country doctors.

Cape Town's harbour was the major trade outlet for the colony and the town was the main market for agricultural produce until the 1850s, experiencing great commercial expansion from the later 1830s and industrial expansion during the 1840s and 1850s, until it was challenged by the wool-producing areas of the Eastern Cape.[33] Cape Town was also the seat of government, a critical factor for local doctors, especially before a colonial parliament allowed Eastern Cape colonists to influence legislation after 1854. Cape Town doctors could and did influence policy and practice, both as appointees to the Medical Committees and through private representations to government. This was as true of the military doctors based in Cape Town who drafted legislation in 1807 and 1823 and civilian doctors who drafted legislation in 1830 and 1836. The Cape Town medical elite was also able to enhance its public profile by taking up government appointments. These posts were concentrated in Cape Town, where there were the only civilian hospitals in the colony until the 1850s; a fear of infectious disease from port traffic was a great incentive to employ doctors in public health duties in Cape Town and the nearby naval base of Simons Town. The growth of the insurance sector in the 1840s spawned more salaried posts for Cape Town doctors (this will be discussed in greater detail in Chapter 5).

Cape Town doctors thus benefited from its historical primacy, its role as the colonial capital and a major urban trade centre. The gap between Cape Town and country doctors persisted even when other colonial towns began to provide some of the same advantages of scale and when legislation was altered to provide the same protection against intra-professional competition for country practitioners as had been enjoyed by Cape Town practitioners since 1807. The historical primacy of Cape Town doctors and the long tradition of poor regulation in country districts made any levelling of the playing field difficult to achieve. The contrast between professional opportunities in town and country should not be overstated, however. Practitioners migrated between country areas and Cape Town, taking their professional ambitions with them. It is also important to remember that even Cape Town, the largest town in the colony for much of the century, was fairly small compared to other colonial towns like Melbourne at this time.

A Cape Town doctor: Dr Peter Chiappini's case book

Peter Chiappini (MD and MRCS, both Edinburgh 1832) was the son of a prominent Italian immigrant merchant in the town and a member of the Cape Town medical elite.[34] His social and educational profile is characteristic of the leading members of the profession at this time; a man of European ancestry, educated in Europe, he practised in Cape Town where he found time to serve on the Council of the South African Literary and Scientific Institute and on the Medical Committee. Unusually for a Cape-born doctor in the first half of the nineteenth century, however, he trained in Edinburgh rather than Leyden.[35]

We know more about Chiappini's medical practice than about most of his contemporaries' because detailed records of his practice are preserved in the University of Cape Town's Medical School Library.[36] He was one of the many Cape Town doctors who supplemented his income from private practice with commercial employment, attending cases on behalf of an insurance company as well as a friendly society. Chiappini had an extensive and varied private practice too, tending not only wealthy settlers in the town and its growing suburbs, but also working-class immigrants from Europe, poor laundresses who had probably been slaves before emancipation in 1838, and Muslim religious leaders. To accommodate this spread of clients he charged three different rates for consultations.

Chiappini, like many other Cape doctors of his time, was interested in practising midwifery. It is probable that doctors like Chiappini were beginning to take on more normal deliveries in urban areas by the 1840s. Cape Town doctors, the most powerful sector within the Cape profession, were paradoxically the most interested in expanding their practice into what was still considered in Europe to be a low status occupation: man-midwifery. Because of the legal restriction against selling medicines outside of their practice and the attempt to distance themselves from 'tradesmen', Cape Town doctors in particular, and urban doctors more generally after 1830, were particularly eager to take advantage of the trend towards seeking male medical attendance at normal births in middle- and upper-class confinements in America, Britain and her Empire.

Chiappini's accounts show that most of the deliveries he attended were followed up by a number of subsequent visits. While this may indicate that these were difficult cases, referred by a midwife, it was not uncommon for doctors to pay a few post-partum visits to their clients even when the delivery had gone well. Chiappini specifically mentions two difficult cases for which he charged more than the usual rate for deliveries,[37] which suggests that the other cases were not difficult. Chiappini's Muslim clients, however, definitely only called him in for particular duties such as the removal of the afterbirth after the midwife had done what she could.[38]

The slowing pace of professionalisation

Although it was clear to the profession and government by mid-century that greater professional regulation was required in growing country towns, no professional regulatory legislation was passed between 1836 and 1891. The demise of the Medical Society and the short-lived medical journal in Cape Town during the 1840s and the failure of Cape doctors to achieve better regulation of competition in country areas in the 1850s were symptoms of a stalled professionalisation process. The Cape Town elite, the most powerful and numerous in the profession, had a deeply ambivalent attitude towards more effective professional regulation in the country districts. Because the difficulties experienced by country doctors were felt to lower the status of the profession as a whole, Cape Town doctors encouraged legislative controls to reduce competition between doctors and druggists after 1829. But there was little political will from Cape Town doctors and merchant-apothecaries to enforce these regulations in country districts. The maintenance of the professional status of the Cape Town doctor depended partly on the distinction between tradesman and gentleman discussed above, but also on a distinction between the professional elite of the town (which did not include all Cape Town practitioners) and country practitioners. For much of the century, country doctors were left to struggle against druggists and shopkeepers without significant assistance from urban doctors.

Cape Town doctors benefited from the fact that poor

enforcement of regulations enabled immigrant doctors to move out of the city and sustain small practices in country towns with income from dispensing medicines. Cape Town merchant-apothecaries did not wish to limit the sale of medicines to country shopkeepers and druggists from their warehouses, but did want to prevent shopkeepers in Cape Town from competing with their own retail outlets.[39] These pressures became more important by mid-century when the Cape Town medical market became over-supplied at the lower levels and Cape Town druggists suffered a rise in bankruptcies.[40] The colony suffered economic depression in the early 1860s, while the number of wealthy patients coming to recuperate at the Cape from British service in India decreased after the opening of the Suez Canal.[41] The depression reduced paying clientele generally and many medical practitioners (still mostly the more vulnerable country doctors based outside Cape Town) went bankrupt.[42] Cape Town doctors were better able to weather the vagaries of private practice during this period by turning to collective employment in government hospital posts, benefit society and insurance work, but this distanced them further from the professional interests of practitioners elsewhere.

The 1840s and 1850s saw the demise of Cape Town as a centre of professional organisation which was possibly related to economic difficulties. After 1834 the Medical Committee (MC) 'declined in influence and activity';[43] it was swamped with institutional administration in the 1840s and was more tightly controlled and supervised under the administration of John Montagu (Colonial Secretary, 1843-53).[44] The Medical Society in Cape Town, which had liaised with (and temporarily replaced) the MC, folded in the early 1840s.[45] Internal conflicts plagued Cape Town doctors during the 1830s and 1840s.[46] The *Cape Town Medical Gazette* which was started in 1847 had a short life, and its editor's calls for a new medical society were not heeded.[47] In the 1850s, Collis Browne, a military surgeon quartered at the Cape Town Castle and a keen inventor himself, complained that the other military doctors failed to keep up with the 'progress of modern science' in the medical field;[48] it was little better among civilian doctors. By this time, Cape Town had to compete for economic and social status with the booming wool-trade towns of the Eastern Cape – Port Elizabeth and Grahamstown. There were a number of well-educated and ambitious doctors in Grahamstown, who were keen to emphasise the scientific nature of their skill and their membership of a professional middle-class[49] rapidly developing in the town. It is significant that a Medico-

Illustration 3.1
Cape Town Medical Gazette

Contents page of one of the first Cape Town Medical Gazettes, published in 1847. It was edited by a member of the Cape Town medical elite, Dr Henry Anderson Ebden (1824-1886). In the 1850s Ebden became a member of the Medical Committee, and served as its president from 1862. He was also the first president of the South African Medical Association.

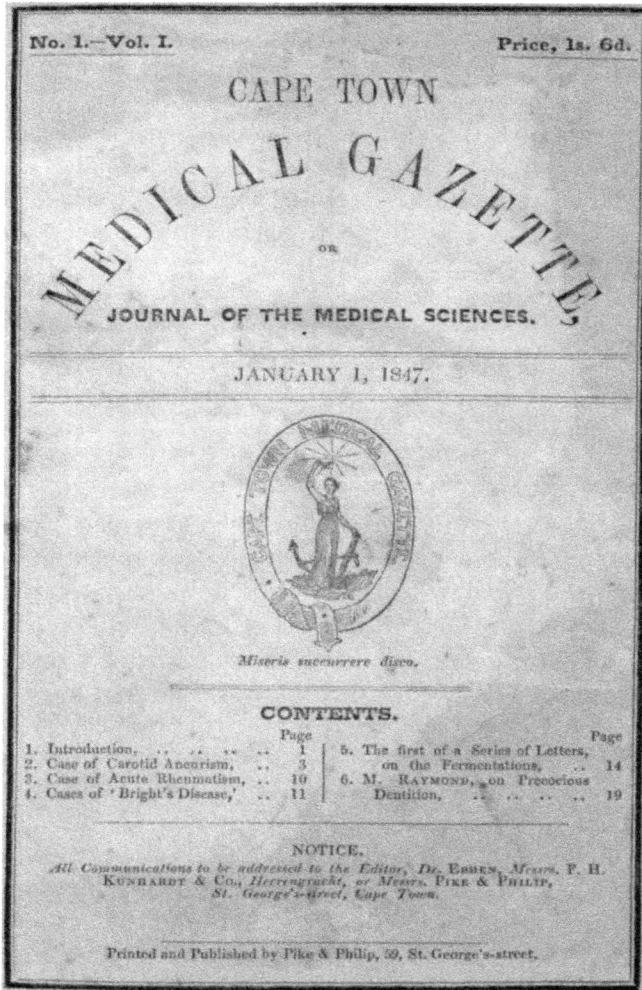

Chirurgical Society was soon founded in Grahamstown to discuss medical and scientific matters.[50] Although this society soon broadened its concerns beyond medicine (see Chapter 6)[51] the Eastern Cape was in some ways a new geographical locus for professional ambitions centred around market regulation and maintaining the public face of a medical profession primarily engaged in private practice. A unified lobbying platform through a national professional organisation was not, however, formed until the late-nineteenth century.

Conclusion

The beginnings of the Cape medical profession can be traced to the early years of the nineteenth century, when government regulation of medical practice was first implemented, licensing requirements were laid down and Cape doctors began to organise themselves professionally. For the first few decades after 1807, as in Britain, the leaders in this quest for professional status focussed more on achieving the status of medical gentlemen (as distinct from tradesmen) than on representing themselves as scientists or public health administrators. These latter roles were to become more important to the profession during the latter part of the nineteenth century.

Drawn up by military doctors under a military government in 1807, the first professional regulations for doctors at the Cape helped to delineate the profession as essentially both European and masculine. Unlicensed practitioners could be fined if they charged for their services. To be licensed, practitioners had to have had a European medical education, which at the time did not offer openings for women and whose expense discouraged all but the wealthier Cape-born men. Local training was allowed only to low-status practitioners: midwives (after 1810) and apothecaries (after 1829). The professional regulation of medicine at the Cape thus helped to reproduce the patterns of gender, race, culture and class within the licensed profession which were being established by professional training and organisation in Europe.

But whereas surgeons in Britain stood closer to apothecaries than to physicians within the profession at the beginning of the nineteenth century, the Cape regulations of 1807 distinguished primarily between doctors (surgeons and physicians) and druggists (apothecaries, chemists and druggists), underlining the distinction between gentlemen (who provided medical services) and tradesmen (who sold medicines). As happened in Britain and some of the other settler colonies, however, urban and rural divisions within the profession became increasingly important in the first half of the century. The initial form and subsequent application of the Cape regulations also served to differentiate between the relatively well-regulated medical market of Cape Town (and later other large towns) and the poorly regulated and less hierarchical medical market of the country districts. Cape Town doctors initially dominated the drive for professional advancement and gained greater benefits from this process, but by the 1850s Grahamstown doctors began to challenge them for the leading position within the Cape's professional hierarchy.

Notes

1. E. Friedson, *Profession of Medicine: A Study of the Sociology of Applied Knowledge, 2nd edn* (New York: Harper & Row, 1988), 72.
2. See R.D. Gidney and W.P.J. Millar, *Professional Gentlemen: The Professions in Nineteenth Century Ontario* (Toronto: University of Toronto Press, 1994), xi–xii; G. Ritzer, *Working, Conflict and Change*, 2nd edn (Englewood Cliffs: Prentice-Hall, 1977) cited in S.R. Quah, 'The Social Position and Organisation of the Medical Profession in the Third World: The Case of Singapore', *Journal of Health and Social Behaviour*, xxx (1989), 451; S.E.D. Shortt, 'Physicians, Science and Status: Issues in the Professionalisation of Anglo-American Medicine in the 19th Century', *Medical History*, xxvii (1983), 51–2.
3. S. Marks, *Divided Sisterhood: Race, Class and Gender in the South African Nursing Profession* (London: Macmillan, 1994); E.B. van Heyningen, 'Agents of Empire: The Medical Profession in the Cape Colony, 1880-1910', *Medical History*, xxx (1989), 450–71; S. Swartz, 'Colonialism and the Production of Psychiatric Knowledge in the Cape, 1891-1920' (unpublished Ph.D. thesis, UCT, 1996).
4. E. Burrows, *A History of Medicine in South Africa* (Cape Town: Balkema, 1958), 116.
5. Compare the date of comprehensive professional legislation at the Cape, for example, to that in Britain (1858) and in India (1912): M. Harrison, *Public Health in British India* (Cambridge: Cambridge University Press, 1994), 35. Even in 1858, British legislation did not ban alternative practice.
6. H.J. Deacon, 'Cape Town and Country Doctors in the Cape Colony During the First Half of the Nineteenth Century', *Social History of Medicine*, x, 1 (1997), 25–52.

7. P.J. Corfield, *Power and the Professions in Britain, 1700-1850* (London: Routledge, 1995), 12, 18, 23.

8. Gidney and Millar, *op. cit.* (note 2), 12.

9. *Ibid.*, 3–11.

10. J.H. Warner, *The Therapeutic Perspective: Medical Practice, Knowledge and Identity in America, 1820-1885* (Princeton: Princeton University Press, 1986), 1, 15–16.

11. H.J. Deacon, 'Midwives and Medical Men in the Cape Colony, 1800-1860', *Journal of African History*, xxxix (1998), 271–92.

12. See for example T. Gelfand, *Professionalising Modern Medicine: Paris Surgeons and Medical Science and Institutions in the Eighteenth Century* (London: Greenwood Press, 1980), xi. See also W. Frijhoff, '"Non Satis Dignitatis": Over de Maatchappelijke Status van Geneeskundigen Tijdens de Republiek', *Nederlandsche tijdschrift voor Geschiedenis*, xcvi (1983), 380–1.

13. I. Loudon, 'Medical Practitioners 1750-1850 and the Period of Medical Reform in Britain' in A. Wear (ed.), *Medicine in Society* (Cambridge: Cambridge University Press, 1992), 229.

14. Gidney and Millar, *op. cit.* (note 2), 6.

15. B. Gandevia, 'A History of General Practice in Australia', *Medical Journal of Australia*, ii (12 August 1972), 381.

16. S.N. Eaton, 'A Housewife at the Cape in 1818', *Quarterly Bulletin of the SA Library*, viii (2) (December 1953), 46.

17. Gelfand, *op. cit.* (note 12), xii and Frijhoff, *op. cit.* (note 12), 382.

18. See for example CMC Minutes 1834-42, CA, MC 2.

19. SMC to CO, 28 January 1830, MC Minutes 1825-31, CA, MC 1.

20. Government Proclamation, 26 September 1823, Proclamations for 1823, CA, CO 5824.

21. Gidney and Millar, *op. cit.* (note 2), 55.

22. Loudon, *op. cit.* (note 13), 246.

23. Government Advertisement, 5 November 1829, Government Proclamations for 1828-31, CA, CO 5829.

24. On Barry's career, see Burrows, *op. cit.* (note 4), 80–2.

25. Vendors' Memorial in Brink to Barry, 20 May 1824, Letters from CO to Medical Inspector 1821-25, CA, MC 7.

26. Barry to Brink, 24 September 1824, Letters from Sundry Committees, 1824, CA, CO 204.

27. Report of the SMC for December, 27 December 1825, Letters from Sundry Committees 1825, CA, CO 226.

28. Government Advertisement, 5 November 1829, Government Proclamations for 1828-31, CA, CO 5829.

29. Burrows, *op. cit.* (note 4), 154.

30. J. Bradley, A. Crowther and M. Dupree, 'Mobility and Selection in Scottish University Medical Education, 1858-1886', *Medical History*, xl (1996), 3.
31. R.D. Gidney and W. Millar, 'The Origins of Organised Medicine in Ontario, 1850-1869' in C.G. Roland (ed.) *Health, Disease and Medicine: Essays in Canadian History* (Toronto: Hannah Institute, 1984), 65–95, 72.
32. Gidney and Millar, *op. cit.* (note 2), 88.
33. D. Warren, 'Merchants, Commissioners and Wardmasters: Municipal Politics in Cape Town 1840-1854' (unpublished M.A. thesis, UCT, 1986), 26.
34. On Chiappini's career, see Burrows, *op. cit.* (note 4), 148–9.
35. *Ibid.*, 149.
36. Account book of Dr Peter Chiappini 1842-46, UCT Medical School Library, Cape Town, MHA 610.6 SOU.
37. *Ibid.* 1845, 14, 81.
38. Deacon, *op. cit.* (note 11), 287, note 86.
39. Memorial of C. Orpen, 20 September 1849, Memorials N-P, 1849, CA, CO 4048, doc.57.
40. Thanks to Wayne Dooling for this information.
41. Burrows, *op. cit.* (note 4), 139. See also R. Noble (ed.), *The Cape and its People, and Other Essays* (Cape Town: Juta, 1869), 38.
42. Thanks to Wayne Dooling for this information. Doctors (especially those outside Cape Town) suffered much greater risk of insolvency than apothecaries in 1864-69 compared to the previous period of economic stress in 1839-45 when doctors and apothecaries were more equally vulnerable.
43. P. Laidler and M. Gelfand, *South Africa: Its Medical History* (Cape Town: Struik, 1971), 211.
44. See Letters from CO to CMC 1837-54, CA, MC 10.
45. Burrows, *op. cit.* (note 4), 133.
46. *Ibid.*, 127. See also the *Cape Town Medical Gazette*, i (1) (1847), 1.
47. *Cape Town Medical Gazette*, i (3) (1847), 32. See also Burrows, *op. cit.* (note 4), 350 and C. Blumberg, 'The South African Medical Society and its Library', *Cabo*, ii, 4 (1978), 18–25.
48. T.J. Lucas, *Camp Life and Sport in South Africa* (Johannesburg: Africana Book Society, 1975), 33–5.
49. N. Erlank, 'Letters Home: The Experiences and Perceptions of Middle-class British Women at the Cape, 1820-1850' (unpublished M.A. thesis, UCT, 1995), 111.
50. See records of addresses to the society, Miscellaneous Collections, CA, M 132(b).

51. L.G. Couch, *A Short Medical History of Grahamstown* (Grahamstown: Grocott & Sherry, 1976), 20–1.

4

Home Taught for Abroad:
The Training of the Cape Doctor, 1807-1910

Howard Phillips

Given that the Cape (or for that matter South Africa) did not have a full medical school until 1920, all Cape doctors before then were trained outside of Africa, the vast majority in Britain and Continental Europe. Accordingly, this chapter examines the kind of training they received in these countries, as this fundamentally shaped the kind of medicine they subsequently practised at the Cape. It concludes by exploring why medical training was so slow to develop at the Cape, and what the long-term effects of this were on these medical schools and their curricula.

The foundations of formal biomedical practice in the nineteenth-century Cape were laid 10,000 km away in the medical schools of Europe, for it was here that almost every Cape doctor received his or her basic training in medicine. Though experience, emulation and the acquisition of further knowledge and skills may have subsequently altered or refined such learning, it was rare for these to produce a paradigm shift in methods of practice or a complete departure from the tenets inculcated during student years. Medical training in Europe – 'the process that makes a practitioner', as it has recently been described[1] – thus played a seminal role in shaping medical practice in the nineteenth-century Cape. Consequently, an examination of what it entailed lies at the root of understanding the nature of that practice. Susan Lawrence has made this point very precisely, noting that 'teaching a particular theoretical position on physiological or pathological processes shapes how practitioners think they might alter those bodily mechanisms.'[2]

Of all the medical training offered in Europe, it was that available in three countries, Britain, Germany and Holland, which most significantly moulded Cape medical practice, for it was in these countries – and in Britain in particular – that almost all nineteenth-century Cape practitioners were trained, since no full medical school existed in South Africa until 1920. Most therefore had a training of a piece with that of their European contemporaries, which, in the case of those trained in Britain, meant that they usually had a formal licence to practise from one or more of the Royal Colleges of Physicians or Surgeons of England, Scotland or Ireland or from an Apothecaries Society, which they had received after being trained by one of the three methods then operating in that country, viz. the traditional system of apprenticeship, the strongly practical training given at hospitals or private medical schools in a large city or the formal medical degree course offered by some universities.

On the other hand, almost all licensed nineteenth-century Cape doctors who had been trained in Holland or Germany (they comprised about thirteen per cent of all the Cape's doctors between 1810 and 1910) had received their training at a university there. Normally this was the only type of non-British medical qualification that the Cape's medical licensing body, the Supreme (later Colonial) Medical Committee (later Council), was prepared to accept, though after mid-century it had to be supplemented by a recognised British College/Apothecaries' licence to practise too.

The overwhelming majority of all these practitioners were male migrants from Europe; only a small percentage were Cape-born men (at most ten per cent), but, in the absence of a local medical school, they too were overseas trained. In the first decades of the nineteenth century most of the latter had chosen to study in Holland or Germany, mainly because of longstanding family, cultural or commercial ties with these lands dating back to the days of Dutch East India Company rule at the Cape – indeed, after the British takeover of the Cape in 1806, several prominent Cape Dutch families deliberately chose not to send their sons to be educated in Britain lest they become too anglicised in the process.

However, by mid-century Holland was becoming distinctly unpopular as a study destination, and Britain (and Scotland in particular) was replacing it as the favoured place of study for Cape-born men.

Neatly encapsulating this shift during the century is the different locales where three generations of one Cape family of doctors, the Fraenkels, studied medicine. Sigfried Fraenkel (1778-1846), who practised in Cape Town from 1808 to 1846, received his initial medical training in the Duchy of Mecklenburg where he had been born, before going on to the Royal Academy of Surgery in Copenhagen where he completed most of the courses required for the degree of MD. He then joined the Danish merchant navy, and it was as a ship's surgeon that he came to the Cape in 1807. His eldest son, Diederich Heinrich (1811-1861), was born in Cape Town and, after a prize-studded schooling at the South African College there, left for Europe in 1832 to study medicine. A year at Leiden University was followed by three years at his father's alma mater, the Royal Academy of Surgery in Copenhagen, before he completed his training at the University of Leipzig, where he gained the degrees of MB and MD in 1837. He returned to the Cape in 1837, where he practised at Colesberg and Worcester. Diederich's younger son, Heinrich Siegfried (1855-1897), who, significantly, anglicised his name to Henry, emulated his father and grandfather in choosing a medical career, but, unlike them, trained not on the Continent, but at the University of Edinburgh where he was awarded the degrees of MB, MC in 1878. He returned to the Cape Colony the next year, and thereafter spent most of his professional life practising in Clanwilliam.[3]

As this experience of the Fraenkels underlines, the Cape differed markedly from other British colonies like Australia and New Zealand, for not only did its medical profession contain a significant minority of doctors who had been trained on the Continent, but throughout the nineteenth century it remained wholly dependent on overseas institutions to train its doctors. Attempts to establish a medical school in Cape Town persistently proved unsuccessful, unlike local efforts which produced medical schools in Melbourne, Sydney, Adelaide and Dunedin by 1900 or the imperial initiatives which created three medical colleges in British India and one in Ceylon by 1870. Thus, while some thirteen per cent of Australia's doctors had been trained locally by 1900, not one Cape doctor before 1922 was a wholly local product. The reasons for this and their long-term implications will be discussed towards the end of this chapter.

The 'long' nineteenth century was the single most revolutionary century in medicine until then. Fundamental innovations in understanding the body and its operation and disease and its transmission, as well as the discovery of new diagnostic tools and surgical procedures, were gradually incorporated into both the teaching and practice of medicine during the nineteenth century so as to render them wholly transformed by 1910. W.F. Bynum correctly observed in 1994, 'the medicine of 1900 [is] closer to us almost a century later than it was to the medicine of 1790'.[4]

The examination of the training received by Cape doctors which follows takes into account these revolutionary changes, but never so as to artificially forget the simultaneous persistence of old beliefs and practices right through the century, in both medical practice and training. As a recent overview of British medical history tartly put it, '[M]edical education always seems to have been deeply nostalgic – instead of educating for the future it hankers for the past.... The system of medicine has evolved slowly... dragging medical education – kicking and screaming – behind it.'[5]

Of the three modes of training prevalent in nineteenth-century Britain, apprenticeship had the longest pedigree and was the means by which a number of pre-1850 Cape doctors were trained. While teenagers, these men had served a period of at least five years indentured to a practising surgeon or apothecary, during which time they had absorbed from their master the rudiments of his trade, especially with regard to the preparation, application and display of medicines and drugs and the performance of everyday tasks like cupping, bandaging and the re-application of splints. A conscientious master would have backed this up by prescribing classical medical texts for study and by allowing a senior apprentice to accompany him on his rounds, thereby affording him an opportunity to observe and even participate in practical work. All training therefore emanated from one man, the master, and thus his knowledge and methods shaped that of his youthful apprentice to an inordinate degree. For instance, to the end of his career in 1848 the Grahamstown surgeon, J.N. Atherstone, still based his practice on a humoral premise he had imbibed from his master in Nottingham in the first decade of the century, namely that 'the blood is the source of all energy and power. Curative treatment should therefore be directed to restoring the purity of the blood by all available means either by reducing the force of the circulation [i.e. by bleeding] or by medicines acting through the lungs or skin.'[6] Nor did the influence of the Nottingham master's sanguinary approach to treatment end there: J.N.'s son, the distinguished physician W.G. Atherstone, testified at the end of his career in 1897 that the views of his father on treatment he had heard in his youth 'influence[d] my own in after life.'[7]

However, not all apprentices had their training confined to just one instructor. From 1815 an apothecary's licence in Britain required the latter part of the apprenticeship period to be spent in a hospital or (later) at a recognised medical school, while would-be surgeons had to attend lectures on anatomy and surgery before being allowed to sit for a Royal College of Surgeons (RCS) licence, a requirement which some masters were willing to allow their apprentices to meet during the last two years of their apprenticeship. Where this was permitted, much of their time would have been spent in nearby hospitals, where operations were frequent and fast, cadavers abundant and individual visiting surgeons more than ready to accept fee-paying spectators.

The late-eighteenth-century apprenticeship system thus tended to produce doctors whose training was narrow and conservative, probably little different from that which the master himself had received decades earlier. Its emphasis was thus still on how to match the symptoms described in detail by a patient with those set out in contemporary taxonomies of disease, and then how to treat these according to well-established custom. Such superficial physical signs as could be detected in those pre-stethoscope, pre-thermometer days were noted, but physical examination beyond these was rare; consequently, the fact that an apprentice could gain little clinical experience while indentured was not seen as a serious deficiency. Indeed, the 1815 Apothecaries Act still insisted on the need for would-be apothecaries to serve a five-year apprenticeship under one master. It was not until the 1850s that these inherent weaknesses in the apprenticeship system were made so patent by, inter alia, the new approaches and techniques in medicine that it became no longer sustainable in its existing form, and it was formally dropped as a requirement by the 1858 Medical Act. The last Cape doctor to qualify by this method was Robert Phillips, a medical missionary who was licensed to practise at the Cape in 1838.

What rendered training by apprenticeship so inadequate was the emergence during the eighteenth century of new medical sciences, especially physiology, morbid anatomy and pathology, which required disease to be closely monitored from onset to autopsy, tasks most effectively undertaken in a hospital. Large hospitals, containing a wide array of cases under close observation, were thus increasingly seen as the best site for training doctors, and those who practised there as the best teachers. By early in the nineteenth century, hospitals in London and some provincial English cities were flourishing as centres of medical instruction, initially by their own staff acting independently, but by the 1830s as full-scale medical schools in their own right. With such resources, schools of this sort (like those at Guy's, St Bartholomew's and St Thomas's) were soon outstripping the many small private schools which had grown up near them, and by mid-century hospital-based medical schools dominated medical training in London, their students forming the largest proportion of those writing Royal College and Hall examinations for a medical licence each year.

In Edinburgh, on the other hand, where a university dominated medical education – unlike the situation in England before mid-century – the local hospital had formed the university's clinical arm since the middle of the eighteenth century already, an arrangement which underlay the high quality of the medical training offered by Edinburgh University, for it effectively 'unite[d] medical theory and practice at the bedside'.[8]

To teach clinical medicine in these hospital medical schools, new techniques were developed which owed something to the old master-apprentice relationship; students were now 'attached' to a particular physician or surgeon under whose guidance they walked the wards, receiving clinical tuition at patients' bedsides, preparing case-histories, attending surgical operations and post-mortems and performing minor tasks as clinical clerks. 'It is in ocular and practical demonstrations over the subject in the dissecting-room and in bed-side clinical instruction, that oral teaching does so much', enthused one Cape Town doctor who had been trained in this fashion in London.[9] This 'hands-on' clinical training – what he called 'the private tutor and bed-side instruction system'[10] – was complemented by attendance at lectures on core medical subjects like chemistry, anatomy, physiology, *materia medica*, surgery, the principles of medicine and midwifery. For these, students usually 'shopped around' among local medical schools and private lecturers, picking (and paying) for only those lectures which they felt would best equip them for the specific career they intended; fixed curricula for all medical students were introduced in Britain only at the end of the nineteenth century. Thus, for instance, John Addey, who became a long-practising doctor in the Boland, completed his medical training in London in the 1810s by attending courses in anatomical dissection and hospital practice given by a private lecturer, lectures on surgery by a surgeon at St George's Hospital and a course on the practice of midwifery by an accoucheur from the Westminster Lying-In Institution.[11]

The new emphasis on a clinical approach to medicine rapidly began to transform practice. Thorough physical examinations increasingly became a standard part of all diagnosis in hospitals, aided by the newly invented stethoscope and the technique of percussion, while diseases began to be conceptualised as specific conditions affecting specific organs, which consequently produced distinctive symptoms which could be identified as such and monitored as they developed. Newman well recognised the implications of these fundamental innovations, concluding that 'By

Illustration 4.1
The making of the Cape doctor in Britain

(i) Cape medical (and other) students at Edinburgh University, 1903

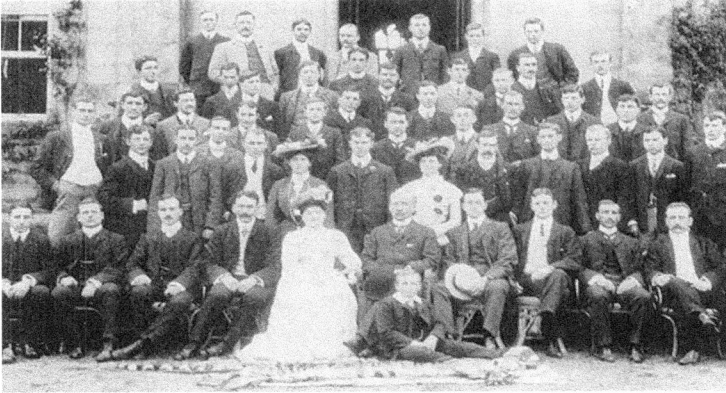

(ii) C.L. Leipoldt (on the left, holding a bottle to his nose) attending an operation while a medical student at Guy's Hospital, circa 1904.

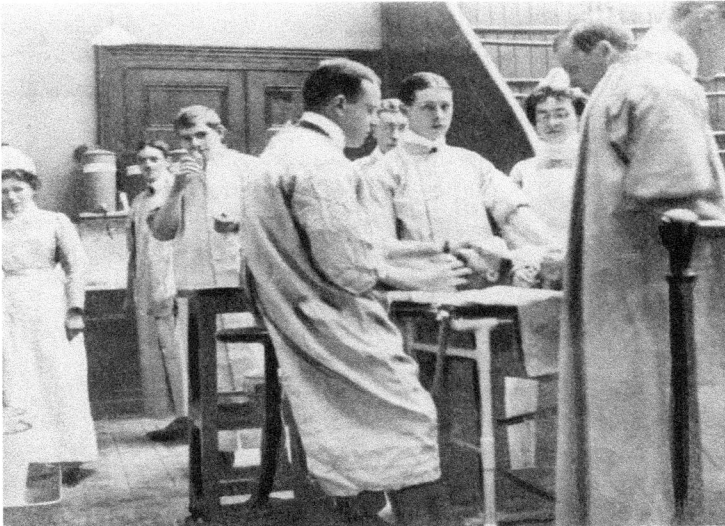

the middle of the nineteenth century the mind of the better doctor was a scientific mind: he may have been relatively ignorant, and he may have been affected to some extent by the remains of respect for an older generation, but his mental processes were modern.'[12]

This new approach can be seen in operation in the account by Henry Bickersteth, a Cape Town surgeon who had been trained at St Thomas's in the late 1820s, of the extensive clinical symptoms he noted when he examined a young sailor admitted to the Somerset Hospital in 1847, short of breath and with acute chest pain:

> Countenance anxious and pale; lips rather livid; tongue covered in the centre with a moist brownish fur; bowels freely open; pulse 120, moderately compressible; respirations 25 in the minute; skin cool and perspirable; left side of the thorax appears fuller than the right, and is almost immovable during inspiration; the whole of this side of the chest dull and resisting on percussion; no breath sound can be appreciated in the lung [on auscultation], with the exception of slight sonorous rhonchus under the clavicle, and faint tubular respiration in the interscapular space; percussion and pressure on the intercostal spaces give pain, particularly in the lateral and inferior regions of the chest, below the nipple. On measuring the relative size of the two sides, the left is found one and a half inches larger than the right.[13]

Empyema (pleurisy) was diagnosed and during the next week physical signs like the patient's pulse, respiration and chest sounds were constantly monitored as one medication after another was tried in vain. Surgery to drain the affected lung produced only temporary relief and he died a few days later. In his report on the post-mortem findings, Bickersteth left no doubt about the specific site of the disease, as he described the 'extensive mischief occasioned by the disease to the lung' and 'the noxious effects of such a collection [of fluid], pent up in one of the most important cavities in the body'.[14] In comparison, J.N. Atherstone's humoral understanding of disease was worlds away, even though the old doctor was still practising (just) in 1847.

However, in the hospital-based training's greatest strength – its emphasis on the clinical – also lay the danger that products of such training might lack sufficient theoretical training to allow them, once in practice, to go beyond the strict clinical regimes they had learnt as students. It was this imbalance in their training and its effects in practice which prompted one critical Cape commentator to complain in 1871:

> Two thirds of the [local] workers in medicine and surgery are mere creatures of routine practice, drudging painfully and ploddingly at

their daily round, and quite unequal, if not positively unfit – to feel
or display any real enthusiasm in the interests of scientific Truth....
[T]he young practitioner in this Colony too often degenerates into
a mere automatic mender of humanity... He is a mere mechanical
drudge, working at so many shillings the job.[15]

Such a lament does not sound all that unfamiliar 130 years later.

The other route of medical training which an increasing
proportion of the Cape profession followed as the nineteenth century
passed lay through a university's faculty of medicine. For most
university-trained Cape doctors this had meant a Scottish or Irish
university degree, for in England, Oxford and Cambridge provided
no practical medical training until the 1890s, while the medical
intake at the new universities in London and the provinces remained
small until well into the later decades of the century. It is not
surprising to find, therefore, that only 5.7 per cent of the Cape's
doctors between 1810 and 1910 held London, Oxbridge or English
provincial degrees.

The source of Scotland's primacy in British university medical
education before 1900 lay, as has already been indicated above, in the
Faculty of Medicine of Edinburgh University, which had adopted a
clinical approach to teaching in the Leiden/Boerhaave tradition
already in the mid-eighteenth century. Utilising the Edinburgh Royal
Infirmary to provide case material for clinical instruction and
complementing this with a systematic course of didactic lectures,
Edinburgh's professors created a system of medical education far in
advance of any other training available in Britain before the 1860s.
Its graduates were therefore men (until 1896 when the first woman
qualified as a doctor there) who had received a broad training in both
medicine and surgery as practical skills rather than theoretical
subjects to be studied from classical texts. This equipped them pre-
eminently as multi-skilled general practitioners, competent to
practise all branches of medicine safely and reliably, irrespective of
the old divisions between physicians, surgeons and apothecaries as to
which medical tasks each 'order' might legitimately perform.
Increasingly, to turn out such an all-round practitioner became the
ideal of nineteenth-century British medical education.

In pursuit of producing such practitioners Edinburgh's formal
medical curriculum was progressively enlarged during the century,
from a wide-ranging three-year course embracing anatomy, surgery,
chemistry, botany, materia medica and pharmacy, the theory and
practice of medicine and clinical medicine in 1800, to a four-year

course in 1825, which included midwifery, practical anatomy, natural history, medical jurisprudence, clinical surgery and military surgery too. In 1889 this in turn was further extended to a five-year course to accommodate advances in scientific and clinical subjects so that Edinburgh could still aver that its graduates knew 'something about everything' on the day they entered general practice. As the proud mother of an Edinburgh student understood it, it was 'a University where every branch of science is regularly taught, and drawn together so... compactly from one to the other'.[16]

A striking example of these broad, Edinburgh-taught skills in a Cape doctor is to be found in the medical practice of Dr James Barry (1795-1865).

Given popular fascination with Barry's sexual identity – it has even been suggested that Barry was a woman who masqueraded as a man to be able to enter what was then a strictly male medical profession – what is usually overlooked in accounts of his twelve years at the Cape is how truly he represented the Edinburgh ideal of the omnicompetent general practitioner whose extensive clinical skills were sufficiently rooted in an understanding of the theory behind them to allow him to adapt them successfully to new circumstances. What follows[17] seeks to restore that dimension to James Barry's career by focussing on the distinctive Edinburgh training which underpinned his doctoring.

Even though his curriculum as a 'literary and medical student' at Edinburgh from 1810 to 1812 still bore elements of the traditional belief that a gentleman physician's training should be more in the theory than the practice of medicine, it already embraced sufficient practical training to mark it as a distinctive Edinburgh fusion of the two. His three-year course consisted of didactic lectures on a wide array of subjects, which were then complemented by one year's clinical experience in the wards and dispensaries of Edinburgh's Royal Infirmary and the Lying-In Hospital. A list of the courses he took at the university underlines Edinburgh's determination that its graduates should know something about everything. The courses were: Greek, natural and moral philosophy, chemistry, botany, theory of medicine, practice of physic (pathology), morbid anatomy, military surgery, clinical surgery, medical jurisprudence, midwifery and dissection. Moreover, he supplemented these with extra private classes in theoretical anatomy and practical dissection, in which he secured hands-on knowledge of anatomy to complement the theoretical knowledge gained from classical texts.

That he had learnt his lessons well was tested in regular university examinations in all subjects save midwifery and dissection, neither of which was examinable as these were still regarded as 'unbecoming' (i.e. as too hands-on, even for Edinburgh) for a gentleman physician-in-the-making. The final examination was a characteristic Edinburgh combination of the theoretical and the practical, requiring a thesis written in Latin – Barry's was 'On Hernia of the Groin' – on which he was given a gruelling viva by several professors, the explanation and illustration of two Hippocratic aphorisms, and comment on two cases put before him.

Success in all three components won Barry his MD in 1812, which he then augmented by a year as a pupil dresser to a leading London surgeon, Sir Astley Cooper, who operated at Guy's Hospital. This gave him extensive additional clinical experience which stood him in very good stead when he took the Royal College of Surgeons' regimental surgeon's examination and the Army Medical Board's examination in 1813, before joining the army in the midst of the Napoleonic Wars. With these qualifications behind his name, he arrived at the Cape as an assistant surgeon to the garrison in 1816.

The wealth of medical knowledge and clinical skill outlined above, which Barry gained as a student in Edinburgh and at Guy's, lay at the heart of his considerable medical and obstetrical achievements at the Cape. In particular, it should be noted that James Hamilton, with whom he took three courses in midwifery at Edinburgh, gave lectures on performing a caesarean section based on the lessons he had learnt from his two unsuccessful attempts to do so. It is not far-fetched to suggest that these lessons were well learnt by the young Barry and put into highly successful practice by him in 1826 when he performed a caesarean operation on Mrs Wilhelmina Johanna Munnik to deliver her son, the first such wholly successful operation recorded in the British Empire. If Hamilton's lectures lay at the root of this operation, they represented a spectacular triumph for Edinburgh's combination of theory and practice in the medical training it offered.

To Edinburgh's pre-eminence in Britain, Glasgow University could pose scant challenge until the 1870s because of the limited access its professors had to the main infirmary in that city until then, while at Aberdeen instruction was even more piecemeal until university education there was completely overhauled in 1860. At St Andrew's not even piecemeal instruction was possible as that venerable university altogether lacked a medical school until 1897 – yet this did not prevent it offering MD degrees for purchase by post.

Across the Irish Sea the Edinburgh example found closer

Table 4.1
Main qualifications held by newly registering Cape doctors,
1807 and 1810-1910 (as percentage of all new qualifications
registered in year[s] indicated)

	1807	1810–1819	1820–1829	1830–1839	1840–1849	1850–1859
Apprenticeship	83	7	30	2	-	-
Edinburgh degree	-	-	6	8	9	3.6
Edinburgh MRCS/LRCS	-	14	12	12	6.5	3.6
Edinburgh LRCP	-	-	-	-	-	-
Edinburgh midwifery diploma	-	-	-	4	-	2.4
Glasgow degree	-	-	-	-	1	1
Glasgow LFP&S	-	-	-	-	1	1
Glasgow MRCS/LS	-	-	-	2	2	-
Glasgow midwifery diploma	-	-	-	-	1	-
Other Scottish degree	-	14	6	-	3	3.6
Other Scottish midwifery diploma	-	-	-	-	-	-
Dublin degree	-	-	-	2	-	1
Other Irish degree	-	-	-	-	-	-
LRCPI/LKQCP	-	-	-	-	-	1
LRCSI	-	-	-	-	2	2.4
Irish midwifery diploma	-	-	-	-	1	1
London degree	-	-	-	-	2	-
London midwifery diploma	-	-	-	-	-	1
Oxbridge degree	-	-	-	-	-	-
Other English degree	-	-	-	-	-	-
MRCS London/England	-	7	12	18	30	29
MRCP/LRCP London	-	-	-	-	1	1
LAC/LSA London	-	14	-	6	16	18
Dutch degree/diploma	4	14	6	14	16.5	8.4
German degree/diploma	13	21	-	20	6.5	17
Other Continental degree	-	-	-	2	1	2
US degree	-	-	-	-	-	-
Total number of doctors registering in year(s) indicated	24	10	17	37	59	51

Cont....

Table 4.1 (cont...)
(N.B. The data on which this table is based is not without its gaps and uncertainties; consequently, the figures in it should be taken as approximations). Key and Sources overleaf.

	1860–1869	1870–1879	1880–1889	1890–1899	1900–1910
Apprenticeship	-	-	-	-	-
Edinburgh degree	9	6	17	13	16
Edinburgh MRCS/LRCS	3	6.7	7	8	9
Edinburgh LRCP	2.4	11	10	9	10
Edinburgh midwifery diploma	8.5	1	-	-	-
Glasgow degree	-	2.7	2	5	5
Glasgow LFP&S	2	2	4	6	8
Glasgow MRCS/LS	0.6	-	-	-	-
Glasgow midwifery diploma	1.2	0.2	-	-	-
Other Scottish degree	7.4	5	4	4	3
Other Scottish midwifery diploma	0.6	-	-	-	-
Dublin degree	0.6	2	1	2	2
Other Irish degree	-	-	1	2	2
LRCPI/LKQCP	0.6	4	4	3	3
LRCSI	0.6	5	4	3	3
Irish midwifery diploma	1.2	1.9	-	-	-
London degree	0.6	1	2	2	3
London midwifery diploma	3	0.2	-	-	-
Oxbridge degree	-	-	0.2	-	2
Other English degree	-	-	0.2	1	2
MRCS London/England	23	24	18	16	14
MRCP/LRCP London	0.6	5	7	13	12
LAC/LSA London	10	10	8.5	4	3
Dutch degree/diploma	6.5	0.6	-	0.1	-
German degree/diploma	13.5	5	7	4	2
Other Continental degree	2	1.6	1.2	1.5	1.6
US degree	-	1.5	0.8	0.3	0.2
Total number of doctors registering in year(s) indicated	91	217	286	486	509

imitation. At Trinity College, Dublin, clinical lectures were formally included in the medical curriculum as early as 1785, but it was not until 1816 that a sizeable modern hospital was built in which these lectures could be effectively presented. Once this was possible, clinical teaching was extended to allow students to examine patients themselves under the watchful eye of their professor, instead of merely observing the latter's examination as at Edinburgh, an approach readily taken up too by the Irish College of Surgeons' School of Surgery in Dublin, the numerous private medical colleges in that city and the Rotunda and Coombe maternity hospitals, which offered courses of their own for licences in midwifery independently of any university. How essential an adequate supply of clinical material was to this mode of teaching is underscored by the inability of the Queen's University's medical colleges in smaller Irish towns like Belfast and Cork to follow suit when they were set up in the 1840s, to the detriment of their standing.

Yet, however advanced the medical curricula at Edinburgh and its emulators may have been, it was only a minority of nineteenth-

---

Key for Table 4.1

LRCS	=	Licentiate of the Royal College of Surgeons
MRCS	=	Member of the Royal College of Surgeons
LRCP	=	Licentiate of the Royal College of Physicians
MRCP	=	Member of the Royal College of Physicians
LFP&S	=	Licentiate of the Faculty of Physicians and Surgeons
LS	=	Licentiate of Surgery
LRCPI	=	Licentiate of the Royal College of Physicians of Ireland
LKQCP	=	Licentiate of the Kings and Queens College of Physicians
LRCSI	=	Licentiate of the Royal College of Surgeons of Ireland
LAC	=	Licentiate of the Apothecaries' Company
LSA	=	Licentiate of the Society of Apothecaries

Sources for Table 4.1

Cape Archives, various files in CO and MC series.
Cape Archives, A2039 (FJ Boonzaaier Collection), vol. 21.
Cape Medical Registers, 1892/3 – 1910.
E.H. Burrows, *A History of Medicine in South Africa up to the End of the Nineteenth Century* (Cape Town: Balkema, 1958).
P.W. Laidler and M. Gelfand, *South Africa: Its Medical History 1652-1898* (Cape Town: Struik, 1971).

century British doctors (and thus of the Cape's doctors of this period) who could afford to be trained at these universities. With the adequacy of apprenticeship already under question in 1800, the majority of would-be practitioners opted for training at private medical colleges or hospital medical schools in Britain's cities, capping this with the requisite licence to practise from one or more of the country's nine Royal Colleges or Apothecaries' Halls; indeed, so much professional status did these licences carry that it was quite common for even graduates of Edinburgh to sit the necessary examinations so they might add them to the 'MD (Edin)' after their names. Not until the Medical Act of 1858 made it quite clear that a university medical degree was sufficient to secure full registration by the new General Council of Medical Education and Registration of the United Kingdom did this practice begin to wane – among Cape practitioners the percentage holding a British degree only rose sharply from the 1870s, eventually topping forty-five per cent in 1900-1910.

Consequently, which licences were most commonly held by Cape doctors, what gaining these entailed and how this shaped nineteenth-century Cape medical practice require some elucidation.

As Table 4.1 shows, until the 1890s the MRCS of the Royal College of Surgeons of London ('of England' from 1843) headed the list of qualifications held by Cape doctors, sometimes in complementary combination with another licence – before 1884, with the London LSA or LAC, thereby constituting the so-called 'College and Hall' qualification, and after 1884 with the LRCP (London) in the popular 'Conjoint' qualification. To contemporaries both combinations signalled that the holder had had a training in medicine, surgery and obstetrics, as befitted a general practitioner, a category of practitioner which emerged during the first decades of the nineteenth century, straddling the traditional boundaries which still formally separated physicians, surgeons and apothecaries. The fifteen-to-twenty per cent of pre-1880 Cape doctors who held the 'College and Hall' were thus comparatively well-equipped to practise as all-rounders – indeed, the first Cape doctor to be licensed specifically as a 'general practitioner' rather than a physician, surgeon and accoucheur, G.M. Nealds in 1841, held the 'College and Hall'.

From as early as 1827 holders of the LSA were required to have had some training in midwifery which contemporaries considered 'the key to general practice',[18] while the RCS of London added this to its curriculum a year later, though in neither case was a candidate required to pass an examination in the subject. The prerequisite of a pass was introduced by the RCS only in 1869, when it was seeking to make its own qualification more comprehensive to meet the General Medical Council's new condition that all licensing bodies had to examine in all subjects. This goal finally produced the RCS/RCP conjoint in medicine, surgery and midwifery in 1884.

The need to provide an all-embracing training was apparent even earlier in the curricula for the LRCS of Edinburgh and the LRCS of Ireland, for both these colleges were located in cities where renowned university medical schools which could award qualifications of their own were already in existence. Thus, both colleges included midwifery as examination subjects already in the 1830s, when the RCS of Edinburgh was formally proclaiming its conviction that all doctors should be instructed in all branches of the profession 'from the intimate connection which subsists between the principles of the several departments of medicine, and the mutual light which they reflect one upon another.'[19] Putting a like principle into practice in Ireland meant that, in the words of an RCSI professor in 1844,

> This College, although called a College of Surgeons, is... just as much a College of Physicians.... [T]his is a College of Medicine and Surgeons and the Diploma you receive from it is universally accepted as evidence of your fitness to practise every branch of the healing art.[20]

Such omnicompetence was certainly a hallmark of the practice of one prominent Cape Peninsula LRCSI holder, C.F.K. Murray, who recalled being called on in one typical day in the 1870s to undertake extraction of teeth, catheterisation, an operation for a strangulated hernia and a cataract operation.[21]

As in England, once the General Medical Council was set up in 1858 and began to demand that all licensing examinations be comprehensive, both the Edinburgh and Irish Colleges of Surgeons began to collaborate with their local Colleges of Physicians to create a formal qualification embracing both medicine and surgery. In Edinburgh this produced a double RCS/RCP qualification in surgery and medicine in 1859, followed by the 'Scottish triple' in 1884 in association with the LFP&S in Glasgow; in Dublin cooperation between the RCSI and the RCPI yielded the 'Irish conjoint' in medicine, surgery and midwifery in 1886.

Indeed, in that year the General Medical Council finally formalized what had become a distinct trend towards comprehensiveness by laying down that henceforth, legal registration as a doctor would require at least a qualification 'such as to guarantee the possession of the knowledge and skill requisite for the efficient practice of medicine, surgery and midwifery.'[22] Simultaneously it stipulated that the courses for such a qualification should occupy a minimum of five years, recommending which courses should be included in the curriculum and in what order. Thus, in the words of a recent medical historian, 'the official purpose of British medical education became... the production in medical school of a fully prepared, safe general practitioner.'[23] Henceforth, all British-trained doctors – and by extension almost all Cape doctors too – came from a common training mould, though the specific contents of their training still varied, depending on the medical school, its staff and resources.

The two elements in the Cape medical profession which distinguished it from the profession in the rest of the British Empire, namely the significant minority of Dutch- and German-trained practitioners in its ranks, brought to their practice a rather different educational experience. Unlike their British-trained colleagues, all (save those trained in Holland as *plattelands-heelmeesters* or country surgeons) were university trained, for in those countries university medical schools offered the only officially approved path to an unrestricted medical career from c.1820. The cachet which such university training bestowed on them at the Cape is plainly evident in the admiring picture drawn of them by a locally born doctor, Meiring Beck, who grew up in Worcester in the 1860s. 'Educated on the Continent... and coming away with the best traditions of such old schools as that of Leyden, Paris, & c., clinging to them', he recalled, 'they were worthy men of wide reading, good linguists, accomplished classical scholars, and able physicians. As a lad I well remember the hero worship inspired by some of them.'[24]

As this memory suggests, Leiden-trained doctors were most numerous among the Cape's Dutch-trained practitioners, but, in fact, for most of the nineteenth century, the training offered there was but a pale shadow of what it had been a century earlier; clinical teaching had ossified into professorial lectures on the cases shown to students, while the explicitly practical component of the seven-year course was limited to just two years, which the Cape's Colonial Medical Council judged was 'hardly sufficient'.[25] It was perhaps the consequential decline in Leiden's reputation as a centre of clinical teaching, along with the growing British cultural climate at the Cape as the nineteenth century developed, which saw the number of Cape-born medical students at Leiden decrease markedly after the 1850s.

The last Cape student to gain a Leiden MD was R.A. Zeederberg, in 1865; tellingly, the other two Cape-born medical students at Leiden in the 1860s did not remain there, but went on to complete their training in Scotland. Equally instructive is the fact that, for all his hero-worship of Continental-trained doctors, Meiring Beck himself went to Edinburgh to study medicine in 1874.

The reputation of most German medical schools, on the other hand, waxed decade by decade from the 1840s. At universities like Berlin, Gottingen, Leipzig, Wurzburg, Jena and Heidelberg (which produced the bulk of the Cape's German-trained doctors) the close clinical instruction and highly didactic teaching which students received were increasingly informed by advances in biomedical sciences (like physiology and bacteriology) made in research laboratories on their campuses. This Humboldtian 'unity of teaching and research' quickly manifested itself in medical curricula. Heidelberg's curriculum, for instance, as the newly graduated J.R. Robertson proudly pointed out in his application to the Cape's Colonial Medical Committee for registration in 1862, included microscopic anatomy and 'diseases of women' as distinct, examinable subjects from 1852, while in 1858 it had made practical laboratory courses in physiology and chemistry compulsory too.[26] In the words of Susan Lawrence, in Germany's best medical schools laboratory science became 'the *sine qua non* of pre-clinical medical education... elevating the physician-researcher to the peak of medical prestige.'[27]

Deploying such state-of-the-art scientific skills in everyday practice in the nineteenth-century Cape was not so easy, however; nor must it be assumed that every German-trained doctor who arrived at the Cape automatically possessed such capability. Several German universities were notorious – even at the Cape – for conferring MDs as St Andrew's did, by purchase, without requiring attendance or more than a perfunctory examination. Several such graduates from Erlangen and Giessen were refused registration by the Colonial Medical Committee on these very grounds. Giessen degrees were 'sold in Tooley-street in London', stormed the Committee's chairman in 1862. '[I]t is a notorious fact stated in the Lancet... from which you will see that they are absolutely made for sale.'[28] After a rash of such applications in the 1860s, the Committee's secretary angrily railed against 'a class of practitioners whose attainments are too superficial, to procure for them a more honourable position. If the merits of these were as great as their ambition, they ought to make no difficulty about procuring proper qualifications.'[29]

Indeed, so numerous did applications of this ilk become that in

1877 the Committee declared that it would no longer register holders of Continental degrees unless they also held an official licence to practise (*staatsexamen*) issued by the government of the relevant state.[30] As the secretary of the Committee confidently pointed out, 'You cannot buy the Staats Examen. diploma.'[31]

Medical degrees awarded by American colleges were even more suspect to the Committee. 'We are very particular indeed about them,' its chairman admitted, 'as we have had many bogus diplomas.'[32]

Applications from people lacking any kind of medical school qualification whatever usually received even shorter shrift from the Committee from the 1830s, at least officially. In practice, however, as the case of *plattelands-heelmeester* H.J. Fockens demonstrates,[33] until quite late in the century the Committee was often prepared to ignore what actually happened on the ground in country districts once it had delivered its formal decision on such an application.

Plattelands-heelmeesters (country surgeons) and *scheepsmeesters* (ship's surgeons) were a class of men (and they were all men) who were trained in Holland in the middle decades of the century. By virtue of this training, until 1865 they were given the right to practise in Holland only in the geographically bound areas indicated by their titles. Between 1830 and 1869, a number of such 'second-class' doctors found their way to the Cape where they sought registration as full surgeons.

The response of the Colonial Medical Committee to their applications was not uniform. Apparently employing the criterion of whether, in its view, there existed a shortage of doctors in the colony at that particular moment, the Committee approved twenty such applications between 1830 and 1869, but rejected some thirty others. Yet, because the colonial administration was still, as late as the 1860s, inclined to turn a blind eye to practice by unregistered practitioners outside Cape Town, many of the thirty nevertheless opened practices in small country towns, even though this was in clear contravention of the law. Astonishingly, in a few instances, the colonial administrations even appointed such men as district surgeons or engaged them to perform official medical duties. Thus, in the middle decades of the nineteenth century, a significant minority of the colony's rural doctors were men who had been trained as *plattelands-heelmeesters* or *scheepsmeesters* in Holland, some of them practising just within Cape law, others just without.

One of the latter was Hendrickus Jacobus Fockens (1835-1903), a Frieslander who ran a very successful general practice in Wellington from 1858 until the mid-1870s. Between 1850 and 1855 he had pursued the course laid down in Holland for training *plattelands-heelmeesters*, viz. a five-year apprenticeship with a local surgeon and accoucheur in Friesland, during which he had also had lessons in pharmacy from a nearby apothecary and in physiology, anatomy, pathology, therapeutics, materia medica and surgery from a physician and a surgeon in the neighbouring town of Groningen. This training had been sufficient to equip him to pass the *plattelands-heelmeester's* examination of the Friesland Provincial Committee of Medical Examination and Superintendence in 1855, after which he had spent three months attached to the practice of a leading Groningen general practitioner, accompanying him on his rounds 'to witness all sorts of diseases', receiving daily lessons from him in the theory of accouchement and assisting him with a number of deliveries, including two difficult cases of twins. This additional experience had enabled Fockens to earn two further licences from the Friesland Provincial Committee later in 1855, viz. those of *scheepsmeester* and *plattelands-voedmeester* (country accoucheur).

On the strength of the former qualification, he was able to take up a position as a ship's surgeon in 1856 and, during the next two years, he visited the Cape more than once in the course of voyages to and from Java. Liking what he saw on shore, he resigned when his ship called at Simon's Town in 1858, and sought registration from the Colonial Medical Committee so he might practise locally. However, the five men who constituted the Committee in that year took a hard line on his application, presumably judging that the colony had enough doctors then, and turned it down with disdain, declaring that his qualifications were inadequate – applicants of this ilk were 'limited in the extent of their knowledge,' said the Committee's chairman, 'not having had that full professional education which they ought to have had, and which all the medical men in town have had. You do not admit half-educated lawyers or clergymen; and so, also, in the medical profession a certain similar degree of caution should be exercised.' The Committee's advisor on Dutch qualifications, a Leiden MD practising in Cape Town, probably put into words what lay at the heart of the Committee's stance – its fear of competition from 'irregulars' – when he blurted out, '[T]his man is not to be put on an equal footing with myself, or any other who has gone through a regular course of study.' The only concession which the Committee was prepared to make was to allow him, by virtue of the lessons in pharmacy he had had during his apprenticeship, to be registered as a chemist and druggist at the Cape.

124

On this lowly official basis Fockens began what, in effect, quickly became a full general practice in Wellington, apparently with great success despite his lack of formal status as a surgeon and accoucheur. Over the next fifteen years he built up a considerable local reputation in the Boland as a most capable doctor who had 'performed many skilful cases as a medical man', a standing which encouraged him to return to Holland in the 1870s, by which time all limitations on where a man with his qualifications might practise in that country had been removed. Accordingly, he set himself up as a general practitioner in Amsterdam where, according to a later report, he developed a 'first rate practice.'

However, on the far more public issue of providing medical education locally, the Colonial Medical Committee offered virtually no such concessions in theory or in practice. In its role as gatekeeper to the Cape medical profession, all through the nineteenth century the Committee was particularly leery of any proposals to set up a medical school in Cape Town to train the sons [sic] of colonists. In its view, the colony lacked not only the personnel required to provide the necessary training, but also the facilities for adequate clinical instruction. Even the 100-bed New Somerset Hospital (opened in 1862) it judged too small and the range of clinical material it offered too circumscribed for such purposes. Medical degrees, it loftily declared, 'ought only to be conferred on Candidates... who have studied in some school... equal to the Standard insisted on by the recognized Universities of Great Britain', but 'no such school could in the present state of the Colony, be established here.'[34] Consequently, it turned down a suggestion by the Colonial Secretary in 1873 that a medical school be established at the New Somerset Hospital along the lines of a London hospital school like Guy's,[35] while two years later it was equally dismissive of a proposal that the new University of the Cape of Good Hope grant medical degrees to students who passed such examinations as the Committee itself prescribed.[36]

The only local training the Colonial Medical Committee was prepared to sanction was eighteen months at the New Somerset, walking the wards, attending dissections and reading texts under the house surgeon's supervision. Through an arrangement the Committee reached with the Royal Colleges of Physicians and of Surgeons in London in 1872-3, this period spent acquiring 'the rudiments of [the] Profession'[37] would be accepted as counting towards the four years' training required of candidates for their licences. However, few locals took advantage of this concession, and of those who did, most were left decidedly unconvinced of the value of such an experience. In the opinion of one:

> Beyond the advantage gained of trying the nerves, and exercising the olfactory organs, and in that way testing one's personal fitness or taste for the work of his life, the information acquired is of so desultory a nature, and so lacks a solid foundation, as to make the student afterwards feel that the two years thus spent have not been commensurate with the good he might afterwards have done.[38]

Yet, there was more to the Committee's opposition to the establishment of a local medical school than just the lack of suitable teachers and clinical facilities. Made up as it was of senior members of the Cape medical profession, all of whom had been trained in Britain, the Colonial Medical Committee shared views then prevalent in those circles, in particular that a colonial medical education was inherently third-rate and that any medical graduates who followed such a path would ipso facto be what one Cape practitioner dismissively called 'men of defective education'.[39] Such a colonial inferiority complex pervaded Cape doctors' (and others') thinking throughout the century, one after another insisting that only training in Europe could broaden a colonial-born student's horizons sufficiently – as one London-trained doctor put it in 1899:

> [C]ontact with the larger civilization and keener intellects in Europe teaches him a great many things which he would not learn in Cape Town and thereby helps to render him better for... a profession in which a thorough knowledge of mankind is of as great importance as a thorough knowledge of the anatomy of the human frame.[40]

The idea of a Cape Town medical school also raised fears among local doctors of being swamped by a flood of its graduates, inferior practitioners, they claimed, who would lower the standing of the profession and provide unfair competition for them. '[T]he present supply [of doctors] requires to be very carefully supplemented to prevent a glut in the market,' warned one in 1871 in his critique of a scheme to create a local medical school,[41] a sentiment by no means absent nearly fifty years later when a medical school was finally set up in Cape Town. 'I see grave dangers ahead, that of a half-educated medical community which will be, like all half-educated people, low in everything in the shape of tone,' predicted a country GP gloomily in 1919. 'We shall be flooded with half-educated medicos whose only chance of competing with the properly trained men who have been overseas will be by resorting to all sorts of discreditable practices.'[42]

In the 1870s a similar anxiety to preserve the closed medical shop on the colony's eastern frontier and restrict access to the profession there saw the Colonial Medical Committee veto a scheme by Dr J.P. Fitzgerald of Grey Hospital, King William's Town, to offer elementary medical training to selected young Africans as a preliminary to sending them to England (at the colony's expense) to qualify fully before returning to British Kaffraria as district surgeons. '[W]hen returned home here with European Diplomata, they would be Physicians with the fullest Privileges, competent to practise in any country,' the Committee explained.[43] '[N]o Kaffir [sic] young man educated in Europe, would be content to settle down on a small stipend, and pass his life in a Hut in a Kaffir Village; and ...therefore it would be unwise to Educate Kaffir youths, fully for the Medical Profession, at the Public expense.'[44] Safeguarding the vested interests of the Cape profession was too important to permit this.

What eventually overcame such medical resistance to the establishment of a complete medical school at the Cape was the development of a teaching university in Cape Town, just as had happened in Australia and New Zealand, where the medical profession also initially opposed the foundation of a local medical school. Whereas from its inception the University of the Cape of Good Hope had never been more than an examining institution and so lacked the means to initiate medical training by itself, from the 1890s the South African College in Cape Town began to upgrade itself from a small university college into a fully fledged teaching university. In this quest a medical school was a powerful accessory, for, to late Victorians, medicine represented the very cutting edge of science, giving an institution *éclat* in the wider community and academic respectability among scholars.

Already by 1900 the South African College had decided to bypass the University of the Cape of Good Hope and to seek Scottish universities' recognition as external teachers of its professors of physics and chemistry, subjects which constituted half of the curriculum for the first year of the Scottish MB,ChB course. Four years later it had its newly appointed professors in the other two first-year subjects, botany and zoology, similarly recognised, thereby in effect enabling its students to take the whole of the first year of the Scottish MB,ChB locally. '[W]e are today at the South African College in possession of a nucleus which is, I believe, destined to become the first Medical School of South Africa,' forecast a senior member of its council confidently.[45] A year later the South African

College Senate formally proclaimed its goal of becoming an independent University of Cape Town with its own faculty of medicine, 'and that with a view to this end everything be done to promote the development of the college with the least possible delay.'[46]

Achieving this required the backing of the medical profession, its organisations and its journals, however, and this was slow to come and by no means unqualified. Though the socio-economic consequences of the mineral revolution since the 1880s had removed the bases of many of their earlier objections to a Cape medical school, cultural prejudice against such an institution, its graduates and the impact these might have on the Cape profession died hard. As late as 1910 a senior member of the Colonial Medical Council, who was also a member of parliament, took strong exception in public to:

> subjects which were the foundation of medicine being taught in this country where the best conditions were not obtainable. We should only get second rate teachers, and we had not the material for teaching, material which, in older countries had been accumulated for ages. Personally he hoped they would never have a medical college in South Africa. In Australia the people would not trust their home educated men, who consequently only took the inferior positions in practice.[47]

Such entrenched attitudes meant that the South African College could approach its goal only step by step, employing abundant persuasion, tact and compromise on the way. Thus, it was 1911 before it offered courses in the second-year subjects of the Scottish MB,ChB degree, anatomy and physiology, and 1918 before it introduced the three third-year subjects, bacteriology, pathology and pharmacology. Teaching in the main clinical subjects followed two years later, with the first graduates trained wholly in what, since 1918, had been the Faculty of Medicine of the University of Cape Town, qualifying in 1922, eighteen years after the inception of first-year MB,ChB training in Cape Town.

Not surprisingly, given the longstanding misgivings as to the adequacy of any local medical training in the Cape, the University of Cape Town went out of its way to put the standard of its training beyond doubt. Its MB,ChB curriculum required six years' attendance, i.e. one year longer than that in Scotland, a feature which became (and remains) the norm in South Africa. This ensured that the country's four provincial medical councils approved its curriculum in advance and it set up a panel of non-university doctors to advise its medical faculty on matters of general policy. With a similar aim in mind, it filled all eight of its medical chairs with British-trained appointees, five of them graduates of Scottish universities. It was one of these, T.J. Mackie, soon to become professor of bacteriology at Edinburgh, who, in an address to mark the full school's inauguration in 1920, reassured the profession that the University of Cape Town was 'now prepared, with the co-operation of various public medical institutions in Cape Town, to undertake the education of medical practitioners.' Thanks to its endeavours, South Africa could now 'undertake the entire responsibility for this form of professional education... I feel confident in saying that the medical training that is provided in Cape Town will compare favourably with European standards.'[48]

This anxiety to ensure that the training that South African medical schools provided was on a par with that in Europe has persisted till today, raising the question as to whether the training of any of those who practised biomedicine in Cape over the last 350 years has been adequately geared to the local situation. From the perspective of 2004, such training might well be summed up by the title of this chapter, as being primarily 'home taught for abroad'.

Notes

1. S. Lawrence, 'Medical Education' in W.F. Bynum and R. Porter (eds), *Companion Encyclopedia of the History of Medicine,* vol. 2, (London & New York: Routledge, 1993), 1151.
2. *Ibid.,* 1152.
3. All the information on the Fraenkels comes from C. Friedman-Spits, *The Fraenkel Saga* (Pinelands: South African Medical Association, 1998).
4. W.F. Bynum, *Science and the Practice of Medicine in the Nineteenth Century* (Cambridge: Cambridge University Press, 1994), xi.
5. R.S. Downie and B. Charlton, *The Making of a Doctor: Medical Education in Theory and Practice* (New York: Oxford University Press, 1992), 14.
6. W.G. Atherstone, 'Reminiscences of Medical Practice in South Africa Fifty Years Ago', in *South African Medical Journal* (*SAMJ*), (April 1897), 244.
7. *Ibid.*
8. T.N. Bonner, *Becoming a Physician: Medical Education in Britain, France, Germany and the United States, 1750-1945* (New York: Oxford University Press, 1995), 105.

9. H.A. Ebden, 'Colonial Medical Education' in *Cape Monthly Magazine* (November 1858), 258–9, .

10. *Ibid.*, 258.

11. Doc. 399 – Memorandum by J. Addey, 21 August 1820, Cape Archives Depot (henceforth CA), CO 3918.

12. C. Newman, *The Evolution of Medical Education in the Nineteenth Century* (New York: Oxford University Press, 1957), 103.

13. H. Bickersteth, 'Case of Empyema' in *Cape Town Medical Gazette*, i, 2 (1 April 1847), 25.

14. *Ibid.*, 28, 29.

15. Y.Z., 'Cape Doctors' in *Cape Monthly Magazine* (February 1871), 107–8.

16. Cited in L. Rosner, *Medical Education in the Age of Improvement: Edinburgh Students and Apprentices 1760-1826* (Edinburgh: Edinburgh University Press, 1994), 47.

17. This information on Barry is drawn from I. Rae, *The Strange Story of Dr James Barry* (London: Longmans Green, 1958).

18. Cited in A. Digby, *Making a Medical Living: Doctors and Patients in the English Market for Medicine, 1720-1911* (Cambridge: Cambridge University Press, 1994), 254.

19. Cited in C.H. Creswell, *The Royal College of Surgeons of Edinburgh: Historical Notes from 1505 to 1905* (Edinburgh: The College, 1926), 281.

20. Cited in J.D.H. Widdess, *The Royal College of Surgeons in Ireland and its Medical School 1784-1966*, 2nd edn (Edinburgh & London: E & S Livingstone, 1967), 80.

21. C.F.K. Murray, 'Some Reminiscences of Medical Practice in the Cape Peninsula' , *South African Medical Record* (SAMR), (13 January 1912), 10.

22. J. Walton, P.B. Beeson and R.B. Scott (eds), *Oxford Companion to Medicine*, i (Oxford & New York: Oxford University Press, 1986), 718.

23. *Ibid.*

24. British Medical Association, Cape of Good Hope Western Branch, *Presidential Addresses 1888-1908* (Cape Town: The Association, 1908), 85.

25. File labelled 'Correspondence re: Neth. Med. Degree' (Report by Colonial Medical Council, 21 November 1896), CA, MC 24.

26. Document R16, J.R. Robertson to Colonial Secretary, 20 May 1862, CA, CO 4127.

27. Lawrence, 'Medical Education' in Bynum and Porter, *op. cit.* (note 1), vol. 2, 1167.

28. *Report of (Select) Committee on Medical Practitioners,* 1862, C.4-1862, 11.
29. Document R12, Gloss by Secretary of Colonial Medical Committee, 10 May 1862, CA, CO 4127.
30. *Cape of Good Hope Government Gazette* (20 February 1877), 4: Government Notice 133/1877.
31. *Report of Select Committee on Medical Law Reform,* 1883, A.25-1883, 17.
32. *Ibid.,* 2.
33. The information on Fockens is drawn from *Report of (Select) Committee on Medical Practitioners,* 1862, C.4-1862; and *Report of (Select) Committee on Medical Practitioners Bill,* A.6-1890.
34. Colonial Medical Committee to Colonial Secretary, 24 September 1875, CA, MC 30.
35. *Ibid.,* Colonial Medical Committee to Colonial Secretary, 25 April 1873.
36. *Standard and Mail* (9 September 1875); Colonial Medical Committee to Colonial Secretary, 24 September 1875, CA, MC 30.
37. W.H. Wood to Colonial Secretary, 29 April 1873 (appended to Colonial Medical Committee to Colonial Secretary, 2 May 1873), CA, MC 30.
38. *Standard and Mail* (21 September 1875), letter from 'A Graduate'.
39. M.D., 'Colonial Medical Education' in *Cape Monthly Magazine* (March 1859), 172.
40. *SAMJ* (February 1899), 210, letter by Dr Edw. C. Long.
41. Y.Z. 'Cape Doctors' in *Cape Monthly Magazine* (February 1871), 111.
42. *SAMR* (26 July 1919), 224, letter by 'More Anxious'.
43. Colonial Medical Committee to Colonial Secretary, 2 February 1877, CA, MC 30.
44. *Ibid.,* Colonial Medical Committee to Colonial Secretary, 9 March 1877.
45. E.B. Fuller, *The Beginning of Medical Education in South Africa* (Cape Town: n.p., 1917), 3.
46. South African College, *Report of the Committee of Senate on University Education* (Cape Town: The College, 1905), 11.
47. Union of South Africa, *Debates of the House of Assembly,* 15 December 1910, columns 830–1.
48. T.J. Mackie, *Some Remarks on Medical Education in South Africa* (Cape Town: Townshend, Taylor and Snashall, 1920), 4.

5

Opportunities Outside Private Practice before 1860

Harriet Deacon and Elizabeth van Heyningen

This chapter discusses the restrictions and opportunities which salaried employment offered Cape doctors in the pay of government and charitable organisations during the first two thirds of the nineteenth century. Although Cape doctors often acted as agents of the colonial state there were many nuances within this relationship. While military doctors played an important role in the profession during the first few decades of the century, by the 1840s civilian doctors were beginning to assert greater influence in Cape Town, if not yet in the Eastern Cape. Hospital posts and an expanding network of charitable organisations and government-funded district surgeoncies provided part-time employment for some doctors throughout the colony. This helped urban-based doctors to sustain practices and encouraged more doctors to practice in the smaller country towns serving large farming areas.

Introduction

Elizabeth van Heyningen has described Cape doctors as 'agents' of empire' after 1880,[1] and we have suggested in Chapters 2 and 3 that Cape doctors had a close relationship with the colonial state during the early-nineteenth century. There were however many nuances within this relationship, and doctors cannot simply be understood as handmaidens of colonialism. Circumstances did not always make it easy for them to have a substantial impact on the process of colonisation. In colonial India, for example, a different disease environment made it difficult for British doctors to aid colonisation by stabilising army or settler mortality and sickness, and because of government recalcitrance and popular resistance, doctors' roles in surveillance and social control were small and often ineffective.[2] At the Cape, basking in a temperate climate that suited Europeans, and supported by an interventionist government, doctors may have been more active in helping to establish the settler population through public health measures and playing a role in social control through, for example, the institutionalisation of the leprous and insane and the development of racist ideology and practice. Doctors would have been more likely to act overtly as 'agents of empire' in the colonial justice system, institutions and policy-making than in their private practice, however. Only a small number of black clients wanted to, or could, consult the few Western-trained doctors at the Cape, and the relationship between private client and doctor would have been different from that in an institution, court or public health programme.

While most colonial doctors would have shared the civilising dreams and prejudices of settler society, and many would have been in a position to enforce policies of the colonial state, they had other concerns too, most important of which would have been professional advancement and making a medical living. Nineteenth-century Cape doctors enjoyed varying degrees of autonomy and status within the civil service. Before the establishment of a colonial parliament in 1854, those who enjoyed full-time employment as military doctors were used by the autocratic imperial governors of the Cape before the establishment of a colonial parliament in 1854 to control civilian activity and opposition. There was a constant struggle between military and civilian doctors, and between Dutch- and English-speaking doctors, who were appointed, often for political reasons, in advisory positions on the Medical Committee and Vaccine Institute and as hospital surgeons. The civilian doctors who took government appointments like these were usually based in Cape Town or, by the 1850s, in other urban centres, and used the appointments to expand their private practice and provide a basic salary. Through this work, they would have had a greater opportunity to influence institutional practice and public health policies. Urban doctors also benefited disproportionally from part-time employment in the charity and self-help sectors. In outlying areas district surgeoncies provided a basic salary, some extra rights of practice (e.g. a vaccination monopoly) and a chance to expand a doctor's private practice. British doctors dominated the ranks of district surgeons, but candidates were so scarce in some areas that government sometimes resorted to employing unlicensed practitioners instead (see Chapter 4). The prominence of the district surgeon within the two-tier social structure and small bureaucracy of country towns meant that he would have played a key role as one of the representatives of the colonial state and the enforcers of its policies.

While opportunities for furthering the aims of the colonial state and achieving its broader imperial ambitions were often limited by circumstance, and only sometimes prioritised by the Cape medical profession, Cape doctors shared many imperial hopes and racial prejudices with their fellow settlers and the colonial bureaucracy. In this chapter, we will examine the ways in which government employment in military, hospital and district surgeon posts, and private employment in the charity and commercial sectors, provided opportunities for Cape doctors to further their professional and personal ambitions, while simultaneously influencing the process and progress of colonisation at the Cape.

The influence of military doctors in the Cape profession

In the early part of the nineteenth century, military posts were the most common means by which Cape doctors found influence and economic security outside of private practice. The most important full-time employment for doctors was, at least initially, with the military. Military doctors helped to draft professional legislation in 1807 and 1823 and dominated early private practice on the eastern Frontier. While some practitioners were attached to the British army, frontier conflicts also created opportunities for colonial doctors who served temporarily with the volunteer forces.[3] During the course of the nineteenth century, tension arose between military and civilian doctors, especially in Cape Town and Grahamstown where they competed for political advantage and private business. Civilian doctors gradually gained ascendancy in the Western Cape, although on the frontier military doctors continued to exert considerable influence for much of the century. By the 1880s, military doctors were in a numerical and political minority within the profession at the Cape.

During the first British occupation (1795-1803) and the period of Batavian rule (1803-6) a number of regularly trained military doctors were brought to the Cape with the occupying forces. The armies provided free passage and certain employment in the colony. Significantly for the profession, military doctors were also able to practise privately from their secure base; many left the military in mid-career and went into private practice full-time. Their involvement in private practice, while enjoying close contact with military governors, had a significant impact on the regulation of the medical profession. Military training and experience were also an important element in the careers of many Cape doctors. Most of the first wave of British immigrant doctors after 1806 were demobilised military surgeons who came to the Cape once the ending of the Napoleonic Wars in 1815 created an increasingly competitive medical market in Britain.[4] An army medical career was a useful stepping stone into private practice and enabled medical immigrants to survey the field before they entered the colonial medical market.[5]

After the Treaty of Amiens in 1802 the Principal Medical Committee in Holland had tried unsuccessfully to introduce general professional medical regulation at the Cape.[6] Locally based doctors were more successful, with the assistance of military doctors appointed to government committees. After the introduction of smallpox vaccine to the Cape in 1803 a *Geneeskundige Commissie* (Medical Commission), under the leadership of the Director-in-Chief of the Military Hospital, was formed to make regulations on vaccination and to vaccinate. Following protests from other Cape Town doctors, the twelve doctors on the Commission agreed to extend the right to vaccinate to others, but only those with proven ability to vaccinate and in possession of a 'Diploma or Testimonial from any qualified person or College'.[7]

The Cape regulations of 1807 (see Chapter 3) were drafted by military doctors appointed to a Supreme Medical Committee (SMC) by the military governor. The regulations were passed by two powerful and authoritarian governors[8] who wanted to emphasise the progressive nature of British rule in imposing a new order on the backward and disorganised former Dutch colony.[9] They saw the Cape as a place where strict regulations could and should be passed to ensure the good of society and the efficient practice of medicine. The SMC was asked to advise the governor on complaints about poor-quality medicines being sold at high prices by Cape Town shopkeepers, doctors and druggists.[10] As we have seen, its proposed regulations echoed the concerns of doctors in Britain about competition from unqualified practitioners and dispensing druggists. The three British military doctors on the committee also had an interest in better regulation of the medical market in Cape Town, where they probably practised privately. In the regulations of 1807, the SMC was made into a permanent advisory and licensing body, staffed by government-appointed doctors from Cape Town.

As Burrows has suggested, the creation of the SMC represented 'the control that a military government felt constrained to exercise over a civilian medical profession in an occupied country'.[11] Military doctors initially controlled the SMC; two of the first three members of the SMC, Alexander Baillie, the Deputy Inspector of Hospitals, and A.L. Emerson, had been on the *ad hoc* committee of 1807. The first two presidents were military men and the only civilian member until 1821 was L.G. Biccard, who had formerly been a physician in the Batavian army. In 1821 the Governor replaced the committee with a Colonial Medical Inspector (James Barry, who was a military doctor).[12] After the establishment of a Colonial Medical Committee (MC) in 1825 military members outnumbered civilians by three to two.[13] Civilian doctors began to play a greater role in formally advising government after November 1831, when the South African Medical Society, an association of civilian Cape Town doctors, was asked to stand in for the newly formed MC, which had been abolished on the orders of the Secretary of State.[14] When the committee was re-formed in October 1834,[15] civilian members outnumbered military members by five to two.[16] Under John Montagu (Colonial Secretary, 1843-53), however, more military men were appointed to the MC.[17] Both military and civilian doctors saw the MC as an instrument of professional advancement, but there was growing tension between the two groups. Members of the Medical Society voted in 1828 not to call in military men to consult on patients as, they complained, 'it has generally been observed that the compliment is not returned'.[18] When, on the death of Dr Louis Liesching, he was replaced by a military doctor as president of the MC in 1842, three civilian members resigned in protest.

By mid-century, therefore, there was a growing divide between increasingly career-minded military doctors, many of whom were on the conflict-ridden eastern frontier, and civilian doctors in the Western Cape. This conflict was evident in the appointment of a surgeon superintendent to the Robben Island General Infirmary in 1855, after the dismissal of Dr Birtwhistle for mismanagement. The Governor asked an Eastern Cape official to make recommendations for the post and told the Cape Town-based MC, by then dominated by Western Cape civilian doctors, to do the same. By some mistake, however, the military man recommended by the Eastern Cape was immediately appointed to the post, ignoring the application of Dr John Laing, a respected Cape Town doctor, who was the MC candidate. The MC protested to no avail against the sidelining of the civilian, Western Cape candidate.[19] Special circumstances continued to favour military doctors until well past mid-century. The Contagious Diseases Act of 1868, which the War Office had forcibly persuaded the Cape government to pass in order to control venereal diseases, led to a new medical appointment, with a doctor to examine prostitutes in and out of the Lock Hospital in Cape Town. To the anger of local civilian doctors in Cape Town, the position was initially given to a military man.[20]

Dr Friedrich Ludwig Liesching and his son Louis

The careers of the two doctors, Friedrich and Louis Liesching, illustrate the tension between military doctors and the civilian profession, and the importance of extra-professional activities and government appointments in securing financial stability for even the most well-regarded of the Cape Town medical elite. Liesching senior was a military doctor under the DEIC who later rose to a powerful position within the civilian profession under the British. He had immigrated to the Cape in 1787 as a surgeon of the Württemburg Regiment, a mercenary regiment recruited by the DEIC. His training in Germany at Württemburg's Military Academy, under the authoritarian aegis of the Duke of Württemburg, had been at least as thorough as that of the British military doctors who came to the Cape a few years later.[21] Once he was established at the Cape, Liesching petitioned the Duke in 1795 to be allowed to remain there to practise privately. Private practice did not provide Liesching with the income he needed to support a household of twenty-eight people (including slaves), however, and he opened an apothecary's shop. He traded a variety of goods from his home, selling anything from tobacco to haircombs and sewing thread. Other activities such as teaching sometimes added to his income, and he rented out three properties in Dorp Street.[22] Liesching also established a medicinal herb garden at Botany (later Bantry) Bay, just outside Cape Town.[23]

The large Liesching family's persistent financial problems meant that the two doctors found government appointments very useful, although they ultimately faced financial ruin through the insolvency of William Liesching and his brother-in-law, Joachim Stoll, in the 1830s.[24] The two doctors' university-level qualifications, so rare in Cape Town, meant that they were particularly eligible for such posts. Under the Batavian government Liesching senior was called in to assist with vaccinations and, after the *Geneeskundige Commissie* (Medical Commission) was convened, he became a member. He continued to assist with vaccinations after the arrival of the British, until civilians were replaced by British military doctors in 1811.[25] Liesching senior was licensed by the SMC in 1807 as one of four physicians in the colony but he was now both a civilian and a foreigner under a government which favoured British military doctors. In spite of this, Lord Charles Somerset, Governor of the Cape, lent a sympathetic ear in 1825 when Liesching junior asked for a government appointment to ease his financial difficulties (his private practice had suffered because of recent ill health). For the same reason, both Lieschings took out an advertisement in the local newspaper, asking patients to pay their debts for visits and medicines, threatening legal action and refusal of further services.[26] It is not known what response they received from the advertisement, but Liesching junior was soon appointed as surgeon to the Slave Lodge (£40 per annum) and as prison doctor to the Town gaol (£75 per annum, plus £10 because he did his own dispensing); he also served on the Medical Committee (£50 per annum) and had worked at Somerset Hospital for five years (£100 per annum, but for three years he had received no salary).[27] These posts were often short-lived, however, and Louis' most long-lasting government appointment seems to have been the £45 per annum he earned running the midwifery school between 1828 and 1838.[28] With the rise of insurance companies in the 1830s and 1840s, he was appointed as one of three doctors serving the Protecteur Fire and Life Assurance Company.[29]

The boundary between profession and trade was a sensitive one, rigorously defended by professional bodies, at least in Cape Town. When it was first established, the Medical Committee complained that, 'At present Dr Liesching engrosses every branch of the profession (surgery excepted) and trade, wholesale as well as retail.'[30] As recounted in Chapter 3, Dr James Barry later took up the cudgel against the licensing of apothecaries who had been locally trained (like Liesching's son Charles) and against Cape Town doctors who traded in medicines (like Liesching senior). Liesching was asked to close down his apothecary's business, but no action was taken against him, and the business flourished. He may have escaped prosecution because he did not dispense himself, employing apothecaries for this purpose,[31] but the legislation was famously toothless (see Chapter 3) and Liesching was one of the most powerful doctors of the Cape Town elite. He served as the first president of the South African Medical Society in 1827, and his son was one of only three civilians to serve on the Supreme Medical Committee before 1830 – Liesching junior became president of the Colonial MC in 1838. On Liesching senior's death in 1841, the pallbearers represented the medical elite of Cape Town: Drs Chiappini, Ahrens, Herzog, Somervaile, Fehrszen, Brown, Bickersteth and Lee Wright.[32] Two of Liesching's sons went into medicine, one as a physician (Carl Ludwig 'Louis') and the other as an apothecary (Carl Friedrich 'Charles'). While most of his children married into the Dutch elite of Cape Town, a number of Liesching's grandchildren married into British army and navy families, representing the shifting and permeable boundaries between Cape Dutch, British, military and civilian medical families by the end of the century.[33]

The civilian profession and civilian hospitals

The first hospitals in the Cape were built in Cape Town and Simon's Town by the DEIC for their sick employees and slaves. These institutions were staffed by ship's surgeons, many of whom had no professional qualifications. The first civilian hospitals (the Somerset Hospital and the Merchant Seamen's Hospital in Cape Town) were founded privately by a surgeon, Samuel Bailey, who surrendered control of the institutions to the municipal authorities when he ran into financial difficulties during the 1820s. Through reforms in the 1840s, doctors began to take over administrative control of the Cape Town hospitals from laymen and -women. There were few hospitals outside Cape Town before the 1850s, but the extension of the hospital system in mid-century gave doctors a greater platform for professional advancement. By mid-century, doctors had access to a number of salaried government positions outside the military establishment, such as hospital posts and district surgeoncies. They were also able to seek salaried employment with insurance companies and charitable institutions, in specialist institutions such as mental asylums, and in industry, which will be discussed in Chapter 8. Importantly, most of these posts allowed them the flexibility to maintain a private practice on the side. Indeed, a salaried post seems to have enhanced doctors' reputation and financial security as private practitioners.

Civilian hospitals provided a secure base for civilians to pursue their careers and private practice. The early Cape hospitals, both civilian and military, were all in Cape Town or at the naval base nearby at Simon's Town. Outside Cape Town, many country jails had hospitals attached to them, where poor patients were sometimes housed. A mission station at Caledon was asked by government to run a nearby leprosy settlement at Hemel-en-Aarde in 1821, with the medical assistance of the Caledon district surgeon. But besides these establishments, and a 'pauper and leper asylum' in the Port Elizabeth area, there were few civilian medical institutions outside Cape Town. In 1846, a General Infirmary for leprosy patients, the insane and the sick poor was opened on Robben Island, an island just off the coast of Cape Town, and in the 1850s several hospitals were built in the eastern Cape: at Grahamstown, Port Elizabeth and King William's Town. The New Somerset Hospital (situated near the modern

Illustration 5.1
The New and Old Somerset Hospitals, Cape Town

After the building of the New Somerset Hospital in the 1860s, the Old Somerset Hospital became Cape Town's institution for the chronic sick poor, like the black patients depicted here. The OSH provided useful, if ill-paid, employment to a struggling medical profession. Below is the New Somerset Hospital as viewed from the waterfront. (UCT, Mss & Archives, Macmillan - Hospitals: Photographs)

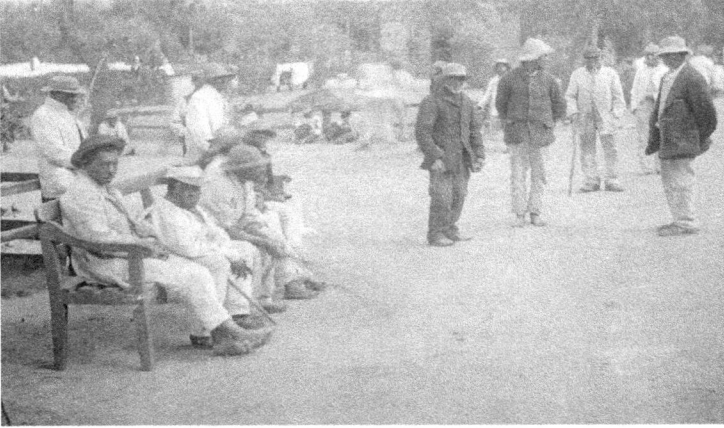

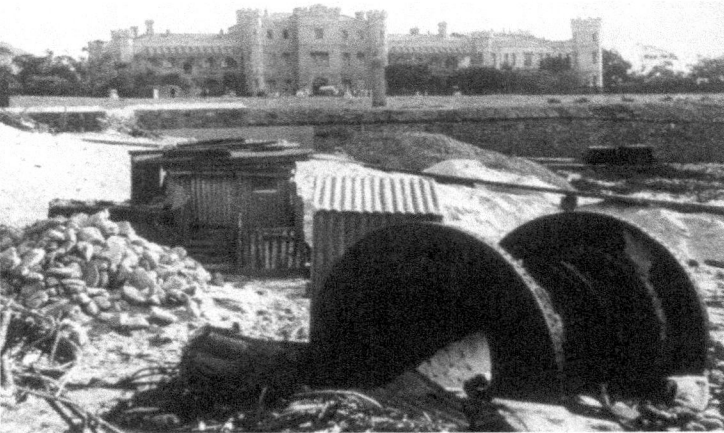

Waterfront development in Cape Town), was opened in 1862.

The Old Somerset Hospital and Robben Island

The first civilian hospital at the Cape was built in 1818 by an ex-military doctor, Samuel Bailey, for poor seamen and slaves. Initially, it operated as a private concern, although built on land donated by the military Governor, Lord Charles Somerset, and named 'Somerset Hospital' in his honour. Because of financial difficulties Bailey was forced to sell the hospital to Cape Town's Dutch-controlled Burgher Senate in 1821, however, and on the dissolution of the Burgher Senate (Town Council) in 1828, the responsibility for the hospital passed to the British colonial government.

The various conflicts over management within the hospital provide a good illustration of the tensions within the Cape medical profession and their struggles for professional status above that of laymen and laywomen. Tension between Dutch- and English-speaking doctors in Cape Town flared up at various times during the course of the century. The change in ownership and control of the hospital in the 1820s had an impact on the ethnic composition of the doctors in charge, for example. Samuel Bailey, the founder, was the first surgeon-superintendent, but he had to relinquish his post to Louis Liesching (who was of German origin – see above) when the Dutch-controlled Burgher Senate took over the hospital. Bailey was reinstated once the (British) colonial government took control of the hospital again in 1828.

In the 1840s the Somerset Hospital was also a site of conflict between laymen and doctors for the control of hospital administration. New rules for the administration of the hospital were drawn up under Medical Committee advice, which gave greater authority to the medical personnel and took away some of the duties and responsibilities of the steward. This caused some conflict within the institution. Similar changes were brought about in the 1850s at the General Infirmary on Robben Island, which had been established in 1846 for 'lunatics', 'lepers' and the 'chronic sick'.[34] The Robben Island Steward felt sidelined by changing power relations and began to complain to government about the surgeon's management abilities – the surgeon was dismissed in 1855 for gross misconduct.[35] The power balance had shifted towards the doctor, however, and it was not until 1895 that a layman commissioner took over administrative authority from the surgeon-superintendent at Robben Island.[36] Throughout the century, conflict between lay and medically trained hospital administrators affected the position doctors held within hospitals. In general, the trend was towards greater medical control over the administration of hospitals, especially as they began to perform teaching as well as curative functions. But in the latter part of the century the appointment of lay boards of governors and lay managers threatened medical control over some government institutions.

Another management issue close to the hearts of Cape doctors was the role of external assessors, or 'official visitors' who came to inspect government hospitals. In some cases these people, usually doctors themselves, overlooked mismanagement of institutions in the interests of political and professional harmony. An example of this was the flagrant misrepresentation of the very poor management of the Robben Island Hospitals in Medical Committee inspections between 1846 and 1853.[37] The MC had to inspect this and other institutions periodically on behalf of the government. In other cases however, such as the inspections by Dr James Barry as Inspector of Hospitals in the 1820s, and those by Dr Jane Waterston from the 1890s, official visitors were much more vigilant about conditions in government institutions. Barry was, for example, very concerned about the personal comfort of leprosy patients at the Hemel-en-Aarde station in the 1820s, and ordered sheepskin mattresses for them.[38] These improvements in living conditions were however accompanied by stricter rules about non-leprosy sufferers staying at the station, and the fostering of healthy children in nearby settlements, which caused many inmates to run away and join their relatives off the station.[39] While Barry effected many improvements in local medical institutions, his interventions were not always welcomed within the medical profession. This was partly because of what some contemporaries referred to as his 'petulant hauteur'[40] and partly because of his uncompromising attitude in support of (British) 'standards'. His strict control over the licensing of doctors and apothecaries caused some friction with those who wished to educate their children as doctors in the Cape (as discussed above and in Chapter 3).[41]

By the middle of the nineteenth century the hospital was acquiring a new importance in the eyes both of the medical profession and the educated public. Despite the strong influence of British medicine the Cape hospital tradition as it developed in the second half of the nineteenth century was often a response to local needs and differed in significant respects from British hospitals. While the Albany Hospital in Grahamstown and the Port Elizabeth Provincial Hospital owed their origin and part of their funding to local endeavours, the Grey Hospital in King William's Town and the Somerset Hospital were entirely government controlled and financed. The absence of Poor Law institutions meant that all the general hospitals became to some extent shelters for the aged and chronic-sick poor, although only the Old Somerset Hospital was formally designated as such. A major factor in retarding the growth of the Cape hospitals and in limiting professional medical interest in them was the absence of a medical school at the Cape. As Granshaw has observed, late-nineteenth-century hospitals were the profession's training ground, the place where scientific medicine could most effectively be explored.[42] Without an educational function, Cape general hospitals remained nothing more than provincial institutions, lacking facilities for research or for the sophisticated treatment of patients.

The New Somerset Hospital

By the 1850s Bailey's hospital had become little more than a refuge for the Cape's chronic-sick poor; most of the other patients were in transit for Robben Island and only a minority were medical or surgical cases.[43] Work was increasingly onerous, with nearly 600 in-patients and about 1,500 out-patients per annum. The building was dilapidated and operations had to be performed in the wards or in the dispensary.[44] The pleas of the resident surgeon, Henry Bickersteth, that the government provide a new hospital found a responsive supporter in the Governor, Sir George Grey.[45] For the Governor, Western medicine was a manifestation of modern civilisation, at once scientific and beneficent and, apart from the Grey and Somerset Hospitals, he also promoted both the Albany and Port Elizabeth hospitals.[46] But Grey's enthusiasm for hospital buildings went further – for him, they were also the physical expression of the dignity and altruism of the state. Both the Grey Hospital in King William's Town and the New Somerset Hospital in Cape Town were intended to be visible symbols of Britain's philanthropic colonial mission. The Colonial Medical Committee was equally determined that the new hospital should reflect the status of the town and the colony. [47]

The cornerstone of the New Somerset Hospital was laid on 18 August 1859 with full Masonic honours, Grey's last act before he left the colony. It was an extraordinary building, crenellated and towered, located near the docks, the first public edifice which new arrivals to the colony would see when they landed at the quayside, then also under construction. As in British and American hospitals, miasmic theories were still widely accepted and adequate ventilation was the chief consideration in a building which was soon to prove less than adequate in other respects.[48] Yet, although the Colonial Medical Committee had been anxious that the hospital should be designed in accordance with the most modern thinking, the pavilion design which was popularised in Florence Nightingale's *Notes on Hospitals*, published in 1859, was not adopted. Only its site, on the shoreline, exposed to the sea breezes, conformed to these ideas.[49]

Although it was officially a national infirmary, accepting patients from the rest of the colony, from its inception the New Somerset Hospital was pre-eminently a Cape Town institution. Its relationship with the municipality and the public was often uneasy, but it was always a consideration in shaping policy. The fear that proselytising Christians would alienate Muslims who were, in any case, wary of Western medicine, was one reason for Dr A.L. Chiappini's determination that Anglican Sisters nursing at the hospital should be subordinate to his authority rather than that of any religious superior.[50] When the Colonial Medical Committee recommended changes in the management of the hospital, it was the failure of the hospital to command the confidence of the public that it cited as a reason for doing so. [51]

The distinction between the two Somerset Hospitals remained blurred. In theory the Old Somerset Hospital retained its role as the infirmary for the chronic-sick poor while the New Somerset Hospital primarily treated the short-term ailments of the poor; increasingly, the out-patients' function was ceded to the publicly funded Free Dispensary, which had been started in the 1850s. But a hard and fast line could never be drawn between the three institutions, all of which were exposed to the same crises of public health in the town. By the 1880s the New Somerset Hospital's function as a general infirmary was frequently lost sight of as Cape Town's growing population and poor sanitary state filled the wards with cases of typhoid and other fevers and it became impossible to carry out any but the most necessary operations.[52] The government felt that the municipality should shoulder more responsibility for its own failings and was only prepared to contribute financially to such diseases as smallpox, cholera or yellow fever which were not directly the result of preventable insanitary conditions.[53]

At the end of the nineteenth century a reformed central government Health Department turned to the model of the English provincial hospitals in order to strengthen the responsibility of the town for its general infirmary. [54] The problem of overcrowding, if not of infectious diseases, was solved partly by the building of a new wing, the Victoria Wing. With the opening of this section, from the beginning of 1898, the government announced that the New Somerset Hospital was to be managed by a local committee chosen by donors and subscribers and subsidised by a government grant.[55] Out-patients were to be transferred entirely to the Free Dispensary.[56] The reorganisation of the New Somerset Hospital transformed its relationship with the town. Fundraising hospital days became a regular feature of Cape Town life. Most significant of all, perhaps, the establishment of the Women's Board of Aid gave Cape Town women one of their first public roles of any real significance.[57]

If the New Somerset Hospital was a local institution in the eyes of the Cape Town public, providing for the sanitary and social failings of the town, for the medical profession it had other roles to perform. In the first place, it enabled local practitioners to broaden their clinical experience in the medical wards and the operating theatre. Such a function was never entirely separated, in the minds of local doctors, from the need to establish a medical school at the Cape; the teaching hospital was for them the epitome of the great hospital.[58] By the end of the century there had been little change. In 1904 the *South African Medical Record* was still harping on this theme:

> In hospital work it is far easier to observe and record twenty cases than it is to do the same by five in private. It is one thing to go round a ward at a stated period with a calm mind, and deal with patients whose temperatures and other clinical points have been carefully noted for you in their proper order... quite another to see a patient to-day at 10am., to-morrow at noon, with all your information based on what you can observe during a call curtailed by the necessity of getting through a visiting list extending over some miles.[59]

The consultant, 'in the main the creation of the hospital', was particularly vital to the profession and a necessary preliminary to the establishment of a medical school. To the *Record* the larger hospitals should be opened to general practitioners, rather than confining cases to the salaried men who ran the hospitals.[60]

The Colonial Medical Committee, often representative of local Cape Town medical opinion, viewed the possibilities jealously and in 1869 they recommended that the salary of the resident surgeon be halved. The remaining money should be used to pay a physician and surgeon appointed from the leading practitioners of the town. All appointments were to be limited to three years, allowing other doctors in the town access to these facilities if necessary. Operations would be conducted on a specified day and time and opened to the medical men of the town for observation.[61] After some prevarication, the system was introduced and a case book recorded the 'highly interesting cases' which were seen in the hospital.[62]

But the value of the New Somerset Hospital went beyond this. As one of the few general infirmaries in the colony, it also provided almost the only opportunity for the training of medical students. In 1873 the Royal College of Physicians and Surgeons announced that it would accept Cape students with a third class certificate in literature and eighteen months in the wards of the hospital as part of the four years' medical training. Local doctors received the news with mixed feelings. The Colonial Medical Committee did not feel that there should be any kind of medical school at the New Somerset Hospital, while W.H. Woods, now resident surgeon, considered that the exchange of eighteen months study in Cape Town for a similar period in an English school of medicine would not be advantageous for students. Nevertheless he was willing to receive them in the wards. By the middle of 1875 medical pupils were working in the wards of the New Somerset Hospital (see Chapter 4).[63]

The decision to introduce a visiting physician and surgeon into the New Somerset Hospital did little to relieve the burden on the resident surgeon. Ill health, contracted in the course of their duties, and inadequate remuneration dogged the careers of the first resident surgeons. Henry Bickersteth died suddenly before he had even taken over the new hospital, after complaining bitterly about the arduous nature of his proposed duties. In addition to the hospital work, he was also surgeon to the Vaccine Institution, which supplied lymph throughout the colony, and was *ex officio* a member of the Colonial Medical Committee. For all this he was paid £400 a year, a sum which he regarded as insufficient given the recent inflation in the Colony.[64]

Conditions of work in the new hospital were uncomfortable. The hospital wards were hot and noisy: 'The echo and reverberation through the wards and corridors are so loud, as to amount to a real inconvenience both to the surgeons and patients and often so great as to prevent conversation in a low tone being audible.' The lighting in the operating theatre was faulty, it had no water supply and the surgical instruments were useless. Bickersteth had had to provide his own, but, with some difficulty, the Colonial Office was prevailed upon to buy these after his death.[65]

By 1876 W.H. Woods was also feeling the demands of the job. He asked diffidently for an increase in pay, for he was getting only £200 a year with quarters and another £132 as surgeon of the Breakwater Convict Station.[66] Although Woods received an increase to £300 a year, he was not well and over the next few years put in for long periods of leave of absence on grounds of ill health, a disease contracted during the course of his duties, he explained. Financial difficulties and ill health dogged the rest of his days at the hospital.[67] By 1881 the pressure of work had become so great that the resident surgeon was pleading for an assistant as he was unable to get away even for an afternoon or evening without neglecting the patients.

While the resident surgeon worked with the visiting medical officers without friction, he was very conscious of other infringements on his authority. The problem of nursing staff made this very clear. The very low salaries paid to nurses and the lack of training meant that nursing was always a problem at the hospital. By 1870 the Cape practitioners were also well aware that the standards of modern hospital care demanded better trained nurses.[68] In 1871 Dr A.L. Chiappini (son of Peter Chiappini), now resident surgeon, decided to employ Sisters of Mercy from England, a thrifty move since they were unpaid. But Chiappini soon found himself embroiled in the kind of conflict over authority that had been a feature of other hospitals employing Anglican sisterhoods.[69] Eventually the female superintendent resigned abruptly, taking the sisters with her. Chiappini received the news with mixed feelings for he was aware that colonial staff would be untrained and, given their ludicrously poor remuneration, unsatisfactory. If authority had been differently allocated, he believed, the system could have worked. [70]

For a time, local nurses seemed adequate. They were working well and taking a real interest in their duties, the board of inspection reported optimistically in 1874.[71] But doctors were conscious that the New Somerset Hospital lacked the professionalism in nursing which was now the standard in English hospitals; 'a superior and educated woman, thoroughly interested in the sick, as the Chief nurse or Matron is a very great consideration,' an inspection report noted in 1875.[72] Woods, asked to comment on the Colonial Medical Committee recommendation, agreed:

> It is in my opinion essentially necessary that she should be a Lady, to gain the respect and cheerful obedience of the nurses and servants; no lady could be induced to undertake the duties of such an office

save one thoroughly interested in the work; and there might be some difficulty in finding one whose interest was not tinctured or dictated by a religious zeal which, if at all sectarian might prove productive of much inconvenience and impair the usefulness of the institution. For this reason I should think it would be better that no person connected with any sisterhood either here or elsewhere should be considered eligible, and that a suitable salary be attached to the office.[73]

The impetus to acquire a female superintendent was hastened when Mrs Bibby, the matron, proved 'unequal to the requirements of office' and resigned.[74] It was decided to return to the earlier system and eventually Sister Helen Bowden was appointed from the Order of All Saints, an experienced woman who 'thoroughly understood the principles and ideals of the Nightingale Scheme.' She earned £60 a year compared with the resident surgeon who was now getting £300 a year. [75]

Race, class and gender segregation in hospitals

The separate and intersecting trajectories of race, gender and class discrimination and segregation has been a key analytical focus of historical writings about colonialism in the past few decades. The role of doctors and intra-institutional pressures in the emergence of discriminatory practices has been underplayed because discrimination has often been explained with reference to broad socio-economic trends in colonial societies, for example the emergence of a labour-hungry mining industry in South Africa.[76] These macro-level theories, while important, do not help us to explain the differential timing of segregation or the intersections and relationships between race, class and gender discrimination. They are also inaccurate. Some institutional racial segregation occurred before the dominant-class consensus in the 1890s that racial segregation was important, and before the local socio-economic crises of the 1880s, both of which have been used to explain its emergence.[77] As early as 1863, government schools (free at elementary level) had already generally excluded coloured children because of pressure from white parents.[78] Some institutions outside government control, such as the Dutch Reformed Church, had been partially segregated by the 1860s.[79] The granting of responsible government to the Cape in 1872, which reduced official barriers to segregation within public institutions, may have been more important in encouraging further institutional segregation than the economic and social pressures of the 1880s or 1890s.[80]

In order to understand how the micro-context affected the emergence of discriminatory practice a distinction needs to be made between different types of discrimination. Deacon has distinguished between patterns of national (territorial), urban (residential) and institutional (organisational) racial segregation.[81] Key events in the territorial racial segregation of the Cape (through, for example, the Land Act of 1913), occurred later than the segregation of living areas in Cape Town (Ndabeni township was created for Africans in 1901 under public health legislation) and the segregation of institutions like Somerset Hospital and Robben Island (1876 to 1893). While racial segregation can occur at national, urban and institutional levels in a society, class segregation tends to be urban and institutional, while gender segregation is largely institutional.

Race, class and gender discrimination can also have widely divergent rationales and require different levels of social acceptance before implementation. In general, racial segregation is thought to have emerged out of class segregation in the western Cape, as opposed to a direct and explicit application of urban and institutional racial segregation in the eastern Cape. Racially differentiated access to socio-economic, legal and political power was well-established in the south-western Cape by the 1830s,[82] and it was only by the 1880s, with the emergence of a small black middle class, that white Capetonians began to enforce racial segregation to the same degree as in other urban centres of the Cape.[83] While informal distinctions around class were introduced from the very beginning at the Robben Island hospitals (where paying patients received better food), and racial discrimination gradually earned these privileges for poorer white patients too, the segregation of patients by gender was implemented much earlier than race- and class-based segregation. The same was true of other Cape institutions like the Somerset Hospitals.

To date, most work has been done on the issue of racial segregation. Differences in the timing of, and rationales for, racial segregation in institutions can illustrate some of the influence exerted over the process by the medical profession, as well as the factors beyond their control. The Old Somerset Hospital chronic-sick wards were racially segregated by 1880,[84] while the chronic-sick hospital at Robben Island was segregated in 1876. Systematic racial segregation of the leprosy hospital at Robben Island took place in 1893, much later than racially discriminatory treatment (which began in the early 1850s) and the racial classification of patients in the annual reports of the institution (which began in the late 1850s).[85] In the 1860s, the surgeon-superintendent used British models of class discrimination in institutions to build informal racial distinctions in the Robben Island asylum while proclaiming the universality of mental illness and reducing formal racial segregation. There were other agents of change too: Robben Island hospital staff requested racial segregation of the chronic-sick hospital during the 1860s, and racial distinctions were often demanded by white patients.[86] With enough patients in each category, segregation could be inexpensively achieved using existing ward arrangements; it was only in the boom years of the 1890s that the colony could afford (and wanted) separate institutions for black and white. Medical theories about the difference between black and white insanity justified and encouraged the emergence of separate institutions for black and white patients in the 1890s.[87] Racist medical theories, doctors', patients' and officials' racism and public health legislation thus influenced the degree and timing of segregatory or discriminatory practices.

The charity and insurance sectors

During the nineteenth century, charitable and self-help organisations proliferated in urban areas like Cape Town, providing doctors with an additional source of income. While societies and charities generally had to employ doctors who spoke the language of their members, sectarian considerations did not unduly limit the employment opportunities of doctors.[88] There were two features which characterised the charity and insurance sectors at the Cape and made them a particularly attractive proposition for Cape doctors seeking part-time salaried employment. First, the Cape government was reluctant to provide poor relief (including medical assistance) or a state welfare programme.[89] Charitable and self-help societies were expected to take on the burden of providing medical and other assistance to the poor, especially after the economic depressions of the mid- to late-nineteenth century. Second, by the end of the nineteenth century these charitable organisations and friendly societies increasingly restricted their aid or membership to those defined as the 'respectable' white poor, who, under better circumstances, might become private patients of their doctor.

There were few avenues through which the poor could seek medical aid during the nineteenth century. A few urban-based hospitals were established for the sick poor, but admissions were limited. Household remedies and community-based care would have been the first resort of the impoverished.[90] Some working people contributed to friendly societies, which provided medical care, but relatively few of the (largely black) poor in Cape Town would have had money to spare for the subscriptions.[91] Wages were very low and irregular employment and underemployment common. Rent and food would have consumed a large proportion of working-class earnings.[92] Those without employers, friends or family, or whose communities were too poor to support them, were most vulnerable.[93] This situation put many Cape residents at the mercy of 'vertical' charitable relief provided by churches and middle-class organisations.[94] Churches, charities and friendly societies often employed doctors to attend to the sick poor under their care, usually on a fee-per-visit basis calculated monthly or annually.

Churches, which had been the mainstay of vertical relief in the eighteenth century, expanded their activities during the nineteenth century. Church relief was, for most of the century, dominated by the DRC, which offered medical care to the poor under various different schemes, such as a system of small payments or through the doctor attending an orphanage established in 1815. Interestingly, although most parishioners would have been Dutch-speaking, they employed a Scottish doctor, James Abercrombie, for the orphanage in the 1860s.[95] On the other hand, Dutch-speaking doctors Wehr, Von Horstok and Pappe attended the members of the European Sick and Burial Society, which mainly served poor Afrikaners.[96] The Ladies' Benevolent Society (LBS), founded in 1822 by the wife of the LMS missionary, John Philip, and other Cape Town women, relieved the poor of all ethnic and religious groups, becoming one of the most long-lived charitable organisations in the colony. In the 1850s doctors Samuel Bailey and James Abercrombie were employed by the Society,[97] which also referred many cases to local state-run hospitals such as Robben Island and the Old Somerset. Dispensing its relief carefully, investigating and supervising the recipients constantly, its provision of relief both ameliorated poverty in the town and created increasing resentment of the 'prying' benevolence it dispensed.[98] By the 1860s, faced with economic depression, more self-help and charitable organisations sprang up in Cape Town to relieve some of the pressures of poverty among its inhabitants. With the increase of British and later Australian working-class immigrants, the unemployed became more vocal.[99] By the end of the century a more militant and articulate working class shunned charitable aid, demanding state welfare instead.[100]

Self-help societies, to which working-class people made small regular contributions, augmented by donations, became important relief agencies for the working class in Britain and in her colonies in the nineteenth century.[101] In Melbourne and numerous country towns in Victoria, Australia, friendly societies provided medical services for up to half the population in the second half of the nineteenth century.[102] In the Cape, self-help was seen as an antidote to the 'pauperisation' of the poor through misdirected charity.[103] The number of friendly societies in the Cape increased from nine in 1845[104] to eighty-three in 1881, mostly in urban areas, with a membership of over 9,500 in the latter year.[105] These societies generally employed doctors to tend to sick members. In the *Cape Town Almanac* for 1840, for example, L. Pappe was listed as being physician to the European Sick and Burial Society and the South African Private Widow's Fund, while D. Somerville was listed as physician to the St. Andrew's Friendly Society.[106] Like mutual aid societies in France,[107] the Cape societies catered mainly for urban working men and tradesmen.[108] While friendly society membership included a significant proportion of the poorer black Capetonians in the period before the 1890s, there was a trend towards a whiter membership thereafter in the registered societies.[109] There were some restrictions on friendly society membership, particularly with regard to age and sometimes religion.[110] The Cape Town-based Catholic St. Mary's Mutual Benefit Society, with 112 members in 1869,[111] refused to give medical aid to drunkards, those outside Cape Town or members of less than a year's duration.[112] The society's doctor, Philip Landsberg, helped in examining prospective members and identifying alcoholic members during the 1870s.[113]

Most of the societies gave short-term relief in times of illness. The DRC-run *Weldadigheidsgenootskap*, for example, provided medicines, medical care from doctors and sick-bed attendants, coffins and sick pay.[114] Doctors working for friendly societies complained that members sometimes feigned illness to get sick benefits.[115] This practice would have reduced doctors' incomes if they were being paid per capita rather than per visit, as some societies seem to have done. Landsberg's salary from St Mary's, for example, was limited to £20 in 1885 because there were only eighty society members eligible for medical aid.[116] Perhaps the low pay increased the tension between his private interests and his role as the society's doctor, as he was scolded by the Secretary of the Society in 1872 for asking a prospective member why he was joining the society when he could pay quite easily for medical care privately.[117] Landsberg did not however serve only one friendly society; in the recession of the 1860s he had been doctor not only to the St Mary's Mutual Benefit Society, but also to the Cape Town English Church Friendly Society, the Odd Fellows Loyal Alfred Lodge, the Trinity Church Mutual Benefit Society, the South African Missionary Society, the Scottish Church Friendly Society, the Breakwater Women and Children's Society, and the Cape Town Free Dispensary.[118] All this was in addition to his paid position as secretary to the Colonial Medical Council.

Most significant of all these mid-century philanthropic institutions was the Free Dispensary, founded in 1860 by Cape Town philanthropists such as the Rev. Thomas Lightfoot and the Rev. Thomas Fuller, to assist those reduced to destitution during the measles epidemic of that year.[119] The Free Dispensary became a significant institution in the town, a marker both of Capetonian beneficence (or the lack of it) and of the town's sanitary condition. Always underfunded, the dispensary struggled to survive, only acquiring its own building in 1906 through a donation from Mrs Florence Philipson-Stow, the wife of a Kimberley mining magnate.[120] Despite its penury, for many years the annual reports of the Free Dispensary provided the only comment on the health of the town, calling constantly for sanitary reform and for the proper collection of statistics. Its publication on the severe fever epidemic of 1867 was a landmark event for it was the first attempt to provide a statistically based analysis of disease in Cape Town.[121] The fever epidemic of 1867 also placed many of the poor in temporary need of aid.[122] While some government- and charity-sponsored medical aid was provided, doctors were expected to contribute their services voluntarily during such epidemics.[123]

The Free Dispensary employed its own doctor to tend to the poor. The work was often onerous. Dr C.E. Piers was paid £120 a year for his attendance at the dispensary every day except Sundays. His surgery usually lasted two to three hours, during which time he saw thirty to forty patients. In addition he had to visit an average of six patients who might be scattered all over the town. In July 1894 he calculated that he had attended 550 patients and visited another 177, an average cost of $3\frac{1}{2}$d per head.[124]

District surgeoncies

Hospital posts (based in large towns) gave doctors less opportunity to practise privately than district surgeoncies, but were better paid. District surgeoncies (based mainly in small country towns) offered the greatest number of posts to immigrant doctors at the Cape. District surgeons, first appointed in any numbers during the 1820s, became important cogs in the administrative structure of the colonial hinterland. Secure annual salaries and monopolies over vaccination gave these doctors an advantage over other country practitioners. District surgeoncies were the country doctor's economic lifeline. They provided a steady income, the right to retail medicines and access to a wide range of potential private clients in the course of their official duties. Such posts had been in existence since the eighteenth century, when the DEIC appointed several *Colonies Chirurgijns* (colonial or country surgeons) to administer medical attention to burghers and employees in the hinterland, but it was only in the 1820s that the British administration at the Cape instituted a formal system of district surgeons. It grew out of a request by the Vaccine Institute in 1820 for government to expedite the vaccination of people living far from Cape Town by appointing district surgeons.[125] Initially, the district surgeons were appointed by and contracted to local magistrates (*landdrosts*), but ten formal appointments of district surgeons were made by the colonial government in 1828. For the rest of the century, it appointed doctors to district surgeoncies and paid (in varying degrees of generosity) for their services to the public.

District surgeons – usually British immigrant doctors – were often the voice of government in local politics. At some level, all medical knowledge is of course constructed and applied within a social context. The connections are, however, particularly stark and definite in times of social conflict. The 1820s were a time of great social upheaval at the Cape, as Dutch farmers' freedom to treat slaves with great harshness was being challenged by British-inspired legislation. District surgeons were drawn into this conflict through their work in examining slaves allegedly beaten by their masters. On the one hand, they had to seek private patients from the local slave-owning community, and on the other hand they were employed by a British government eager to see social reform. In one famous case, the district surgeon of Stellenbosch, a Scotsman named Robert Shand, argued that the slave Joris had been beaten to death, a verdict supported by Barry which countered the testimony by Dr Tardieux that the slave had died of 'bulimia'.[126] Like his successor in 1827, Daniel O'Flinn, whose practice suffered on account of his liberal attitude towards slaves,[127] Shand was probably shunned in his private practice by the slave-owners of the district because of this stance.

District surgeons had a variety of public duties. James Barry drew up the first formal list of instructions for them in 1823. These guidelines gave them exclusive rights to vaccinate and the right to sell medicines as well as give medical advice.[128] New regulations were

Illustration 5.2
Dr Brown's surgery

Photograph of Dr John Brown's late-nineteenth-century surgery in
Fraserburg, showing the Brown family with the visiting Dr Saunders
on the verandah. The surgery was probably the flat-roofed building
on the left of the Brown residence. Note the church in the
background – Brown found that an association with the Dutch
Reformed Church was essential in gaining acceptance in the
predominantly Dutch-speaking farming community.

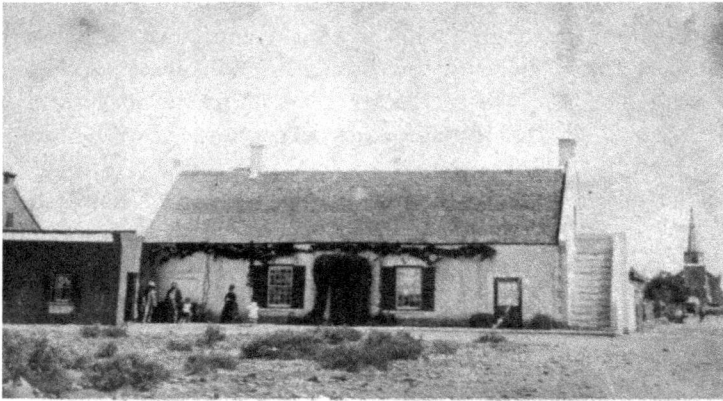

issued in March 1828 by the Medical Committee (reconstituted after
Barry's dismissal). These defined a district surgeon's duties as
embracing several areas: inspections of local prisons, free attendance
on prisoners, paupers and civil servants, observation of physical
punishments, post-mortem forensic duties and inspection of
apothecary shops. They were asked to report to government on
general health matters. Crucially for our discussion here, they were
allowed to have a private practice alongside these public duties.[129]
This flexibility was important for government, as it allowed salaries
to remain low, and it was also important for the surgeons themselves,
as it gave them a buffer against penury while allowing them the
chance to earn a significant income from private clients. In addition,
the position of district surgeon provided appointees with
considerable personal authority and a significant advantage over
other private practitioners (who were not allowed to vaccinate).[130]
There was growing friction between district surgeons and
apothecaries because the district surgeons had to inspect

apothecaries' shops while often continuing to sell medicines themselves (contrary to the regulations of 1829).[131]

While district surgeons enjoyed the advantages of salaried employment, their salary was neither large nor static. The government tried in various ways to reduce the cost of administering public health care. District surgeons were employed on the 'fixed establishment' (i.e. as permanent employees) with a fixed salary (of around £100-150 per annum) from 1828 until the mid-1830s. In 1834 however, they were paid on a tariff system and in 1836 they were placed on the 'supplementary establishment'. These changes were reversed in the early 1840s,[132] but with the cost-cutting measures instituted by John Montagu as Colonial Secretary in the mid-1840s, salaries were reduced by half and district surgeons were paid pro-rata for duties performed outside of a narrower range of required duties.[133] The MC and the district surgeons disliked the tariff arrangement because it added to the red tape surrounding their work. But the government was reluctant to return to the fixed salary system in the 1850s because of the greater cost involved.[134]

Reluctant the government may have been, but once Montagu had passed from the scene, the pressure increased to return to the fixed salary procedure. The Colonial MC was burdened with the task of vetting and passing all claims for payment, and the result was constant friction between the district surgeons, the Colonial MC and the government.[135] The system was easily abused and district surgeons complained about the amount of paperwork involved and the time which elapsed between claim and payment. A regular remuneration, the Colonial MC considered, would obviate the difficulties suffered by all parties and be less expensive for the government to administer.[136] Even when fixed salaries were reintroduced, the parsimony of the central government ensured that complaints continued. The district surgeon of Colesberg was a case in point. Paid only £40 a year, his district included not only Colesberg itself, but two new townships, one ten and the other twenty hours away on horseback. Only one post-mortem a year in each place (a duty likely to be frequent since these rapidly growing townships were populated by 'low and reckless people'), he estimated, would cost him over £26, leaving him only £14 to remunerate him for his other duties which had become increasingly arduous.[137]

It was this inadequate remuneration, the Colonial MC considered, that led to the continuing employment of unqualified practitioners in the remoter districts, for there was no inducement for properly qualified medical men to settle in these areas, a situation which was to the detriment of the colony as a whole. Only in 1855, after a protracted struggle, did the Colonial MC feel that it had achieved an arrangement which was acceptable to all parties.[138] This remained the position until the 1890s when overcrowding of the profession led to renewed examination of the position of the district surgeons.

This did not mean that the role of the district surgeon did not become more significant. During the 1880s the district surgeons became the conduit through which the Colonial Office gained its information about the health of the rural areas. The significance of this for public health reform will be noted in Chapter 7, but here it should be understood that these reports gave the district surgeon a new status in the colony. They indicated, too, that the new breed of district surgeons was more alert to the sanitary deficiencies of their districts and were anxious to play their part in public health reform. Nevertheless, the lives of many district surgeons remained isolated:

> [The country doctor] would perhaps go into practice there as a young man, full of ardour, full of hopes and ambition. He found that, although his time might be fully taken up with his work, in reality he saw very few patients, on account of the great distances he had to travel by cart or wagon; ...if he was the only one in the district, he would have no competition, no medical brethren with whom he could have a chat on medical subjects, talk over difficult cases, and exchange thoughts thereon, thereby preventing his knowledge becoming rusty and himself apathetic.[139]

Limited improvement in salaries did little to remove the grievances for district surgeons. Greater colonial prosperity and immigration only increased the work of the district surgeon, where salaries and allowances remained unaltered for fifty years. Despite some changes which improved the official status of the district surgeon, the situation remained essentially unchanged at the end of the century.[140]

By the turn of the century the district surgeons had formed their own association to lobby for their interests. In 1904 a deputation to the Colonial Secretary reiterated their grievances. Salaries were still inadequate 'fixed many years ago when there was very little competition amongst medical men... and when expenses were very low'. Gratuitous work had increased and district surgeons received no holidays without paying for a *locum tenens* out of their own pockets. Travel allowances were inadequate and the supply of medicines continued to be unreliable. Assaults in urban areas, in particular, were numerous and expensive to treat. There were other problems:

> Science had enormously advanced, and the skill expended on operations was far greater than it used to be, and many more ailments were rightly submitted to operation than was formerly the case. It was monstrous that a man should be called upon to do an operation requiring the highest of skill, and perhaps attend for six or eight weeks, for the paltry fee now given.

There were a host of other complaints about the cost of court appearances, about post-mortems, about the general demands on the time and pockets of the district surgeon in the country districts, all of which he was forced to accept for: 'He dreads losing his appointment because he does not take it for the remuneration, but for the purpose of keeping unfair competition out of his district'. Nor did the district surgeons care to be placed under the authority of the Colonial Medical Officer of Health whom they regarded as occupying too autocratic a position. 'They desired to revert to the practice of the old days, wherein the Colonial Secretary was their actual head.' The Colonial Secretary claimed to be sympathetic but, he pointed out, the government had not, up to now, had any difficulty in securing district surgeons. Any concessions they gained, therefore, were limited.[141] The reality remained that the post of district surgeon was too valuable to the emergent practitioners for them to boycott the posts.

Conclusions

In this chapter we have outlined three types of salaried employment taken up by the Cape doctor in the nineteenth century: military appointments, hospital work and district surgeoncies. While military doctors played an important role in the profession during the first few decades of the century, by the 1840s civilian doctors were beginning to assert greater influence in Cape Town, if not yet in the Eastern Cape. Military influences on the profession were always stronger in the turbulent frontier areas of the colony where most of the military surgeons were posted for official duties (see Chapter 6). In general, military doctors, who tended to have been born and trained in Britain, were less sympathetic to any move towards local medical training and accreditation or examination of apothecaries than locally born men were. Their influence on the licensing regulations meant that apothecaries only gained local accreditation in

1829. Even more importantly, in the first part of the century, the dominant influence of military doctors encouraged a close bond between the Medical Committee and the colonial government which was maintained for the rest of the century. The MC was appointed by government and acted both as an adviser to government on policy matters and as a professional regulatory body. Professional regulation and lobbying was thus not independent of government influence.

For civilian doctors, the first opportunities for salaried employment by government arose in civilian hospitals such as the two Somerset Hospitals (established in 1818 and 1862) and the Robben Island General Infirmary (established in 1846). These opportunities were centred in the larger towns, such as Cape Town, Grahamstown, Port Elizabeth and King William's Town. In these hospitals, doctors fought to claim a dominant role over lay employees as practitioners as well as administrators, a battle which had been largely won by the last few decades of the century. While hospital appointments did not always allow enough time for building up an extensive private practice, they did often provide opportunities for other part-time official medical posts in prisons and harbours. Hospital posts thus offered doctors a chance to define their role within the network of urban administration, and to gain authority as practitioners and administrators within this area, which was later codified by the appointment of Medical Officers of Health.

From the 1820s, an expanding network of charitable organisations and government-funded district surgeoncies provided partial employment for some doctors throughout the colony. This helped urban-based doctors to sustain practices and encouraged more doctors to practise in the smaller country towns which served large farming areas. In the early part of the century, district surgeons performed a key role in vaccinating inhabitants of country districts, providing some of these people with their first contact with the colonial authorities and with western medicine. By the 1880s the network of district surgeons was used by the colonial government to begin collecting morbidity data on key diseases such as syphilis and leprosy, which informed policy decisions made in Cape Town. But at the same time, district surgeons had their own interests and concerns. They had to balance their government duties, such as performing post-mortems on abused farmworkers, with the need to maintain a sufficiently large private practice in the farming community. District surgeons complained bitterly about the poor remuneration they received from government. At the lower end of the status hierarchy among doctors, they were also very sensitive about government policies and pronouncements which did not accord them the desired status as gentlemen professionals. District surgeons were however able to use their position to protect themselves from competition from other practitioners (for example through their legal monopoly over vaccination), and maintain a more secure income than other country doctors. Whatever their disagreements with government, they helped to enforce government health policies in outlying areas and to increase the impact of legislative and judicial changes at a local level.

Notes

1. E. van Heyningen, 'Agents of Empire: The Medical Profession in the Cape Colony, 1880-1910', *Medical History*, xxx (1989), 450–71.
2. M. Harrison, *Public Health in British India* (Cambridge: Cambridge University Press, 1994), 228–9.
3. See the example of W.G. Atherstone in Chapter 6.
4. A. Digby, *Making a Medical Living: Doctors and Patients in the English Market for Medicine* (Cambridge: Cambridge University Press, 1994), 226.
5. See Chapter 6.
6. Caledon to Castlereagh, 25 June 1808, PRO, PRO 48/2, Original Correspondence, 1808. See also E. Burrows, *A History of Medicine in South Africa* (Cape Town: Balkema, 1958), 72.
7. *Ibid.*, 99–100.
8. W.M. Freund, 'The Cape Under the Transitional Governments 1795-1814' in R. Elphick and H. Giliomee, *The Shaping of South African Society, 1652-1840*, 2nd edn. (Cape Town: Maskew Miller Longman, 1990), 345–6.
9. On the impact of British rule on the Cape see M. Boucher and N. Penn (eds) *Britain at the Cape, 1795-1803* (Johannesburg: The Brenthurst Press, 1992). See also Burrows, *op. cit.* (note 6) , 71.
10. Burrows, *op. cit.* (note 6), 72
11. *Ibid.*, 79.
12. *Ibid.*, 80.
13. *Ibid.*, 84.
14. *Ibid.*, 132.
15. *Ibid.*, 133.
16. *The South African Almanac and Directory for 1835*, 135.
17. See Burrows, *op. cit.* (note 6), 300 and Minutes of Proceedings of CMC (Colonial Medical Committee), 1842–8, CA, MC 3; Letters of appointment in 1846, Letters from the CMC, 1837–54, CA, MC 10.

18. Minutes of the South African Medical Society, 6 April 1828, UCT Medical School Library, Cape Town, MHA 610.6 SOU.

19. Bailey (for CMC) to Rawson, 12 March 1855, Letters from Old Somerset Hospital, CMC, and Robben Island for 1855, CA, CO 659. Parliamentary Debate on 'Dr Minto's Appointment', 27 March 1855, in *The Advertiser and Mail*s Parliamentary Debates, CA, CCP 3/2/2, 138.

20. E.B. van Heyningen, 'The Social Evil in the Cape Colony 1868-1902: Prostitution and the Contagious Diseases Acts', *JSAS*, x, 2 (April 1984), 173.

21. P. McMagh, *The Three Lieschings" Their Times and Contribution to Cape Medicine 1800-1843* (Cape Town: The Society for the History of Pharmacy in South Africa, 1992), 49–56.

22. *Ibid.*, 190.

23. *Ibid.*, 78–9.

24. *Ibid.*, 182 ff.

25. Burrows, *op. cit.* (note 6), 101.

26. McMagh, *op. cit.* (note 21), 133.

27. *Ibid.*, 134.

28. *Ibid.*, 136.

29. Burrows, *op. cit.* (note 6), 138.

30. McMagh, *op. cit.* (note 21), 90–1.

31. *Ibid.*, 91.

32. *Ibid.*, 200–1.

33. *Ibid.*, xiv–v.

34. H.J. Deacon, 'A History of the Medical Institutions on Robben Island, 1846-1910' (unpublished Ph.D. thesis, University of Cambridge, 1994).

35. *Ibid.*, 82.

36. *Ibid.*, 233.

37. *Ibid.*, 78.

38. Letter from Barry to Goverment, October 1823, in papers relating to the *Report of the Commission of Inquiry into the General Infirmary and Lunatic Asylum on Robben Island*, G31-1862, 216.

39. B. Kruger, *The Pear Tree Blossoms: A History of the Moravian Mission Stations in South Africa 1737-1869* (Genadendal: The Provincial Board of the Moravian Church of South Africa, 1966), 148.

40. Journal of Samuel E. Hudson, CA, A 602, 3 December 1824.

41. See for example Barry to Brink, 24 September 1824, Letters from Sundry Committees, 1824, CA, CO 204.

42. L. Granshaw, '"Fame and Fortune by Means of Bricks and Mortar": the Medical Profession and Specialist Hospitals in Britain, 1800-

1948' in L. Granshaw and R. Porter, *The Hospital in History* (London: Routledge, 1989), 201.

43. Resident Surgeon of OSH (Old Somerset Hospital) to Colonial Secretary, Letters from OSH *et al.* 1854, 31 December 1854, CA, CO 659.

44. Resident Surgeon of OSH to Colonial Secretary, 27 December 1855, Letters from OSH *et al.* 1855, CA, CO 659; Resident Surgeon of OSH to Colonial Secretary, 15 February 1856, Letters from OSH *et al.* 1856, CA, CO 673.

45. Resident Surgeon of OSH to Colonial Secretary, 28 February 1857, Letters from OSH *et al.* 1857, CA, CO 699.

46. See Chapter 4.

47. Secretary, CMC to Colonial Secretary, 16 April 1858, Letters from OSH *et al.* 1858, CA, CO 724.

48. Secretary, CMC to Colonial Secretary, 6 October 1858, Letters from OSH *et al.* 1858, CA, CO 724.

49. C.E. Rosenberg, *The Care of Strangers: The Rise of America's Hospital System* (Baltimore: Johns Hopkins University Press, 1987), 126–8, discusses the ideas informing hospital architecture in the mid-nineteenth century.

50. A.L. Chiappini to Bishop Gray, 8 February 1872, CA, CO 959.

51. Secretary, CMC to Colonial Secretary, 12 January 1869, CA, CO 905.

52. Annual report on New Somerset Hospital (NSH) for 1888, 28 January 1889, CA, CO 1434–5.

53. Memorandum on the proposed site for and the administration of the infectious diseases hospital, 27 April 1894, CA, CO 7019-16.

54. *Cape Times* 26 February 1890, 15 March 1890, 17 March 1890; *Cape Argus* 6 March 1890.

55. *Cape Times* 29 November 1897.

56. Annual report of the Free Dispensary for 1897, CA, CO 7638, f.1160.

57. *Cape Times* 12 April 1902. See also *South African Review* 23, 25 September 1903.

58. Resident Surgeon of OSH to Colonial Secretary, 16 January 1860, CA, CO 762.

59. *SAMR*, ii, 3 (March 1904), 50–1.

60. *Ibid.*

61. Secretary, CMC to Colonial Secretary, 12 Jan 1869, 30 June 1869, 4 July 1870, CA, CO 905; Secretary, CMC to Colonial Secretary, 22 January 1869, CA, CO 940; A. Chiappini to President, CMC, 27 August 1870, CA, CO 927.

62. Secretary, CMC to Colonial Secretary, 31 December 1874, CA, CO 1008.

63. Secretary, CMC to Colonial Secretary, 7 April 1873, 25 April 1873, CA, CO 972; W.H. Woods to Colonial Secretary, 25 April 1873, CA, CO 972; Secretary, CMC to Colonial Secretary, 20 July 1875, CA, CO 1008.

64. Resident Surgeon to Colonial Secretary, 27 February 1860, CA, CO 762.

65. Surgeon J.E. Dyer to Colonial Secretary, 11 November 1862, CA, CO 797; Surgeon J. Laing to Colonial Secretary, 27 August 1863, CA, CO 817.

66. W.H. Woods to Colonial Secretary, 10 April 1876, CA, CO 1027.

67. W.H. Woods to Colonial Secretary, 25 January 1877, 10 February 1877, 2 May 1877, CA, CO 1045; W.H. Woods to Colonial Secretary, 4 December 1878, CA, CO 1067.

68. B. Abel Smith, *The Hospitals 1800-1948: A Study in Social Administration in England and Wales* (London: Heinemann, 1964), 68. Smith notes that the authority demanded by the matrons to implement the reformed nursing system inevitably led to clashes with the conservative male doctors.

69. A.L. Chiappini to Colonial Secretary, 1 September 1871, 4 November 1871, CA, CO 944. See, for instance, F.B. Smith, *The People's Health 1830-1910* (London: Croom Helm, 1979), 260ff.; A.L. Chiappini to Colonial Secretary, 15 December 1871, CA, CO 944.

70. A.L. Chiappini to Colonial Secretary, 23 March 1872, 7 May 1872, CA, CO 959; H. Badnall to Colonial Secretary, 27 March 1872; Acting Resident Surgeon to Colonial Secretary, 30 December 1872, CA, CO 959.

71. Secretary, CMC to Colonial Secretary, 14 January 1874, CA, CO 989.

72. Secretary, CMC to Colonial Secretary, 20 July 1875, CA, CO 1008.

73. W.H. Woods to Colonial Secretary, 11 August 1875, CA, CO 1008.

74. W.H. Woods to Colonial Secretary, 7 April 1876, CA, CO 1027.

75. Sarah, Sister Superior, St George's Home, to the Resident Surgeon, New Somerset Hospital, 31 July 1876, CA, CO 1027; W.H. Woods to Colonial Secretary 5 September 1876 CA, CO 1027; S. Marks, *Divided Sisterhood: The Nursing Profession and the Making of Apartheid in South Africa* (London: Macmillan, 1994), 20; W.H. Woods to Colonial Secretary, 14 February 1877, CA, CO 1045.

76. For an overview of the debates about the emergence of racial segregation in South Africa see W. Beinart and S. Dubow,

'Introduction: The Historiography of Segregation and Apartheid' in W. Beinart and S. Dubow (eds), *Segregation and Apartheid in Twentieth-Century South Africa* (London: Routledge, 1995).

77. H.J. Deacon, 'Racial Segregation and Medical Discourse in Nineteenth-Century Cape Town', *JSAS*, xx, 2 (1996), 287–308.
78. Thompson, Minutes of evidence, *Report of a Commission to Inquire into and Report upon the Government Educational System of the Colony*, G24-1863, 122.
79. P. le Feuvre, `Cultural and Theological Factors affecting Relationships between the Nederduitse-Gereformeerde Kerk and the Anglican Church of the Province of South Africa in the Cape Colony 1806-1910' (Unpublished Ph.D. thesis, UCT, 1980), 19–20.
80. Deacon, *op. cit.* (note 77).
81. *Ibid.*, 287.
82. R. Elphick and H. Giliomee 'The Origins and Entrenchment of European Dominance at the Cape, 1652-c.1840' in R. Elphick and H. Giliomee (eds), *The Shaping of South African Society, 1652-1840* (Cape Town: Maskew Miller Longman, 1989), 522. The authors suggest that the racial order at the Cape was created by the DEIC in the first decade of colonisation and sustained for various economic and circumstantial reasons thereafter.
83. J.V. Bickford-Smith, *Ethnic Pride and Racial Prejudice in Victorian Cape Town: Group Identity and Social Practice, 1875-1902* (Cambridge: Cambridge University Press, 1995), 23–5, 70–2.
84. Annual report on Old Somerset Hospital for 1880, G3-1881, 2.
85. Deacon, *op. cit.* (note 77).
86. Deacon, *op. cit.* (note 34).
87. H.J. Deacon, 'Madness, Race and Moral Treatment at Robben Island Lunatic Asylum, 1846-1910', *History of Psychiatry*, vii (1996), 287–97.
88. Burrows, *op. cit.* (note 6), 137 lists a number of societies and the doctors employed by them.
89. N. Worden, E. van Heyningen and V. Bickford-Smith, *Cape Town. The Making of a City* (Cape Town: David Philip, 1998), 121–2, 181–3, 248–9, 251; T.O. Lloyd, *The British Empire 1558-1883* (Oxford: Oxford University Press, 1984), 139. The principles of the welfare state were accepted and applied only partially in the twentieth century. See V. Bickford-Smith, E. van Heyningen and N. Worden, *Cape Town in the Twentieth Century* (Cape Town: David Philip, 1999), 33–8, 100–4, 109, 111. For a different perspective see B. McKendrick and E. Dudas, 'South Africa' in J. Dixon (ed.)

Social Welfare in Africa (London: Croom Helm, 1987), 185.

90. E. van Heyningen, 'Poverty, Self-help and Community: The Survival of the Poor in Cape Town, 1880-1910', *South African Historical Journal,* xxiv (1991), 129.

91. S. Judges, 'Poverty, Living Conditions and Social Relations: Aspects of Life in Cape Town in the 1830s' (unpublished M.A. thesis, University of Cape Town, 1977), 46.

92. Treble calculates that up to eighty per cent of the income of the poor in later nineteenth-century London was spent on food and rent: J.H. Treble, *Urban Poverty in Britain 1830-1914* (London: Batsford Academic Press, 1979), 181.

93. A. Bank, personal communication, February 1994.

94. 'Vertical' relief is provided by richer members of society, while 'horizontal' relief is provided by people of the same socio-economic status.

95. *Zuid-Afrikaanse Weeshuis,* Letters 1815-1867, CA, V5 2/1, July 1867.

96. Burrows, *op. cit.* (note 6), 137; J. Iliffe, *The African Poor* (Cambridge: Cambridge University Press, 1987), 101.

97. M. Naude, 'The Role of the Free Dispensary in Public Health in Cape Town' (unpublished B.A. thesis, University of Cape Town, 1987), 13.

98. E. Bradlow, '"The Oldest Charitable Society in South Africa": One Hundred Years and More of the Ladies' Benevolent Society at the Cape of Good Hope', *South African Historical Journal,* xxv (November 1991), 77–104.

99. 'The unemployed', *Cape Chronicle,* 14 September 1860.

100. Worden et al., *op. cit.* (note 89), 248–9.

101. D.G. Green, *Working Class Patients and the Medical Establishment: Self-help in Britain from the Mid Nineteenth Century to 1948* (New York: St Martin's Press, 1985).

102. D. Dyason, 'The Medical Profession in Colonial Victoria, 1834-1901' in R. MacLeod and M. Lewis (eds), *Disease, Medicine and Empire: Perspectives on Western Medicine and the Experience of European Expansion* (London: Routledge, 1988), 199.

103. *South African Commercial Advertiser,* 13 May 1829. Thanks to A. Bank for this reference.

104. Iliffe, *op. cit.* (note 96), 101.

105. Cape of Good Hope *Blue Book for 1881,* 240.

106. *The Cape Calendar and Annual Register for 1840* (Cape Town: 1840), 274, 282.

107. A. Mitchell, 'The Function and Malfunction of Mutual Aid Societies

in Nineteenth-Century France' in J. Barry and C. Jones (eds) *Medicine and Charity before the Welfare State* (London: Routledge, 1991), 173–5.

108. Hoffman, Minutes of Evidence, Commission of 1880 (Friendly Societies), A16-1880, 11.

109. C. Simkins and E. van Heyningen, 'Fertility, Mortality and Migration in the Cape Colony, 1891-1904', *International Journal of African Historical Studies*, xx, 1 (1989), 91. This would have been exacerbated by the fact that subscriptions rose in the 1890s. Even among the largely white membership of the *Weldadigheidsgenootskap* between 1890 and 1907, 180 out of about 250 members (72%) defaulted through non-payment of subscriptions (*Weldadigheidsgenootskap* membership emendations, 1890-1907, Dutch Reformed Church Papers, CA, G1 32/1).

110. For example, see Rules and Regulations for the SAUIO Excelsior of Cape Town, Limited Companies 1888-1920, CA, LC 25.

111. O'Callaghan to Elliott (CO), 10 February 1870, St MMBS Papers, Letterbook 1869-1885, RCA, B1.

112. O'Callaghan to Landsberg, 16 July 1869, 11 October 1870 and 5 March 1870, St MMBS Papers, Letterbook 1869-1885, RCA, B1.

113. O'Callaghan to Landsberg, 16 July 1869 and O'Callaghan to Dooling, 11 August 1873, St. MMBS Papers, Letterbook 1869-1885, RCA, B1.

114. Accounts, December 1856, Dutch Reformed Church Papers, *Weldadigheidsgenootskap* 1847-1893, CA, G1 32/3.

115. Ebden, Minutes of Evidence, *Select Committee of 1880 (Friendly Societies)*, A16-1880, 43.

116. O'Callaghan to Landsberg, 26 August 1885, St. MMBS Papers, Letterbook 1869-1885, RCA, B1.

117. O'Callaghan to Landsberg, 8 July 1872, St. MMBS Papers, Letterbook 1869-1885, RCA, B1.

118. Landsberg, Minutes of Evidence, *Select Committee of 1865 (Old Somerset Hospital)*, A27-1865, 16.

119. Naude, *op. cit.* (note 97), 20.

120. *Ibid.*, 109–10.

121. R. Thornton and T.E. Fuller, *The Epidemic in Cape Town, 1867-'68* (Cape Town: Juta, 1868). It is worth noting that Thornton was a military doctor. See also Worden *et al., op. cit.* (note 89), 180–1.

122. Duminy, Durbanville, to Resident Magistrate of Cape Town, 12 October 1867, Letters on medical matters 1812-1911, Ross to Resident Magistrate of Cape Town, 14 October 1869, Letters from Police Surgeons etc. 1861-1911, CA, 1/CT 11/43.

123. For example in the 1840 smallpox epidemic: Liesching to Bell, 21 April 1840, Letters Received 1840, CA, CO 490.

124. *Cape Times*, 20 September 1894.

125. Vaccine Institute to Colonial Secretary, 11 July 1820, CA, CO 116.

126. Burrows, *op. cit.* (note 6), 87 and Correspondence between Inspector of Hospitals and Colonial Office, 14 September 1822, Misc. Correspondence 1821-25, CA, MC 15.

127. Confidential Reports on Civil Servants 1843-45, CA, CO 8551, 1843-1855.

128. Burrows, *op. cit.* (note 6), 86–8.

129. *Ibid.*, 88.

130. See for example, the complaint by Campbell, 26 June 1826, Memorials 1826, CA, CO 3931, doc.282. The regulations were rarely applied in remoter districts. See Chapter 6.

131. For example, Minutes of SMC, 22 November 1828, SMC Minutes 1825-31, CA, MC 1 and Minutes of CMC, 24 November 1835, CMC Minutes 1834-42, CA, MC 2.

132. Memo by the CO, 23 June 1844, Medical Correspondence 1829-50, CA, CO 4372.

133. Circular from CO, 31 May 1844, Circulars, CA, CO 4921.

134. Colonial Secretary to CMC, 11 July 1853 and 14 September 1853, Letters from CO to MC 1837-39, 1842-54, CA, MC 10.

135. Secretary, CMC to Colonial Secretary, 9 September 1851, CA, CO 606. See also 6 February 1851, CA, CO 606, 25 February 1853, CA, CO 627.

136. Secretary, CMC to Colonial Secretary 9 September 1851, 25 November 1851, CA, CO 606.

137. District surgeon, Colesberg to the resident magistrate, 3 May 1853, CA, CO 627. See also the comments of the district surgeons of Fort Beaufort and Somerset (East), 4 May 1853, 6 May 1853, CA, CO 627.

138. Secretary, CMC to Colonial Secretary, 19 January 1855, CA, CO 659.

139. *SAMJ*, 3, 5 (September 1895), 125.

140. *SAMJ*, 4, 9 (January 1897), 221–3.

141. *SAMR*, 2, 5 (May 1904), 86–8.

6

Medical Practice in the Eastern Cape

Elizabeth van Heyningen

The Eastern Cape developed slightly different medical traditions
from the Western Cape. The majority Xhosa population had
healing practices of their own which they shared only partly with
the Khoi, while Boer medical practice had become more remote
from modern Western medicine. Missionary medicine was
relatively undeveloped in this period but through the Grey
Hospital the Governor, Sir George Grey, promoted Western
medicine amongst Africans. In this frontier territory, British
military doctors encouraged early scientific societies and, in the
absence of other medical men, treated civilians both black and
white. The advent of the British settlers after 1820 placed a
strongly British stamp on the practice of Eastern Cape medicine.

The Eastern Cape presented very different conditions for doctors
from the western province. In the first place the ethnic composition
was very different, numerically dominated by Xhosa-speaking
peoples who were expanding slowly south and west. They occupied
the regions west of the Kei River at least from the late seventeenth
century.[1] White settlement came later. In 1778 eastward-trekking
Boers reached the Fish River, then designated as the boundary of the
Cape Colony. They were thinly scattered but already the expansion
was sufficiently threatening to Xhosa existence to give rise to frontier
war. The eastern frontier remained unsettled for the next century as
white encroachment gradually whittled away black territory and
political independence. But colonial wars bore heavily on the British
exchequer after that country had finally acquired the Cape in 1814,
with the settlement of the Peace of Paris at the end of the Napoleonic
wars. In an effort to find another way of pacifying the frontier, in
1820 the British introduced some 4,000 British immigrants to
provide a buffer against the Xhosa in the Zuurveld (later the Albany
District) between the Sundays and Fish Rivers. When numbers of
Dutch trekked north from the region in 1838, the British settlers

became the most significant white component on the frontier, although the military continued to be a major presence for many years.

This, then, was frontier territory, with small towns, predominantly English in culture, language and institutions, and a large rural hinterland occupied by beleaguered farmers struggling to survive in inauspicious environmental conditions and by a substantial black population whose land, culture and very survival were under increasing pressure as a result of colonial encroachment. It was a region in which these ethnic differences were played out in medical terms as well. Xhosa healing seemed to embody very different traditions from the apparently rational 'scientific' medicine of the Western-trained doctors. Between the two lay the healing systems of the Boer and British settlers, a mix of European folk culture, of assimilated indigenous healing systems and, gradually, the acceptance of the scientific medical culture.

Xhosa medicine

The healing practices of the Xhosa are particularly well-known, frequently described by European travellers and missionaries in the nineteenth century and by anthropologists in the twentieth. D. Hammond-Tooke comments on the essential continuity of beliefs on healing in southern Africa, noting that the descriptions of Xhosa medical practices by missionaries and others in the early nineteenth century appear to be identical with those current amongst the Cape Nguni, as described by Monica Hunter in the 1930s, and by himself in the 1970s. This conservatism, he suggests, can partly be explained by the conscious use of tradition as a symbol of resistance to colonial penetration, but also because these practices were accepted as efficacious therapy.[2]

The Xhosa distinguished between diseases which were susceptible to herbal or animal-based 'drug' therapies, on the one hand, and those such as fevers or internal complaints which were considered to be of supernatural origin or the result of malicious intent.[3] Sharing a common environment with the Khoi, who were often absorbed into African society, there had undoubtedly been an exchange of knowledge between them but their notions of healing were not identical.[4] Amongst the Xhosa certain herbs were widely known and used as 'home remedies', while others were a valuable secret, to be inherited or bought.[5] Those people who were trained in this knowledge had often learned from their parents, so that the knowledge might remain within certain families. Herbalists provided

170

Illustration 6.1
Xhosa diviner

This early photograph of a Xhosa diviner (probably 1850s to 1860s) comes from the ethnographic, photographic collection of Sir George Grey. The gender is not clear but the diviner wears the traditional garb of the diviner, including animal-skin cap, bracelets and necklaces. (NLSA: ALBX 19, 15611)

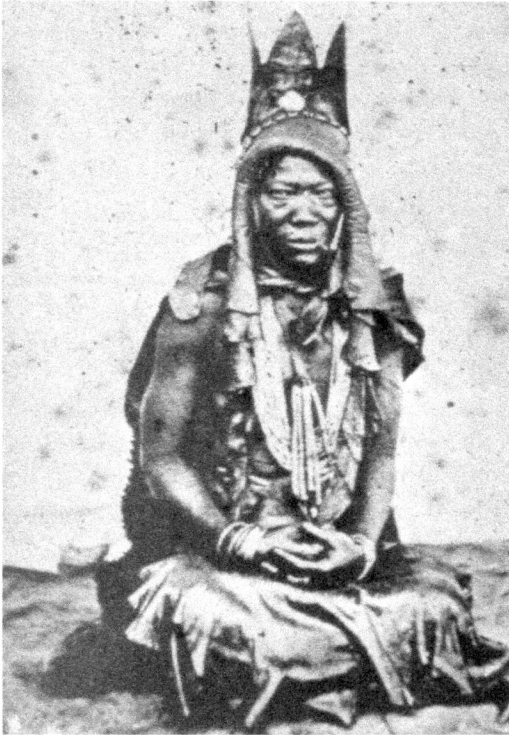

protective and curative medicines. Apart from treating disease, some herbalists gained fame, for instance, as 'lightning doctors', cleansing families and their possessions after a lightning strike.[6]

Reliable informers distinguished between the *ixhwele* (pl: *amaxhwele*) or herbalists and the *igqira* (pl: *amagqira*) or diviner. Although there were elements of magic in the work of the *amaxhwele*, the powers of the *amagqira* were more mystical. The calling of *igqira* was a vocation which was recognised through 'illness' and achieved through a process of initiation.[7] The work of the diviner, frequently a woman, involved the 'smelling out' of an evil-doer or 'witch' as the source of disease or trouble, and was also more directly linked to distribution of power and authority in the society. Since divining was a co-operative effort between the diviner and her support group, traditional healing was 'holistic' in its practice:

> It treats disease not only with powerful medicines, but also with rituals that place the patient at the centre of a social drama in which emotions are highly charged and symbolically expressed. The afflicted person is made to feel important and the object of social concern, while the ritual also relates what is happening to her to wider cosmological and social concerns. These healing techniques, then, enhance positively the patient's psychological state - thus providing a more favourable climate for physical and psychological healing to take place.[8]

As with European or North American witches, those who were accused of witchcraft were often on the fringes of the society and were despised or feared.[9] However, critical nineteenth-century observers sometimes offered a different explanation, claiming that the 'witch' was frequently a person of wealth or standing, whose status threatened that of the local chiefs.[10] While such perspectives may be open to question, there seems little doubt that diviners played an important role in maintaining community structures.[11]

Herbalists interested most European witnesses less than the diviners. Europeans were struck by the apparent cruelty and superstition of the latter, which seemed to them to contrast sharply with the humanity of Christian, European civilisation, and to provide a rationale for colonial conquest and the destruction of Xhosa culture. Their accounts are, consequently, often misleading, especially in relation to gender. Both Hunter and Hammond-Tooke noted that the Xhosa diviners were almost invariably women, and this is borne out by some of the early observers, like the naturalist, Andrew Smith (1832).[12] This was also corroborated by a number of missionaries, for whom a society which allowed a woman to play such a prominent role, was an additional example of the need to convert to civilised Christianity.[13] Others, however, either made no such distinction or described the diviners as men. A particularly striking example is that of J.P. FitzGerald of the Grey Hospital in King William's Town. While he often accorded the 'doctors' professional recognition, he invariably described them as male.[14]

172

Although there may have been striking continuities, as Hammond-Tooke claimed, contact with Western society undoubtedly altered some traditional practices.[15] As the Transkeian territories passed into the control of the Cape colonial authorities, traditional healers fell under Cape law. Although our main focus has been on the way in which indigenous healers limited the markets of Western-trained doctors, to some extent African healers were similarly affected. [16] The medical acts weakened their authority, preventing them from claiming payment for their work, although they might still have the means of extracting it outside the law courts. The availability of patent medicines threatened their incomes as well. Other legislation touched healers more directly, particularly the Witchcraft Act, No 20 of 1895, which forbade the killing of 'witches'. As a result, Hunter noted in the 1930s, 'his word does not mean life or death, as it did formerly. He is now a reactionary rather than an innovator.'[17]

Boer medicine

Boer medical practice has already been partly discussed in Chapter 2. The continuing isolation of frontier Boers from Western medicine meant that the knowledge they had brought from Europe had become extremely attenuated by the nineteenth century. Barrow noted that in the whole district of Graaff Reinet at the end of the eighteenth century, there was only one medical practitioner, an apothecary, who was attached to the Drostdy (the official residence of the magistrate).[18] While the Boers still retained lingering memories of pre-industrial European medical practice – cupping, and sweating in the case of fever, for instance, remained techniques which they favoured – the lack of Western-trained doctors meant that they were largely unaffected by nineteenth-century European medical developments. Perhaps the most striking instance of this was Boer use of animal parts and excreta. Animal excreta were removed from the London Pharmacopoeia in 1788[19] but the Boers continued to make use of such items into the twentieth century.[20] Best known was '*dassiepis*' (dassie urine) or *Hyraceum*, taken from the shelters of dassies (*Hyrax*).[21] The sceptical F.R. Davel, in his unpublished memoirs written in the late nineteenth century, made relatively little reference to herbal remedies; most were animal in origin, ranging from '*koraan maag*' (guinea fowl stomach) to blood or urine of various kinds. Boers used these medicines, he explained, because they were so far from doctors, because the roads were so bad or because the doctors were sometimes so incompetent that jackal liver or crow

173

soup (for rheumatic fever) were preferable.[22]

Isolation may also have meant that the Boers were relatively free of infectious disease – childbirth, snakebite and wounds from misfired guns or animal attacks were the most common hazards they encountered.[23] Survival from wounds inflicted by lions was often recounted with pride.[24] Sometimes the injured victim was nursed at home. Jacobus Bota was saved by his wife who used herbs boiled in water to dress the wound.[25] More often victims used brutal surgery on themselves, as did a farmer who dragged himself home, cut off his lacerated hand with an axe and dressed the stump with cow-dung, tied a bladder over it, and healed his other wounds with a salve made of a decoction of 'odoriferous herbs', lard and wax.[26] The salve may well have included the European sow-thistle or deadly nightshade, both, C.P. Thunberg noted, found growing wild near every farmhouse.[27]

Faith and 'magic' were often essential components of treatment and remained features of rural medicine until late in the nineteenth century. The treatment of snake bite included a mixture of European practice dating back to Pliny, and local methods:

> His hand had been scarified immediately, and a cupping-glass applied, in order to extract the poison from it. After this it was steeped in a solution of vitriol, which was said to have been rendered quite black by it. An onion was next applied, and afterwards tortoise blood. This latter, when laid on the wound in a dry state, was said to dissolve and turn to a fluid blood, that exhibited signs of effervescence; as the poison of serpents has a stronger attraction for tortoise blood than for human blood, so as to attract the poison to itself. [28]

Continuing contact with the Khoi probably meant that the two societies still shared healing practices, while frontier Khoi may well have been agents for the transmission of Xhosa medical knowledge as well. To what extent the Boers acquired knowledge directly from the Xhosa is less clear. The latter's knowledge of local herbs, different from those of the Western Cape, may have been significant, but the tension existing between them may also have hindered such transmission.

By the time British doctors began to penetrate the Eastern frontier, Boers had become largely self-sufficient medically, apart from their attachment to the 'Dutch medicines', providing only a limited market for the British doctors entering the colony. Of these, on the eastern frontier there were three main groups of doctors – military surgeons, English-speaking general practitioners and medical missionaries. Each group had its own concerns although broadly they shared a common medical culture and they were often forced to rely upon one another for support.

Military doctors

The dominant medical presence on the frontier for much of the century was the army, and the thin scattering of settlers and civilian doctors meant that their influence was, in many respects, more far-reaching (see Chapter 5). In the first half of the century the skills of these military surgeons were often limited and the quality of their training seems to have varied. Dr G.A. Hutton, Staff Assistant Surgeon at military headquarters in Grahamstown, had served an apprenticeship with consulting surgeons in his home town of Newcastle, 'qualifying' in 1852. Like many of his contemporaries, he had no formal medical degrees or diplomas and had attended no medical schools. His only official medical qualification was the examination set by the Army Medical Department.[29] Similarly, W.G. Atherstone, whose career is discussed in more detail later in this chapter, had served only an apprenticeship with his father in Grahamstown, but was considered sufficiently skilled to be appointed as Assistant Staff Surgeon to Colonel Harry Smith during the sixth frontier war in 1834.

At this time most army surgeons were recruited directly from the medical schools. In an era when public health measures were beginning to reduce the mortality rates of Britain's industrial towns, such under-trained doctors often lacked this knowledge, which would have enabled them to cope with the sanitary demands of the army or the ability to treat the type of wounds which they would encounter. The medical schools at Netley and Woolwich, which would go some way to remedying these deficiencies, were only established from the mid-1850s, after the Crimean War.[30] Nor did the army attract the best recruits. Rates of pay were poor, and the status of doctors in the army was ill-defined; they were often regarded with scant respect by their fellow officers. Despite these disadvantages, a few outstanding men did enter the service. Amongst those who came to the Cape were the naturalist, Andrew Smith, and his contemporaries at Edinburgh University, Robert Knox and James Barry.[31]

Except in times of crisis, medical work in the army was not arduous. Dr Irwin described a relaxed life:

> I live quietly, take my glass of wine in moderation, ride out my horses, and live quite at my ease, as I have in this post nothing to do but look into my Hospital for five minutes in the morning, and there is hardly any sickness. [32]

But for any young man who had professional ambitions this was a tedious existence and a number of military doctors found stimulation outside the army. Hutton was one of the founders of the Grahamstown Medico-Chirurgical Society in 1855. A prominent member of the society and its first president was Dr Alexander Melvin, the Principal Medical Officer of the forces in the Colony.[33] The secretary was yet another military doctor, Staff Surgeon D.D. McC. McDonald. By 1856, of the ninety members of the Literary, Scientific and Medical Society as it had become, thirty were doctors, including thirteen civil practitioners and seventeen army surgeons.[34]

Army headquarters in Grahamstown also provided a resource for local doctors since their medical library subscribed to the *Medical Times and Gazette* and the *Lancet*.[35] Military doctors participated in local medical accomplishments. Doctors Hadaway of the 91st Regiment and Irwin of the 27th Regiment were both present at W.G. Atherstone's 1847 operation using anaesthetic.[36] It was, indeed, the presence of the army which made Grahamstown a medical centre in the Eastern Cape since the first and second hospitals, both military, were located there from the early 1820s. By 1840 there were four military surgeons in the town.[37]

For a large part of the nineteenth century military doctors also had a more central role to play on the frontier, however, for they were integral to the functioning of local administration. In 1823, while still serving as a military doctor, Andrew Smith was appointed district surgeon of Grahamstown, an office he was given because of the reluctance of civilian doctors to undertake the work. He remained in this position until December of that year when he was posted to Fort Willshire with specific instructions to observe the indigenous peoples and their way of life.[38] Smith was not the only military doctor to act as an ethnographic informant. Nathaniel Morgan, the head of an 1820 settler party who was attached to the frontier forces as a temporary surgeon in 1825, also collected notes on the Xhosa.[39]

Andrew Bank has suggested that there was a more sinister side to the ethnographic interests of men like Knox and Smith; their interest in ethnography and anatomy, and their pursuit of phrenology through the collection of African skulls contributed to early scientific racism. Philip Curtin has, in fact, argued that Knox, who served on the frontier between 1817 and 1820 in the fourth frontier war, was the real founder of British racism.[40]

Burrows suggests that the military surgeons played an active role in promoting Sir George Grey's 'civilising mission' on the frontier.[41] Until the Grey Hospital was established, military surgeons were the only doctors in British Kaffraria,[42] the first being the Assistant Surgeons John Caw of the 75th and William Ford of the 72nd Regiment (1835). Later army surgeons were regularly appointed as district surgeons in the region. Hutton performed this function at Fort Peddie, enabling him, he noted, to become better acquainted with African life. In 1855 William Sall and in 1856 H.J. Schooles, the latter surgeon of the 60th Regiment, were acting district surgeons of King William's Town.[43] Charles Brownlee of the Buffalo Mission at King William's Town noted of the work of Henry Vereker Bindon, Assistant Surgeon of the 6th Regiment stationed at Dohne's Post in 1855, that:

> I have endeavoured to induce as many Kaffirs as possible to place themselves under Dr. Bindon's treatment. (His) successful treatment is much talked of in this neighbourhood, and if he should continue to treat cases brought to him, much will be accomplished towards inducing Kaffirs more generally to place themselves under the treatment of European physicians; thus forwarding an object contemplated by H.E. the Governor, namely the establishment of hospitals for the reception of Kaffirs.[44]

It was testimony of this kind which enabled Grey to persuade the imperial government to fund his ambitious schemes 'for promoting the Civilisation of Native Tribes' and which gave rise to the Grey Hospital.[45]

It was not only the civil administration which had recourse to military doctors on the frontier. For settlers, too, they were often the sole source of medical attention. Particularly in the early days of the settlement the only professional medical care available to the 1820 settler, Jeremiah Goldswain, was the local Wesleyan missionary or, in serious cases, the military surgeon at Bathurst.[46] As late as 1847, when he had moved to Bathurst, Dr Allen of the Cape Mounted Rifles was still Goldswain's only recourse when he was injured in falling off his horse.[47] For many years the missionaries also had to turn to the military doctors when they needed specialist advice and care. Smith, for instance, was called in for the delivery of Helen Ross's baby at the Tyumie mission station in the Ciskei.[48]

Military doctors, then, played a central role on the frontier in introducing a more modern Western medical culture to the region, which emphasised its scientific base, in contrast to the 'superstitious' practices of the Boers or the Xhosa. In doing so, they were active as 'agents of empire', assisting in the implementation of frontier policy in its broader context, and for many years provided the only professional medical care available to civilians and military alike.

Settler doctors

The arrival of the 1820 settlers stimulated the emergence of a civilian medical profession which remained, however, largely urban-based. Amongst the terms laid down by the British government for the immigration scheme was the instruction that all large parties should include a doctor. Nineteen medical men arrived, the first substantial number of civilian doctors on the frontier.[49] As their farming failed, many drifted to the Western Cape, but a few remained, mainly in the emerging towns of Grahamstown, Port Elizabeth and later East London. By the 1830s Grahamstown had at least three civilian practitioners, all fiercely competitive in this small community.[50] The population was still too limited and impoverished to support many doctors and it was only a few who could survive successfully. Quite apart from the size of the population, self-help and the use of folk medicines was still the order of the day amongst the settlers and also limited their recourse to professional doctors.

Jeremiah Goldswain's journals illustrate a blend of traditional knowledge and appeal to current medical practices. Medical care was centred on the household. Home provided careful nursing and a few tried remedies such as emetics, brandy or lavender water. Doctors could set bones or bleed their patients when they were feverish. Vigorous therapeutic intervention was still expected, at least by the patients. In 1847, when Goldswain's broken ribs were set, he was in considerable pain, and Dr Allen of the Cape Mounted Rifles was once again called from Bathurst:

> ...and when the Dr. came he stated that inflemation had taken place and that he must bleed me as quick as posable – 'it may stop it.' I was blead in the wright harm. The Dr. tuck from me two large basons of blood from me: before he had taken the last bason from me he asked me if I felt faint. I said: 'No but if you take much more I shall soon have non left.' 'Is the pain abated?' 'I think it is a little.' Jest as the second bason was full they caught me as I was falling all

tho it moved the broken ribs. My wife and thouse that was standing round me said to the Dr. that they beleved that I should never return to conchesnes again as all restorectives [restoratives] had been applied but to no porpeses. The Dr. then ordred a quantey of water to be thron into my face but my wife interfeared and said that was imposable to do so for if they maid my cloes wet that they could not take if off of me: so he tuck the water in both his hand and bathed my face when I gave a hevey sieth. It was more then an hour before I came to my self.[51]

In addition, settler parties were initially so isolated that, despite the increased numbers of civilian doctors, they had to depend mainly on their own medical skills in the early days. When Thomas Pringle's party reached their final destination of Camp Drift (Glen Lynden) in 1820, the nearest doctor was a military surgeon stationed at Roodewal about forty miles away. A doctor on board the emigrant ship had taught Pringle how to bleed and he had brought a small medicine chest with him; he soon acquired a reasonable degree of skill in dispensing his simple pharmacopoeia and in wielding his lancet.[52] In such circumstances, with such limited resources, patent medicines like Holloway's Pills and Ointment also had an invaluable role to play, more familiar and apparently more 'modern' than the Boer medicines which were the other alternative.[53] They were also more easily available since they could be sold by shopkeepers as well as apothecaries.[54]

Isolation also provided opportunities for a few women who were, in most respects, excluded from the professional practice of medicine on the frontier. Hannah Dennison, an 1820 settler of working-class origins, left her unreliable husband and moved to Colesberg, where she eked out a living as a midwife. She was also contracted to the Methodist Bechuana mission circuit to act as midwife to the mission settlements in the Orange Free State.[55] Dennison had no medical training other than experience but she took great pride, not only in her own proficiency, but in that of midwives as a whole.[56]

The position was rather different in towns like Grahamstown, Port Elizabeth or King William's Town. By mid-century these populations were big enough to sustain a few viable practices. But numbers were not the only factor in attracting doctors to the towns. By the 1850s many of the British settler towns had an infrastructure of literary and scientific societies, museums and libraries, and other cultural institutions.[57] The existence of a society like that of the Literary, Scientific and Medical Society in Grahamstown meant that recent medical knowledge was disseminated amongst the educated lay community as a whole. Rudimentary these organisations may have been, but urban doctors did not have to function in the intellectual vacuum which rural doctors found so stultifying.

The dominance of a literate English culture and an enterprising frontier spirit encouraged a few doctors to try innovative procedures. An occasional outstanding figure also provided a stimulus to the local profession. Dr W.G. Atherstone's use of ether as an anaesthetic in 1847, only a year after its first use in the United States, is too well documented to need repetition here.[58] Above all, this success demonstrated not only the initiative of some individual doctors, but the ease with which pioneering medical techniques could still be adopted in the mid-nineteenth century before scientific advance was laboratory-based or needed an expensive and complex infrastructure of hospitals and research institutions.

Dr William Guybon Atherstone, settler doctor

Dr W.G. Atherstone (1814-1898) epitomised the successful settler doctor. He received his early medical training as an apprentice to his father, Dr John Atherstone, deceased prisoners from Grahamstown jail providing subjects for the study of anatomy. With the outbreak of the sixth frontier war in 1834, since he had completed his apprenticeship, he was examined by a medical board and appointed Assistant Staff Surgeon to Colonel (later Sir) Harry Smith at his Grahamstown headquarters. Subsequently Atherstone trained in Dublin achieving the MRCS (London) in 1837 and then his MD in Heidelberg (Germany).

From his return to Grahamstown in 1839 Atherstone was a leading figure in the development of medicine in the Eastern Cape. He was an active member of the Literary, Scientific and Medical Society, contributing papers on a range of subjects, including geology, which was one of his greatest interests. He was largely responsible for the establishment of the Albany Hospital in 1833 and the later Fort England mental institution in 1878. His hand could also be seen in the establishment of the government Bacteriological Institute in Grahamstown in 1892, making it the first centre for medical research in South Africa. As a member of the Grahamstown municipal council. Atherstone kept a stern eye on sanitation in the town and, when he was later elected to the colony's Legislative Assembly, he continued to support medical reform. Politically Atherstone was conservative, a strong supporter of Eastern Cape separatism and of settler interests against those of the indigenous societies.

Throughout his life Atherstone kept a series of notebook-diaries, recording his many interests which ranged from geology and botany to Boer recipes and women's fashions. He travelled widely throughout South Africa recording geological formations and exchanging information with his friend, the geologist Andrew Geddes Bain. Although he is well known particularly for performing the first operation in South Africa under anaesthetic and for the identification of the first diamond in the Kimberley district, his contribution to learning in the Eastern Cape has never been fully explored.[59]

Although Grahamstown was probably the most intellectually lively of the frontier towns, it was not the only place to produce doctors of such calibre. Dr William Bisset Berry of Queenstown was probably more intellectually daring than Atherstone. He was forced to retreat from Queenstown for a time after a lecture on Darwinism alienated his fellow citizens. Upon his return he built up a remarkable library containing works which reflected a wide spectrum of contemporary thought, ranging from Marx and Freud to Herbert Spencer, Karl Pearson and Francis Galton, to name only a few.[60]

Frontier hospitals

For the first forty years British settler society on the frontier functioned almost without hospitals, although Dr Ambrose Campbell had a small private hospital in Grahamstown by the 1840s. Dr John Atherstone's original appeal in 1829 for a government hospital was turned down on the grounds of 'the salubrity of the climate, the absence of dangerous contagious disease, and the small population'.[61] By the late 1850s several factors encouraged a movement to establish such institutions. The burgeoning wool industry had brought new wealth to the area and increased the population. But the boom-and-bust nature of the economy added to the numbers of the sick poor for whom home care was not available. The governor, Sir George Grey, was a proponent of hospitals and encouraged any initiatives to establish such institutions. Finally, the medical profession wanted hospitals.

The demand for hospitals was not driven by the 'needs and priorities' of the medical profession in the same way as it was in Britain or the United States. There the hospital was at once the classroom for the training of students, who were instilled with the knowledge of recent scientfic advances, and a means of displaying the profession's medical skills.[62] In the Cape the lack of any tertiary educational institutions stunted the development of teaching hospitals. The medical profession was, however, aware that hospitals provided clinical experience which they could not get elsewhere, given the usually limited range of private practice. Hospitals were also a means of caring for the sick poor whose numbers were slowly mounting during the nineteenth century and to a reform-minded profession, they were the mark of a civilised society.

In the late 1850s both Port Elizabeth and Grahamstown acquired hospitals. They shared a number of common features which distinguished them from the Somerset and Grey Hospitals. In both cases Grey endowed them with public lands which were sold to provide funds for the building and running expenses. Both had public boards of management, both were supported by local fund-raising as well as government funding; both were run by lay superintendents (although in the case of the Albany Hospital, the superintendent, T.P.O. Mathew, was a licensed apothecary and later practised as a doctor in Adelaide, Cape).[63] Both hospitals were served by visiting consultants and the first resident medical officer was appointed to the Albany Hospital only in 1891. Other Eastern Cape hospitals – the Frere in East London, the Queenstown Frontier Hospital and the Graaff Reinet Midland Hospital were all establishments of a later generation of Cape hospital development.

The establishment of scientific institutions and medical participation in the creation of hospitals served to reinforce the claims of the professional doctors that the healing they proffered was 'scientifically' based. Like their counterparts in the Western Cape, their incomes were threatened not only by home practitioners, apothecaries and shopkeepers. In addition, as in the case of J.B. Hammerschmidt, medical men whose qualifications were not recognised by the Colonial Medical Committee might claim official acceptance in some other form. Jesse Shaw of Fort Beaufort, who advertised himself as M.D. (USA), Medical Botanist by Diploma, Specialist in Cape Materia Medica; and Member of the Society of United Medical Botanists of Great Britain, approached the Medical Committee for a licence to practise as a herbalist and to dispense herbal medicines. Despite his rejection by the CMC, Shaw continued to practice herbal medicine.[64] He was by no means the only such practitioner in the Eastern Cape. J.E. Hulling of Grahamstown and A.R. Welsh of Herschel also approached the CMC for licences, while G.E. Cook of King William's Town advertised 'Orsmond's Great African Remedy' prepared from 'Cape Roots'. A pamphlet in English, Dutch, German and Xhosa, indicates the extent of the market he hoped to tap.[65]

Religious and secular medical missions

The role of Western medicine in the missionary enterprise in southern Africa has been explored very little. Medicine played a more conspicuous role in some mission societies than in others. The Glasgow Mission Society (GMS) was particularly keen that its missionaries should have some medical training. In his list of talents required of a missionary, the Rev. Thomas Bell urged that '6thly, He should have some acquaintance with the Rules of Physic, as in knowing the pulse, letting of blood, etc.'[66] Somewhat later the Society explained its motivation in making this demand:

> The Caffers [Xhosa] have bodies to be cured of disease, as well as souls to be saved. As in all the barbarous countries, their healers are Quacks, whose cataplasms are revolting in their materials, and who roar, and jump, and drum, to render their remedies efficient. The Missionaries are therefore anxious, that some one of their future fellow-labourers should be a practical Physician, as well as a Minister of the New Testament. They are eagerly solicitous on this point, for the good of the natives, and also for their own domestic comfort. They have wives and children whose health is to be cared for. The medical men stationed on the frontier, have indeed most obligingly paid them several visits, but they are far distant and cannot always leave their post.[67]

Nor was this a paper demand. A number of the GMS missionaries had some medical training, including James Laing who attended classes at the Andersonian University in Glasgow (where David Livingstone had also qualified), studying under Robert Hunter and Robert Knox in Edinburgh, amongst others.[68] In the next generation Bryce Ross also attended medical classes at the Andersonian University,[69] while Dr James Stewart, Principal of Lovedale College, who had followed closely in the footsteps of Dr David Livingstone literally and metaphorically, was a fully qualified doctor. A number of the sons of these missionaries qualified and practised formally as doctors, including William Anderson Soga, the son of Tiyo Soga, the first black Presbyterian minister in South Africa (see Chapter 7 for a more detailed discussion of Soga's career). John Ross, the son of Bryce Ross was an enthusiastic practitioner in King William's Town, making his mark on a town which had a number of outstanding doctors.[70] He brought a missionary zeal to the issue of public health. In 1887 he published a practical little book, dedicated to Dr James Stewart of Lovedale Institution, 'my old teacher, who first gave me a liking for scientific study':

Attention to the laws of health is a public as well as a private duty...
People must be taught that attention to public health is a moral duty,
that cleanliness, avoidance of excess, and health preservation go hand
in hand with mental and moral training, and that morality consists
as much in a hearty submission to the precepts of health as to the
observation of creed.[71]

Medical training was not confined to the GMS however. Dr van
der Kemp, one of earliest missionaries of the London Missionary
Society (LMS), had qualified as a doctor in the Netherlands and the
Rev. Richard Birt of Peelton Mission had studied medicine for three
years.[72] William Girdwood was a licensed but unqualified doctor
while at least three of his sons entered the medical profession.

Despite their medical training and the occasional availability of
military doctors, the missionaries were sometimes still dependent on
local indigenous practitioners for assistance. When Mrs Helen Ross,
the wife of the Rev. John Ross at Tyumie, gave birth in 1824, the
midwife who delivered her baby was a Khoi woman who was 'very
cautious' and 'very attentive'. Andrew Smith, the military doctor
from Fort Willshire, twenty-seven miles away, only arrived when all
was over.[73]

Missionaries regularly co-operated with Eastern Cape district
surgeons in vaccinating the indigenous people. At Pirie mission
station the Rev. John Ross reckoned:

A thousand natives were vaccinated here. Of these three hundred
were done by my kind hearted, & clever helpmate, some by the
lancet, but likely more by or with a darning needle. She vaccinated
herself too; chiefly, I believe, as an encouragement to the people to
use the sole means of warding off the hideous disease.[74]

In spite of their medical training, in the first half of the century the
attitudes of the missionaries to African healing were shaped as much by
religious belief as by scientific knowledge. Their views were little
different from those of Mrs Harriet Ward who commented of the Xhosa
that, 'All disease is looked upon as the effect of magic, from their total
ignorance of a Providence.'[75] While missionaries ascribed to Providence
the miraculous healing which they encountered within their own sphere,
in their encounters with African healers they demanded rational
explanation. James Backhouse's account of the work of a 'doctress' is a
striking example. Gender is a significant element in the description. To
nineteenth-century Europeans the immorality of the healing process was
increased by the sex of the doctor and by her nakedness:

On another occasion, a man was taken ill with a violent pain in his side, and a Fingo[76] doctress was sent for, to charm him. As this woman was quite naked, except having a rope around her waist, Richard Tainton[77] declined going into the hut where she was, but requested his wife [Ann] to go. The doctress applied her mouth to the young man's side, and sucked, and then spit out a few grains of Indian-corn; these, she said, she had sucked out, and that they were what occasioned the sickness.

Ann Tainton insisted that a fraud had been committed and forced the woman to continue despite her growing anger, until the secret was revealed:

In the end, the doctress spit out a piece of a tobacco-leaf, rolled up, which explained the whole matter. She had swallowed the tobacco-leaf to produce nausea, and had afterwards swallowed the Indian-corn; by the help of the rope round her waist, she had been able to keep such a command over her stomach, as only to bring up a few grains of the Indian-corn at a time.

Despite this success in exposing the fraud, the missionaries had no better cure to offer and the young man was removed to another *kraal* 'where they might not be interfered with by Christians'.[78]

Although healing was an element in their mission work, the Eastern Cape missionaries were slow to establish mission hospitals. The first such institution was the dispensary which Dr Jane Waterston established at Lovedale in 1882. Lovedale Hospital itself was established in 1898, but it really developed only in the twentieth century when Dr Neil MacVicar was appointed as the superintendent.[79]

Dr John Patrick FitzGerald – secular missionary

The missionary dilemma, that they might expose superstition but could offer nothing better themselves, made their medicine relatively ineffective and gave Dr J.P. FitzGerald at the Grey Hospital in King William's Town his opportunity. The Grey Hospital was an overtly proselytising institution, instigated by Sir George Grey, to 'civilise' the Xhosa and to weaken the power of the chiefs by eliminating the diviners who, Grey believed, were a source of chiefly influence. At the Grey Hospital, FitzGerald offered not only the best of Western medicine but also a coherent healing system and dedicated care which was more convincing than anything the limited resources of the missionaries could produce. FitzGerald's personal conviction and

Illustration 6.2
The Grey Hospital, King William's Town

From the same page of the Grey collection, the Grey Hospital, opened in 1859, was intended to undermine the authority of the diviners by marketing the powers of Western medicine. (NLSA: ALBX 19, 15612)

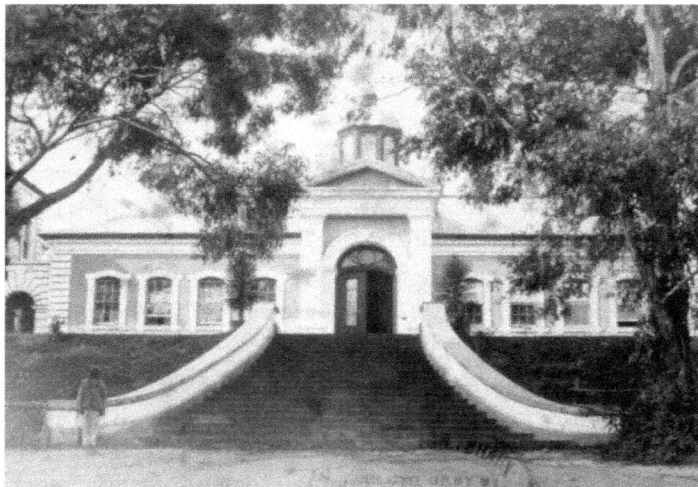

his genuine benevolence added a another dimension to his work. He offered to the Africans of the Eastern Cape a secular mission which in some respects rivalled that of the Christian missions, as it was intended to do.

FitzGerald's practice of medicine in the Eastern Cape was shaped by his previous experience in Wellington, New Zealand, and by his association with the Governor, Sir George Grey, which also dated back to New Zealand. In New Zealand FitzGerald had been particularly concerned about the plight of the Maoris whose numbers, it was believed, were being decimated partly through tuberculosis, but also, FitzGerald considered, because of their style of life. The hospital would not only provide them with clean surroundings, pure air and a nutritious diet, but would also be a significant aid in encouraging the Maoris to adopt European civilisation. FitzGerald's ideas complemented those of the Governor, Sir George Grey, who possessed a broader vision of the imperial role amongst indigenous peoples, but whose liberal, scientific bent led him to see modern medicine as a significant tool in attaining his

186

ends. FitzGerald's work at the Grey Hospital has to be seen, then, in the context of his loyalty to Grey and Grey's objectives in the Eastern Cape.[80]

Grey's complex and vicious personality has been analysed by others.[81] FitzGerald, however, seems to have been oblivious of Grey's ruthless agenda to incorporate the Xhosa into the labour structures of the Cape. In the Eastern Cape, where he arrived in 1856, FitzGerald devoted his life to providing a healing system for Africans which was to be a showpiece of European civilisation – scientific, benevolent and just.

At the centre of FitzGerald's endeavours was the hospital itself.[82] In his design FitzGerald was influenced by contemporary thinking on the central importance of ventilation.[83] Building before the publication of Florence Nightingale's influential *Notes on Nursing* (1859), FitzGerald evolved his own unique solutions to the problem with a 'ventilating device' based on the Hall of Baths in the Alhambra in Spain, through which 'heated air and impurities' could escape.[84] Later on FitzGerald added permanent canvas marquees, where he could remove all 'foul smelling cases' and surround them 'with pure air day and night whereby they have a better chance of recovery... when we go in for saving human life we should go the whole way'.[85] In the wards FitzGerald attempted to provide a pleasant and cheerful atmosphere with landscape pictures 'and there can be no doubt that anything which tends to cheer the sick and keep up their spirits contributes much towards the recovery of their health';[86] this 'improving' environment was part of the coherent health care system which he offered.[87]

The hospital had another function. Here, skilled assistants could be more thoroughly exposed to Western ways, groomed to spread the message amongst their countrymen. An optimistic plan to train 'Native Surgeons' never materialised but the interpreters and assistants, some of whom, such as Ned Maqoma, son of a senior Xhosa chief, were men of some status, played this intermediary role. They were also, Gordon suggests, colonial collaborators who encouraged Xhosa healers to trust FitzGerald during the early period of his mission in the Eastern Cape.[88]

FitzGerald's concept of hospital management and of the role of the hospital in society, were in keeping with current medical notions, although his solutions to his problems were sometimes individual. In the 1850s his hospital was in marked contrast to the Old Somerset Hospital with its overcrowded wards and damp, crumbling fabric, or with Robben Island.

FitzGerald's early medical career preceded the era of biomedicine. The emphasis which he placed on care, on a pleasant atmosphere, on the appropriate behaviour of the healer, on the total environment of the hospital, were all part of a system of healing in which the culture was as significant as the therapeutic skills. At the same time, however, FitzGerald subscribed to a therapeutic system which was based on the notion of progress, in which knowledge was dynamic.[89]

FitzGerald was also a skilled surgeon and gained a considerable reputation in this field, particularly in eye surgery. He was quick to make use of techniques suggested by the Colonial Office. When the department circulated an article on the virtues of carbolic as an antiseptic in 1869, he seized upon it enthusiastically.[90] Like many of his contemporaries, however, he probably did not fully understand the implications of antisepsis; in other respects his therapies remained old-fashioned, as in his lavish use of alcohol as a stimulant.

FitzGerald's attitude to African healers was by no means straightforward. Fundamentally, like his patron, he regarded traditional healing as uncivilised and, worse still, cruel, detrimental to the patients and society.[91] Despite these views, in his dealing with healers FitzGerald treated them with courtesy as peers, equal colleagues in the profession – a reason, perhaps, why he found women unacceptable in this role. He always referred to diviners as 'doctors' and he addressed his closest associate, Gota, brother-in-law of the deceased Xhosa chief Ngqika, as 'Dr Gota'.[92]

It is probable, however, that FitzGerald had little real understanding of the context of Xhosa healing. He made no distinction between the diviners and herbalists, nor does he seem to have been aware that the *amagqirha* were predominantly women while herbalists were more usually men.[93] It must be borne in mind, however, that FitzGerald's observations were meant, above all, as propaganda, intended to demonstrate the value of the Grey Hospital to a colonial government which, after Grey left, was parsimonious and uninterested in this project of 'civilising' though medical care.

FitzGerald arrived in King William's Town in 1853, only months before the start of the millenarian cattle-killing movement which decimated the Xhosa population and led to their incorporation into the colonial labour system.[94] Gordon suggests that the initial popularity of the hospital waned as the cattle-killing prophecies spread.[95] If so, it became a refuge for the starving in the months that followed. A greater problem for FitzGerald after British Kaffraria was incorporated into the Cape Colony, was his relationship with the colonial government. Not only was funding less generous but the

Colonial Office officials were unenthusiastic about Grey's project. Nevertheless, FitzGerald's diligence and persistence ensured that King William's Town remained a significant medical centre in the Eastern Cape for most of the nineteenth century.[96]

Conclusion

Although the institutional structures of the Colonial Office and Colonial Medical Council governing the practice of medicine in the Eastern Cape were the same as those of the western province, there were marked differences between the two regions. No town was as dominating as Cape Town, so the urban-rural divide was less sharp. The scattered nature of white settlement perhaps opened the way for the competition of unlicensed practitioners to a greater extent than in the west. Because they were so far from Cape Town, professional doctors lacked the immediate support of the Colonial Medical Committee or other government departments, so that they were forced to rely far more on themselves to assert their 'scientific' professional status. This may partly explain their central involvement in scientific societies and organisations. The presence of a large and, to colonial eyes, an unruly and barbaric indigenous population, as well as military surgeons and missionaries meant that the Eastern Cape doctors could more obviously act as 'agents of empire'.

On the other hand, despite the leading role which a few doctors played in introducing and using the most modern medical procedures, the practice of medicine in the Eastern Cape was retarded in comparison with England or even the Western Cape. A significant missionary presence meant that in some quarters, at least, a providential explanation of disease and healing continued to have a place well into the nineteenth century.[97] British and Boer settlers clung to a humoral discourse and even in the second half of the century some doctors, like FitzGerald, made reference to notions which had fallen out of fashion elsewhere in the colony by the beginning of the nineteenth century.

Where Cape Town had a hospital from the start of settlement, hospitals in the east of the colony were established only after mid-century. Unlike the Cape Town institutions, most were implicitly segregated, with the Grey Hospital as the only general asylum devoted to the black population. Unlike their counterparts in India and China, before the late nineteenth century missionaries failed to fill this gap in the provision of health care for Africans, despite the early emphasis of some on the value of medical training. Eastern Cape doctors were beacons of 'modernism' in a relatively retarded region, but their culture usually served to reinforce the prevailing racism of white settlers.

By the start of the twentieth century then, the Eastern Cape was significantly less developed than the western province and this relative backwardness would be reinforced with the establishment of the Cape's first medical school in Cape Town and the emergence of that region as the centre of medical teaching and research. Twentieth-century management of health care reinforced these differences with the result that, at the millennium, the Eastern Cape remained the most impoverished province in South Africa, still with an inadequate health care system.[98]

Notes

1. G.H. Hofmeyr, 'King William's Town and the Xhosa, 1854-1861. The Role of a Frontier Capital During the High Commissionership of Sir George Grey' (unpublished M.A. thesis, University of Cape Town, 1981), 2–3.
2. D. Hammond-Tooke, *Rituals and Medicines: Indigenous Healing in South Africa* (Johannesburg: Ad. Donker, 1989) 8; see also M. Wilson and L. Thompson (eds), *The Oxford History of South Africa*, i, *South Africa to 1870* (Oxford: Oxford University Press, 1969), 128–9 on the essential 'conservatism' of Xhosa society.
3. Hammond-Tooke, *op. cit.* (note 2), 48, 73–85.
4. J.B. Peires, *The House of Phalo: A History of the Xhosa People in the Days of their Independence* (Johannesburg: Ravan, 1981), 64.
5. M. Hunter, *Reaction to Conquest: Effects of Contact with Europeans on the Pondo of South Africa* (London: Oxford University Press, 1936), 320, 341.
6. Hunter, *op. cit.* (note 5), 342, 344; Hammond-Tooke, *op. cit.* (note 2), 103–13.
7. Hunter, *op. cit.* (note 5), 320–35.
8. Hammond-Tooke, *op. cit.* (note 2), 123.
9. *Ibid.*, 73–85.
10. J. Backhouse, *A Narrative of a Visit to the Mauritius and South Africa*, (London: Hamilton Adams, 1844), 243.
11. Peires, *op. cit.* (note 4), 64–78; J.B. Peires, *The Dead Will Arise: Nongqawuse and the Great Xhosa Cattle-Killing Movement of 1856-7* (Johannesburg: Ravan, 1989).
12. Hunter, *op. cit.* (note 5), 320; Hammond-Tooke, *op. cit.* (note 2), 104; P.R. Kirby (ed), *Andrew Smith and Natal: Documents Relating to the Early History of that Province* (Cape Town: Van Riebeeck Society, 1955), 113. Backhouse identified three categories of healer;

Backhouse, *op. cit.* (note 10), 230.

13. See, for instance Backhouse, *op. cit.* (note 10), 284–5.
14. Amongst many other examples see FitzGerald letter book, Vol. 1, 14 April 1856, 2 March 1857, King William's Town Museum.
15. See, for example, Peires, *op. cit.* (note 4), 64–78.
16. Hunter, *op. cit.* (note 5), 347.
17. *Ibid.*, 347. Note that in her general discussion Hunter also describes the *amagqira* as male.
18. J. Barrow, *An Account of Travels into the Interior of Southern Africa in the Years 1797-1798* (London: T. Cadell & Davies, 1801), 159.
19. P.W. Laidler and M. Gelfand, *South Africa: Its Medical History 1652-1898* (Cape Town: Struik, 1971), 71.
20. For a discussion of this issue and the British response see E.B. van Heyningen, 'Women and Disease: The Clash of Medical Cultures in the Concentration Camps' in G. Cuthbertson, A. Grundlingh (eds), *Writing a Wider War: Rethinking Gender, Race and Identity in the South African War, 1899–1902* (Athens: Ohio University Press, 2002), 186–212 .
21. C.P. Thunberg, *Travels at the Cape of Good Hope 1772–1775*, ed by V.S. Forbes (Cape Town: Van Riebeeck Society, 1986), 73.
22. Unpublished memoir of F.R. Davel in private possession.
23. It should be noted, however, that almost nothing is known of Boer mortality rates, although a belief in the healthiness and fertility of the eighteenth- and nineteenth-century Boer families became an ingredient of Afrikaner ethnic identity.
24. The lion attack on Paul Kruger is probably the best-known example, passing into folk memory.
25. Thunberg, *op. cit.* (note 21), 207.
26. *Ibid.*, 296.
27. *Ibid.*, 66.
28. *Ibid.*, 301–2. See also 43, 104–5. On the use of 'snakestone' see Chapter 2.
29. G.A. Hutton, *Reminiscences in the Life of Surgeon-Major George A. Hutton* (London: H.K. Lewis, 1907), 8–10
30. A.R. Skelley, *The Victorian Army at Home: The Recruitment and Terms and Conditions of the British Regular, 1859-1888* (London: Croom Helm, 1977), 41.
31. P.R. Kirby, *Sir Andrew Smith: His Life, Letters and Work* (Cape Town: Balkema, 1965), 2–8.
32. E. Burrows, *History of Medicine in South Africa* (Cape Town, Balkema, 1958), 174; Minute book of the Literary, Scientific & Medical Society of Grahamstown, Albany Museum.

33. Burrows, *op. cit.* (note 32), 174–5;

34. *Ibid.*, 175.

35. *Ibid.*, 174; Hutton, *op. cit.* (note 29), 22 *et seq.*

36. Hutton, *op. cit.* (note 29), 22–3; Burrows, *op. cit.* (note 32), 174.

37. L.G. Crouch, *A Short Medical History of Grahamstown* (Grahamstown: Grocott & Sherry, 1976), 6–7.

38. Kirby, *op. cit.* (note 31), 17–22. Smith's ethnographic work has never been published.

39. *Ibid.*, 29.

40. A. Bank, 'Of "Native skulls" and "Noble Caucasians": Phrenology in Colonial South Africa', *JSAS*, xx, 3 (Sept. 1966), 392–3; P. Curtin, *The Image of Africa: British Ideas and British Action, 1780-1850* (London: Macmillan, 1965), 377.

41. Burrows, *op. cit.* (note 32), 180–1.

42 . British Kaffraria was the region betweein the Keiskamma and Kei rivers, which was ruled directly by the British government between 1847 and 1866, when it was incorporated into the Cape Colony.

43. Burrows, *op. cit.* (note 32), 180; Imperial Parliamentary Papers, Blue Book presented to Parliament on 6 June 1856, Bindon to Brownlee, 28 May 1855.

44. *Ibid.*, Brownlee to Maclean, 30 May 1855.

45. *Ibid.*, Maclean to Brownlee, 4 June 1855.

46. J. Goldswain, *The Chronicle of Jeremiah Goldswain* (Cape Town: Van Riebeeck Society, 1946), Vol. 1, 69–70.

47. Goldswain, *op. cit.* (note 46), Vol. 2, 83.

48. Kirby, *op. cit.* (note 12), 22.

49. Burrows, *op. cit.* (note 32), 162.

50. A number of publications describe the quarrels amongst early Grahamstown doctors; see for example, Crouch, *op. cit.* (note 37), 10–19.

51. Goldswain, *op. cit.* (note 46), Vol. 1, 83–4. Goldswain's phonetic dialect form of English has interested linguists.

52. F.C. Metrowich, *The Valiant but Once* (Cape Town: 1956), 82.

53. F.C. Metrowich, *Assegaai over the Hills* (Cape Town: 1953), 20–1.

54. M. Ryan, *A History of Organised Pharmacy in South Africa 1885-1950* (Cape Town: The Society for the History of Pharmacy in South Africa, 1986), 3.

55. R. Edgecombe, 'The Letters of Hannah Dennison, 1820 Settler, 1822–1847' (unpublished M.A. thesis, Rhodes University, 1968), 54–5.

56. *Ibid.*, 168.

57. See, for example, B.M. Randles, *A History of the Kaffrarian Museum*

(King William's Town: The Museum, 1984).

58. Burrows, *op. cit.* (note 32), 127, 171. This experiment was published in the *Grahamstown Journal,* 26 June 1847 and the *Cape Town Medical Gazette*, i, (1846), 56.

59. Burrows, *op. cit.* (note 32), 168–9; Crouch, *op. cit.* (note 37), 36–40, *DSAB*, Vol. 1, 25–7. Atherstone's notebooks have been idiosyncratically and unhelpfully edited by N. Mathie, *Dr W.G. Atherstone 1814-1898: Man of Many Facets... Pseudo-Autobiography*, 3 vols (Grahamstown: Grocott & Sherry, 1998).

60. *DSAB*, Vol. 2, 55–6. Berry's library has been donated to the Cory Library, Rhodes University, which also holds the catalogue.

61. Crouch, *op. cit.* (note 37), 24.

62. C.E. Rosenberg *The Care of Strangers: The Rise of America's Hospital System* (Baltimore: Johns Hopkins University Press, 1987), 7, 189.

63. Crouch, *op. cit.* (note 37), 25–6.

64. Ryan, *op. cit.* (note 54), 5–6.

65. *Ibid.*, 6. A number of German military men had been settled on the eastern frontier.

66. Glasgow Mission Society, *Quarterly Paper*, ii, 3 (1828) RUCL.

67. Glasgow Missionary Society, *Report for 1826* (Glasgow, 1926), 15–6, RUCL.

68. *Journal of the Rev. J. Laing*, Vol. 3, RUCL, MS 9043. My thanks go to Sandy Rowoldt of Cory Library for this reference.

69. *Lovedale Christian Express* (January 1898), Obituary.

70. *Kaffrarian Watchman* (11 September 1891), Obituary of Dr John Ross.

71. J. Ross, *A Few Chapters on Public Health, Adapted for South Africa* (King William's Town: 1887), 1.

72. A.W. Burton, 'The Life and Times of John Patrick FitzGerald', 16, RUCL, MS 14,614(2).

73. Helen Ross's letterbook, 8 February 1824, RUCL, MS 2637.

74. John Ross to Mrs Main, Edinburgh, 10 May 1866, RUCL, MS 2836.

75. H. Ward, *Five Years in Kaffirland* (London: Colburn, 1948), I, 127–9.

76. The Mfengu were Xhosa-speaking peoples whose social structures had been destroyed in tribal wars. Many of them drifted into the Ciskei where they were usually more amenable to missionary instruction than other Xhosa societies.

77. Wesleyan missionary at Mount Coke near King William's Town.

78. J. Backhouse, *op. cit.* (note 10), 284–5.

79. *DSAB*, Vol. 1, 492–3.

80. J.P. FitzGerald to Sir G. Grey, 10 April 1886, SAL, MSB 223, Grey collection 2(61).

81. Peires, *op. cit.* (note 11), 46. His footnotes provides an introduction to this issue.

82. The 'Native Hospital' was only named the Grey Hospital in 1888, SAL, MSB 223 Grey collection 2(61), J.P. FitzGerald to Sir G. Grey, 26 February 1888.

83. Rosenberg, *op. cit.* (note 62), 124.

84. *Ibid.*, 148–9; J.P. FitzGerald, *A Short History of the Native Hospital and Permanent Canvas Marquees* (King William's Town: n.p., 1885), 3–4.

85. FitzGerald to Grey, 16 July 1886, SAL, MSB 233, Grey collection 2 (61).

86. FitzGerald, *op. cit.* (note 84), 7.

87. D. Gordon, 'Science, Superstition and Colonialism: Disease and Therapy at Kingwilliamstown, Xhosaland, 1847–91', unpublished paper 1996.

88. Gordon, *op. cit.* (note 87), 13–14.

89. Rosenberg, *op. cit.* (note 62), 72, 101, 104.

90. Annual Report of the Grey Hospital for 1968, 3 June 1869, CA, CO 905.

91. *Ibid.*

92. Fitzgerald, *op. cit.* (note 84), 17.

93. M. Hunter, *op. cit.* (note 5), 321; Hammond-Tooke, *op. cit.* (note 2), 8.

94. For a full account of this episode see Peires, *op. cit.* (note 11).

95. Gordon, *op. cit.* (note 87), 14.

96. Unlike many of these nineteenth-century projects for the 'civilising' of Africans, the Grey Hospital has not been allowed to deteriorate. It has recently been renovated and now serves as an administrative centre for health care in the impoverished Eastern Cape province.

97. In Afrikaner society such explanations were still prevalent at the time of the 1918 influenza epidemic. H. Phillips, '"Black October": The Impact of the Spanish Influenza Epidemic of 1918 on South Africa' *Archives Year Book for South African History*, 1 (1990), 137–53.

98. R.M. Packard, *White Plague, Black Labor: Tuberculosis and the Political Economy of Health and Disease in South Africa* (Berkeley: University of California Press, 1989).

7

'Regularly Licensed and Properly Educated Practitioners': Professionalisation 1860–1910

Elizabeth van Heyningen

This chapter explores the later professionalisation of medicine at the Cape, particularly after the discovery of diamonds and gold, when the number of doctors increased. As the demand for an improved public health system grew, and the Colonial Medical Committee was unable to cope with the more complex demands of the colony, legislation was gradually set in place to transform the practice of medicine. This legislation included a Public Health Act, improved censuses, the registration of births and deaths, and a more effective registration of nurses as well as doctors and pharmacists. By the time the Cape entered the Union in 1910, it possessed modern, well-organised medical structures.

The mineral revolution, sparked by the discovery of diamonds in 1868 and of gold in 1886 (discussed more fully in Chapter 8) penetrated almost every aspect of life in South Africa. Immigration and urbanisation altered the demographic structure of the country. The Cape medical profession and the practice of medicine in the colony did not escape change. The increase in the number of doctors created fiercer competition but promoted the organisation of the profession. In the growing towns mortality rates rose as infectious diseases such as typhoid and diphtheria threatened the lives of the residents, placing new demands on the medical profession. The depression years of the 1860s and the 1870s were a period of limbo as the new influences in the colony took root. It was then that the colony gained greater control over its own affairs. Representative government was granted in 1854, but it was the attainment of responsible government in 1872 which gave the colony much greater financial control over its own affairs, and the ability to institute independent public health measures. While Britain and, to a lesser extent, Australia, were the main models to which the Cape continued to look, local conditions shaped the decisions which were made and the structures which were established. Broadly speaking, the organisation of the profession and the process of professionalisation were very similar to those of other British colonies, such as that of Victoria in Australia, although the Cape tended to lag both in numbers and in the pace of legislative change.[1]

The Colonial Medical Committee and professionalisation

At mid-century, the Colonial Medical Committee, formally established in 1830, continued to have the main responsibility for maintaining standards in the profession, as well as advising the government on sanitary matters.[2] Throughout its existence the Colonial Medical Committee was a Cape Town-based organisation, drawing its membership from local practitioners; the interests of the Eastern Cape were, in consequence, under-represented in the making of medical policy.

Until the reversion to fixed salaries, much of the work of the Colonial Medical Committee was taken up with vetting the claims of district surgeons and it was through this contact that the Colonial Medical Committee was confronted with the problems of professionalisation in rural practice, particularly in the Eastern Cape which was still dominated by military doctors, and, where there was no military presence, unqualified practitioners tended to find space.[3] In the absence of suitable medical practitioners, such men were often appointed as district surgeons by the Colonial Office.[4] The result, the Colonial Medical Committee complained, was 'a great injustice both to the public and to the regularly licensed and properly educated medical practitioner' and it urged the government to 'render its powerful aid in upholding the dignity and respectability of the Medical Profession... by offering a sufficient inducement to its members to settle in those country districts where none are at present to be found', rather than allowing unqualified pharmacists to spoil the field.[5] Nor could the Colonial Medical Committee prevent the widespread sale of drugs by 'ignorant traders and pedlars' with £3 licences, who were 'perfectly ignorant of the composition and nature of medicines'.[6]

From the late 1850s the Colonial Medical Committee made greater efforts to protect the interests of the qualified practitioners. When an enquiry to resident magistrates in 1853 revealed that 'several persons, of low character and of still lower status of education' were 'imposing upon the credulity of the farmers', and exacting 'the most exorbitant remuneration', the Colonial Medical

Committee compiled a list of all those practising medicine in the country districts of the Cape.[7] From 1862 a fuller list of qualified practitioners was published regularly in the *Government Gazette*.[8] But the list had no official standing and its *ad hoc* status meant that over the years it became increasingly inaccurate as doctors moved away or died.[9] Nor did it end the appointment of chemists as district surgeons. As late as 1888 the Colonial Medical Committee was still protesting against the practice, for the shortage of qualified practitioners in the rural areas continued as long as district surgeons were inadequately remunerated.[10]

Moreover, just what constituted a 'regularly licensed and properly educated' practitioner was by no means clear. As we have noted in Chapter 3, the distinction between physician and surgeon had not been enforced in the colony. As competition increased, however, the situation became more uncertain. In 1871 'Mr Hall' was licensed to practise only as a surgeon and a few years later the Colonial Medical Committee protested against the misleading formula, 'Physician, Surgeon and Accoucheur', used in the *Government Gazette*, since doctors who only had a surgeon's diploma should not be licensed as physicians.[11] The distinction between physican and surgeon was the object of further debate when, in 1884, the Griqualand West High Court ruled against Dr F. Rutherfoord Harris, associate of C.J. Rhodes in Kimberley, for claiming fees for giving advice as medical practitioner. (Harris held the Edinburgh LRCS and midwifery diploma.)[12] In Kimberley's fiercely competitive medical world a number of doctors supported this decision, arguing that 'a manifold injustice will be done to those Professional Men who have been put to the trouble and expense to qualify themselves in both branches of the Profession' if English law were not followed.[13]

Harris, however, considered that the Scottish diploma qualified him to practise as a physician since it included substantial medical training. He asked to be put on the same footing as his brother professionals of the London College who were licensed to practise as surgeons and physicians with the Licenciate of the Society of Apothecaries.[14] Confronted by these complex anomalies, the Colonial Medical Committee supported Harris's claims:

> The Board are greatly surprised that your full right to practise and charge as a physician should ever have been called in question, for all through South Africa Physicians practise as Surgeons and Surgeons as Physicians, charging legally in each case, and their perfect right to

197

do so, has never before been called in question by anyone or disallowed by any court.[15]

The government was asked to clarify the position in the *Government Gazette*.[16] Subsequently the Colonial Medical Committee urged that all applicants for licence as medical practitioners in the colony should be required to produce two diplomas, or the double qualification, or a certificate of the *Staats Examen*.[17]

If the translation of British qualifications in the colonial context proved problematic, that of foreign qualifications was even more difficult. Over time the Colonial Medical Committee became more stringent in its demands. Because the possession of medical degrees in Holland and Germany did not entitle a man to practise until he had passed the *Staats Examen*, the Colonial Medical Committee had begun to demand this certificate as well.[18] But this decision worked against colonial doctors who found it cheaper to train in continental Europe than in Britain, which was reckoned to be at least twice as expensive. R.J. Reinecke had taken the MD from the University of Berlin. He could not, however, present himself for the *Staats Examen* without also attending a German gymnasium and passing the finishing examination, an impossibility on the £65 a year at his disposal. He asked that, as he was a colonial, the *Staats Examen* requirement be waived, but the Colonial Medical Committee was obdurate.[19]

One means of solving the problem of foreign qualifications was to look to the British example. French and Swiss qualifications would not be accepted, the Colonial Medical Committee announced in 1890, since the Swiss and French governments did not recognise the respective British qualifications (although the qualifications of the Swiss-French missionaries were accepted).[20] Medical qualifications from other British colonies were also considered suspect, and the Colonial Medical Committee demanded that they be registered in London before they were accepted at the Cape.[21] American diplomas and degrees were regarded with profound suspicion and few were licensed to practise in the colony.[22]

While these decisions went some way to formalising the status of the medical profession, they had little standing in law. Nor was the position of the Colonial Medical Committee itself entirely clear. For much of its life most of the members were unpaid and it was years before its pleas for remuneration were granted..[23] The absence of adequate public health legislation also undermined the position of the Colonial Medical Committee. However much it might advise the government to take action, it could enforce nothing and, in the face of rising mortality rates, its advice was purely palliative. It was clear from the debates on the budget votes of the Colonial Medical Committee that its prestige stood very low in the eyes of parliamentarians.[24] The growing hostility to the Colonial Medical Committee filtered through to the press as well.[25] By 1889 James Rose Innes, one of the most educated and liberal parliamentarians, made a scathing attack on the Colonial Medical Committee. This was, he said:

> [A] most effete and useless body.... What had the Medical Committee done? It consisted of four or five gentlemen resident in Cape Town who examined certificates of lunatics, and during the last year they visited Robben Island once, and went down to the beach to examine the seaweed which had been washed up. For this they were paid nearly £500 per annum. This was an important question; instead of a useless body we should have a useful body. There should be a Department of Public Health – no country wanted one more. The reports of the district surgeons were quite appalling.[26]

Innes, however, failed to address the issue of the regulation of the medical profession, increasingly also a matter of concern to pharmacists who wanted greater autonomy.[27]

Two parliamentary commissions of inquiry, in 1883 and 1890, examined the problem. Practitioners who gave evidence pressed for qualifications in all three branches of medicine before registration.[28] They were unwilling to subordinate the medical profession to pharmacists who might be represented on the proposed medical council. [29] At the same time, they demanded the right to control independent midwives, whom they wanted examined and certified by the colonial medical profession as they had been in the early years of the century. [30] In all respects, they asserted the superiority of the medical profession over and their autonomy from pharmacists, nurses and midwives.

Unlike New South Wales, where there was substantial resistance from the lay public to medical professionalisation, the Cape Colony saw little active opposition to the improved registration of doctors. The delay in passing a new bill arose, rather, from dilatoriness in parliament where the medical profession, unlike lawyers, was poorly represented before the 1890s. Finally, in 1891, a new act was passed without undue difficulty – Act No 34-1891, the Medical and Pharmacy Act. The affairs of the pharmacists and doctors were separated with the creation of an eight-member Colonial Medical Council, consisting of four members elected by the medical profession and four (including a dentist) nominated by government, to represent the profession. The functions of the council were confined largely to the regulation of the profession and to the certification of nurses and midwives. A medical practitioner was defined as anyone licensed as a physician, surgeon or accoucheur before the passing of the Act, or, afterwards, as 'every person duly qualified by licence and registration under the Act to practise as a physician and surgeon in the Colony', including the right to work as an accoucheur. In a colony not noted for its advanced feminist views, Clause 33 explicitly stated that no person should be disqualified merely because she was female – almost certainly a tribute to Cape Town's respected Dr Jane Waterston. As in Britain, laypeople were not prevented from practising medicine, but they could not recover charges in a court of law, hold any official appointments or sign medical certificates.

Much has been made of the novel features of the 1891 Act, particularly of the registration of nurses and midwives, which was well in advance of British legislation.[31] This was, however, less a step in the professionalisation of women in health care than a means of ensuring their subordination to doctors. By the passing of the act the Cape medical profession acquired the attributes of professionalism which were to remain features of the South African medical profession – the right to regulate itself, the legal authority to enforce its decisions, the ability to protect the practice of medicine from lay encroachment, and its superiority in the medical hierarchy. In one striking respect, however, it remained an adolescent. As long as there was no medical education available at the Cape, the Cape medical profession remained a colonial dependency, surbordinated to European standards (see Chapter 4).

Despite its new-found status, the Colonial Medical Council remained somewhat insecure, jealous of its independence from central government control and uncertain of its position. When the Health Department at the Colonial Office began to stretch its wings early in the twentieth century, the Colonial Medical Council campaigned vigorously against the transfer of the administration of the Medical and Pharmacy Acts to the colonial medical officer of health. Dr Darley-Hartley, the editor of the *SAMR*, explained:

It submits that the change alters the status of the Council from that of an expert advisory committee to the lay Minister, to that of an advisory committee to a medical official who *is ex officio* one of its own body, and further that this latter status is not one contemplated by the Act which called the Council into existence, and is not compatible with its position as a body representative of the medical profession.[32]

If the clash was partially resolved in 1893, the Colonial Medical Council remained sensitive about its official status. In June 1893 it protested to the Colonial Office that no representative from the Council had been included in official invitations, for instance to the Governor's dinner in honour of the Queen's birthday. Other branches of the public service were recognised and the Colonial Medical Council had always previously been invited: '...and these acts of courtesy have always been accepted by the profession in this Colony as a mark of official recognition'. The Under Colonial Secretary, H. De Smidt apologised hastily for the oversight.[33]

The informal organisation of the medical profession

The formulation of the 1891 Act had been assisted by the local branches of the British Medical Association which, it claimed, had 'watched the Bill carefully through all its stages, and was able very appreciably to influence the legislature'. Two of its nominees had been appointed to the new Colonial Medical Council.[34] The presence of the BMA at the Cape reflected a new spirit within the larger medical profession in the colony, at once more entrepreneurial and more imperialist.

In 1883 a South African Medical Association had been founded in Cape Town, largely at the instigation of two colonials, Drs C.L. Herman and J.H. Meiring Beck, with the support of Dr Henry Ebden (the editor of the defunct *Cape Town Medical Gazette*). Despite its title and the formation of several country branches, the association never got off the ground. The associations established in Kimberley, Grahamstown and elsewhere soon exhibited fissiparous tendencies and the membership of the South African Medical Association failed to grow. In 1889 it was ousted by the British Medical Association.[35]

In an illuminating article T.J. Johnson and M. Caygill commented on the imperial role of the BMA.[36] Military doctors, who felt professionally isolated in their regiments and lacked the authority and status accorded to regular officers, were often responsible for the

BMA's expansion in the colonies. These men were familiar with the work of the BMA at home in protecting the rights and professional status of general practitioners. They hoped to enlist its support in negotiations with the London government and at the same time they expected that it would draw together a group of colleagues who would aid in enhancing their status and authority.[37] The BMA itself actively encouraged such expansion. It prided itself on being an imperial institution which linked members of the profession in one body, animated by a common purpose – 'the advancement of scientific medicine and the social well being and dignity of its associates'.[38]

The Cape of Good Hope branch of the BMA (later the Cape Western branch) conformed remarkably closely to the broad picture drawn by Johnson and Caygill. It was founded largely at the instigation of a military doctor, Surgeon-General J.G. Faught, the Principal Army Medical Officer. The membership consisted mainly of the more active and imperially-minded British doctors, Sir Edmund Stevenson, Jane Waterston and Darley-Hartley among them, although the presence of such men as the Afrikaner, Dr J.H. Meiring Beck, one of the most distinguished of the Dutch-speaking doctors, testified to a somewhat wider membership.

Undoubtedly the BMA in Cape Town enhanced professional standards. In the early 1890s it established a library, although its use was hampered by the lack of an adequate home until it finally found a place in the new university buildings in 1907.[39] Its meetings allowed doctors to discuss a range of professional issues. At a typical meeting of the Cape Town branch of the BMA in 1895, Dr L. Beck described a case of compound fracture which he had recently treated, while Dr Fuller read a paper on 'New methods of diagnosis and treatment of diphtheria' which aroused considerable discussion on the value of the use of 'antitoxines'.[40] A couple of months later Dr E. Sinclair Stevenson read a paper on 'Some points in the progress of surgery and medicine observed during a recent tour in Europe', commenting particularly on the value of aseptic surgery. Six years ago, he noted, a great war had been raging in Europe between two camps favouring antiseptic versus aseptic surgery. His recent visit demonstrated the wonderful results to be obtained by the latter – 'No rise in temperature, no inflammatory complications; nothing but a smooth and continuous course leading to recovery'.[41]

But the BMA also had its limitations. Despite the proliferation of branches in the British colonies, its imperial character prevented it from achieving wider South African acceptance.[42] In 1892 the first

Illustration 7.1
Members of the South African Medical Congress, 1910

By the time of Union in South Africa, the medical profession in
South Africa, had become fairly well-organised. National medical
congresses were a regular feature. This group photograph represents
the cream of the South African medical profession. The woman in
the front row is Dr Jane Waterston, South Africa's first woman
doctor. Fifth from the right in the second row is Dr Darley-Harley,
editor of the *SAMR*. (*SAMR*, 12 November 1910)

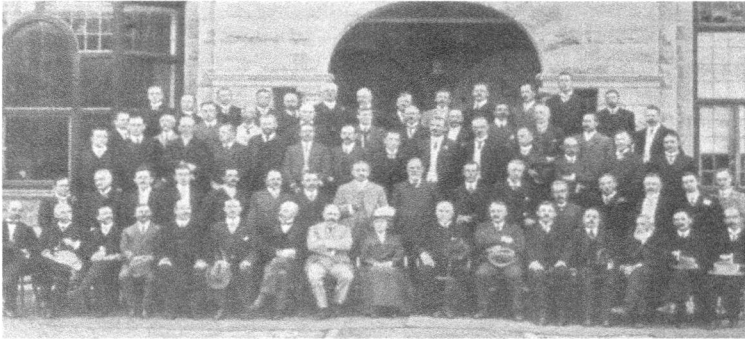

South African medical congress was held in Kimberley in
conjunction with the Kimberley Exhibition in an attempt to
overcome these divisions. Two motions were put forward – to form a
South African medical association and to publish a South African
medical journal, the latter to be the medium through which 'obscure
facts in medicine and surgery, of colonial interest, might be placed on
record and made available to others'. The move to create a larger
association was abandoned 'as being liable to interfere with the
working of the various branches of the British and other medical
associations' but the *South African Medical Journal* was launched a
few months later in May 1893 with Dr Alexander Edington, the
Cape government bacteriologist in Grahamstown, as editor. [43] He was
succeeded later by Dr George Eyre of Cape Town. The *South African
Medical Journal* remained in existence until the South African War
brought about its demise. Its obvious success and the clear need for
such an organ encouraged Dr Darley-Hartley to found the *South
African Medical Record* in 1903 as a business venture and this
continued until 1926 (see Chapter 9). [44]

As the Cape medical profession became more self-conscious, it began to express the belief that it had a special function to perform in colonial society. In his presidential address to the first South African medical congress in 1892 Dr Alfred Hillier, later a member of the Uitlander Transvaal Reform Committee which was to promote Jameson's inauspicious raid into the South African Republic, saw Britain's imperial role in medical terms:

> Throughout this country, in town and village, we are continually seeing the doctor speaking out or 'rubbing it in' in the cause of civilisation; and I feel most strongly that here, where the number of men of liberal education is small, the function of medical men is often wider than in the older countries of Europe.[45]

Dr Darley-Hartley, editor of the *South African Medical Record* and founder of the South African League, Milner's agency for imperial expansion, was an equally ardent imperialist. In the journal Darley-Hartley explicitly championed the political cause of the medical profession. He drew attention regularly to the activities of those doctors who were engaged in politics and continually emphasised the need for the profession to be represented in parliament.[46]

But less imperialistically minded men also thought that the work of the profession should be performed on a larger stage. Dr J.H. Meiring Beck, who was a leading member of the Afrikaner Bond party in the Cape House of Assembly for many years, in a rousing presidential address to the Cape Western branch of the British Medical Association, remarked on the extent to which everything was being democratised. This threw a responsibility on all:

> it is impossible, undesirable, and wrong for an educated and intelligent profession like that of medicine to keep aloof from doing its share of public work... we should... bear in mind that, in the shaping of the destinies of a new country like this we ought to bear no inconsiderable share.... We must see to it, gentlemen, that this medical influence as the years roll on is not lessened. In an age when public health legislation is rapidly and recognisably pushing its way as a first essential in good government, it would be disgraceful for us as a profession not to assist in shaping the laws.[47]

On a number of fronts by the 1890s doctors were more vocal than they had previously been. In part a better official status and better organisation gave them new self-confidence; but, as the

Table 7.1
Population of the major towns in the Cape Colony 1875-1904[48]

	1875	**1891**	**1904**
Cape Town	45,000	79,000	170,000
Port Elizabeth	13,000	23,000	33,000
East London	2,000	7,000	24,000
Kimberley	13,600	29,000	34,000
Colony Total[49]	72,000	1,500,000	2,400,000

number of doctors in the country increased, they also had to fight harder for their turf.

The creation of a public health movement

The emergence of a public health movement gave doctors greater prominence in local and central government affairs, although they continued to chafe against their lack of status in the eyes of the authorities. The demand for sanitary reform in the Cape Colony was largely a product of the effects of immigration and urbanisation. While there were no figures to support them, it seemed clear to informed observers that mortality rates were rising and that major causes of death were the infectious diseases associated with urbanisation.

It has been estimated that immigration accounted for thirty-nine per cent of the total growth of the white population in the colony between 1891 and 1906 – a total of 88,236 people.[50] Most were urban dwellers. Black people, especially African men, were also urbanising.

Public health reform at the Cape was never a popular movement. Local authorities were dilatory, hampered by inadequate legislation but even more by the ignorance and incompetence of local officials. The district surgeon of Caledon commented pungently in 1887, 'I can only attribute this spread of typhoid fever to the incompetency of the Public Health Board at Caledon. This board consists of the members of the Caledon Municipality without the addition of a medical man, and the board as now constituted is as obstinate as it is ignorant of the rudiments of sanitation.'[51] Above all, local élites feared the costs which might be involved. Nor did parliament show any initiative. For almost thirty years after representative government was granted, legislation at the Cape catered almost entirely to the interests of the farming sector.

205

Reform initiatives came mainly from a small body of enlightened opinion which, influenced by the British example, pressed for similar legislation and public services in the colony. The English language press self-consciously attempted to mould public opinion, constantly exhorting colonials to adopt the civilised standards of the metropolitan. At times, however, sanitary rhetoric was infused with bigotry and used as a weapon to create ethnic prejudice and division.[52] The pulpit was another platform for sanitary publicity, influenced by such movements as the Christian Socialists, of whom the best-known was Charles Kingsley. In Cape Town press and pulpit came together in the founding of the Free Dispensary in 1860, to provide outpatient care for the 'deserving poor'.[53]

The value of the dispensary was forcibly demonstrated during the fever epidemic of 1867 when it undertook the only serious investigation into the state of Cape Town during the middle decades of the century.[54] The results were published in a pamphlet written by R. Thornton, Staff Surgeon Major, and the Rev. Thomas E. Fuller, a Baptist minister and editor of the *Cape Argus* from 1864.[55] This remarkable little work revealed only too vividly the deficiencies of the town, and of the collection of statistics. Even after the municipality had introduced a regulation in 1868 that births and deaths in Cape Town should be registered at the Town House, returns from the harbour signalman on the hill above the cemeteries, who could count the burials, remained the most reliable figure.[56]

But the most obvious group to press for health reform was the medical profession. Galvanised by the reorganisation of the profession, they were a much more effective pressure group but their role was necessarily subordinate. They could not, of themselves, initiate legislation or public works programmes. It was, in the first instance, those public-private hybrids, the district surgeons, who provided ammunition for government reformers. They were best placed to monitor the health of the colony although for much of the century their reports were submitted irregularly and never published.[57] The real initiative, however, came from the Colonial Office.

In the early 1880s the Colonial Office had no programme for fundamental reform. Improvements which were introduced were usually *ad hoc* responses to local crises or occasional public demand. In 1882, however, the decision was taken to collect and publish the reports of the district surgeons, possibly as a response to the calamitous smallpox epidemic in Cape Town and Kimberley in 1882-3. The early reports were brief, unco-ordinated and impressionistic but they drew attention to the more spectacular deficiencies in the colony. Lacking any other data, district surgeons tended to emphasise the most visible health problems. The first report, in 1882, drew attention to the prevalence of syphilis and leprosy.[58] Evidence of the existence of such disfiguring diseases with such emotive connotations was one of the few things that aroused enough public concern to persuade parliament to pass the Contagious Diseases Act No. 39 of 1885 and the Leprosy Repression Act No. 8 of 1884, promulgated in 1892, introducing the compulsory segregation of leprosy sufferers, usually on Robben Island.[59]

Integral to health reform in Britain had been the statistical movement. There, collection and dissemination of data had made it possible for reformers to put their case with what appeared to be incontrovertible clarity. At the Cape, however, apart from rudimentary censuses in 1865 and 1875 and the incompetent registration of births and deaths in Cape Town, there had been very few professional, or even amateur, attempts to record demographic details of Cape society. The 1891 census coincided with the decennial imperial censuses. By 1891, also, colonial revenues had improved sufficiently to make it possible to finance a thorough census and, in the person of the newly appointed Under Colonial Secretary, Henry De Smidt, for the first time the Colonial Office had an officer with the skills to conduct the survey. Married to the daughter of Dr J.Z. Herman, one of Cape Town's more notable doctors, De Smidt may have been particularly sensitive to the need for improved health administration in the Colony.[60] To deal with the vital statistics in the census he employed a newcomer to the colony, Dr Alfred John Gregory.

Gregory was to prove a stormy petrel in the Colonial Office – ambitious, energetic and unpopular. Although he only became colonial medical officer of health in 1901, he was the dominant figure in the Colonial Office from 1891. Determined to centralise the organisation of health care at the Cape, his view of public health encompassed aspects of social life beyond that of the purely medical. The British medical heritage was clearly a vital influence in shaping his frame of reference, which was also permeated with a mild jingoism.[61] Published government reports suggest that Gregory and De Smidt enjoyed a considerable rapport. While Gregory praised De Smidt's 'admirable administrative foresight' in the 1893 public health report, De Smidt prefaced the report of the following year with an extraordinary eulogy of Gregory.[62]

207

Elizabeth van Heyningen

Table 7.2
Urban mortality rates in the Cape Colony 1890–1892

		1890	1891	1892
Cape Town	All races	24.08	24.94	24.99
King William's Town	European	13.55	10.68	14.37
	Coloured	36.08	20.37	25.89
Kimberley	All races	36.61		
	European		25.69	5.38
	Coloured		41.14	55.27

Under De Smidt the Colonial Office was reorganised. Two new branches, Statistics, and Health and Local Government, were established in December 1891.[63] These reforms in the Colonial Office also encouraged more rapid developments in public health legislation in the 1890s. Changes in the department were first reflected in the district surgeons' reports which began to be shaped into a vehicle for initiating change. After 1890 the reports appeared with a general introduction, written by Gregory, which attempted to analyse the contents and which underlined the criticisms and suggestions the district surgeons made.

The reports emphasised three features above all. One was the need for an adequate births and deaths registration act. As far back as 1874 the *Cape Monthly Magazine* had pointed out that the Cape was, in this respect, well behind New South Wales or any other colony of importance.[64] Ten years later the district surgeon of Albert was forced to explain:

> I regret very much to state that I am not able to furnish a statistical report of the health of the district with the slightest approach to any correctness. As there are about a dozen medical men practising in this district, and as a consequence my practice is almost entirely confined to the town, I have very little knowledge of the state of health of the district beyond the immediate neighbourhood of Burghersdorp.[65]

Such information as could be gleaned suggested that mortality rates were abnormally high. Gregory attempted some analysis in 1892.

As Gregory explained, these figures were unreliable but it was obvious that infant mortality was devastating. If appeals to the consciences of the legislators did not work, Gregory could emphasise melodramatically the danger of undetected crime. In the existing circumstances, he suggested, mothers could rid themselves of any

208

inconvenient baby without fear of detection.[67]

Related to the high mortality rate was the need for improved sanitation in most districts. In a country which was plagued by drought, water was frequently in short supply and pollution was a constant hazard. Typhoid was widely prevalent. Even when the Colonial Office took up the matter with individual local authorities, their representations were usually ignored.[68] It was for this reason that Gregory pressed his third point so hard: the need for a central public health department which could galvanise municipalities into some action.[69]

The following years saw further stages on the road to sanitary reform. Three events, closely linked, occurred at this time. The first was the appointment of a medical officer of health for the colony. Provision had been made in the estimates for such a post as far back as 1890 but only in December 1893 was it filled, in a part-time capacity, by Dr Alexander Edington, the colonial bacteriologist. It was an unsatisfactory appointment and in 1895, therefore, the post was re-advertised.[70] Dr George Turner, a man of impeccable qualifications and extensive experience, was appointed with Gregory as his assistant.[71] Turner, however, was soon involved in rinderpest and leprosy research. When war broke out in 1899 he was seconded to the British Army and afterwards settled in the Transvaal. Except for a brief period, to all intents and purposes, therefore, Gregory remained the dominant figure in the Colonial Office.

The second related event of this period was the introduction of the first comprehensive public health bill into parliament.[72] This remarkable document was probably the joint work of Henry de Smidt and Gregory. Drawing principally on British and Australian (Victorian) legislation, and above all on the English Public Health Act of 1875 – 'the father of all acts' – it was intended to be a thoroughly comprehensive local administration bill. It was distinguished by the compulsory powers granted to the central government. It provided for the appointment of a battery of officials to watch over the health of the colony, including a civil engineer who should be an expert in sanitary matters, district health officers responsible to the government, and locally appointed medical officers of health. The bill also consolidated all the scattered local authority legislation on adulterated food, cemeteries, dairies, sewerage, water supply and disposal of refuse, spelling out the powers and duties of the local bodies with a precision which went far beyond anything attempted before. Further than this, in keeping with Gregory's belief that health legislation had a social function, it ventured into the delicate field of 'native affairs', legislating also for urban locations and the 'native territories'. Most novel, perhaps, were the clauses providing for the regulation of lodging houses and tenement buildings, and for establishing and maintaining poor-houses for the accommodation of paupers. Finally, the bill introduced the compulsory notification of infectious diseases and the vaccination of children within three months of birth, and it ameliorated the quarantine restrictions on ships.

The bill was not well received in parliament. Opposition hinged on the issues of compulsion and centralisation and came largely from the representatives of the local authorities. In the House of Assembly the MLA for Grahamstown, Mr Arthur Douglass, complained that it struck at the roots of self-government; that it bore the mark of an autocratic mind.[73] Three common strands ran through the criticisms. One was the fear of the cost of the reforms; the second was hostility to the expert, the professional; and the third, more muted, was suspicion of the newcomer from Europe. Dr Hoffman of Paarl also wanted a medical board: 'I think they [the board] must be better acquainted with the wants of the Colony than a stranger fresh from Europe, who would take a long time to get rid of his European ideas and notions.' Colonel Schermbrucker, MLA for King William's Town, expressed himself most volubly:

> The result of that will be that you will have a general health officer and a general engineer, thirty-six district medical officers and thirty-six engineers, and every one of these seventy-two will make it their business to worry you day after day. He will detect nuisances here and nuisances there, and naturally so, because a professional man has no regard for the circumstances of cases, but will proceed on his peculiar scientific opinion in the way he thinks right. You would have these thirty-six doctors and thirty-six engineers worrying every municipal council and divisional council of the country, day after day, and in the end such will be their united power presided over by the chief medical officer, that the Government would be obliged at the expense of the taxpayer to make works of sewerage and waterworks, which are actually unnecessary, and will necessitate a great deal of taxing beyond what properties can stand.[74]

Even in its amended form the bill was too drastic to be acceptable to parliament. But a major reason for the failure of the Colonial Office officials to fight for it successfully was their inability to furnish convincing facts and figures, especially on the rise of typhoid in the towns.

The third great step of the period, the passing of the Births and Deaths Registration Act No. 7 of 1894, went a long way towards rectifying this deficiency. As with other health reforms, the act had been mooted for years but successive governments had been reluctant to introduce it, fearing the expense involved and ignorant of the value of such statistics.[75] Fortunately parliamentary members were generally too uninterested to block its passage, and the act came into force at the beginning of 1895. The effect was immediate. For the first time it was possible to record with relative accuracy, not only the mortality figures in the colony, but also the causes of death. The initial report at once pointed to the very high number of deaths among children. In the first three months of 1895, of the total number of 3,950 deaths, 2,036 were of children under five.[76] The newly appointed medical officer of health, Dr George Turner, also made ready use of the information in his annual reports.[77]

Even with these alarming figures to back it, and considerably modified, the Public Health Bill did not have an easy passage through parliament. It failed in 1896 and was eventually enacted only in the following year as the Public Health Amendment Act No. 23 of 1897. In its final form it differed vastly from the original draft; almost all the coercive powers had been abandoned. The medical officer of health for the colony was firmly entrenched and locally appointed health officers were permitted, with certain functions specified under the act. A measure of uniformity was imposed on the widely varied local regulations and the local bodies had their powers extended. The notification of infectious diseases was made compulsory and the government undertook to subsidise the full costs of combating an epidemic introduced from outside the colony.

The 1897 Public Health Act put new powers into the hands of the colonial medical officer of health. As the voluminous files of the Colonial Office indicate, little escaped the attention of an energetic man like Gregory. Bye-laws were scrutinised and health problems carefully investigated. More than this, his opinion was sought in the investigations of major commissions of enquiry – the Native Locations Commission of 1900, the Cape Peninsula Commission of 1902, the South African Native Affairs Commission of 1905, to name only three – and carried a weight which enabled him to have a major voice in the formation of social policies of the period.

Yet the position of the medical officer himself was somewhat anomalous, dependent on the goodwill of the Colonial Secretary and the Under Colonial Secretary for his executive authority. De Smidt and Dr T.W. Smartt, the Colonial Secretary in 1898, had both intended that Turner should have the rank and status of a head of department.[78] Gregory, however, complained that this policy was ignored and that he was subordinated, not only to the UCS, but even to junior clerks in the department.[79] He envied Dr G. Pratt Yule, the medical officer of the Orange Free State, who had started with 'a fair field', with no vested interests to deal with. He had been faced with 'the old story of the Lay Administration clinging with jealous tenacity to all power and patronage... and... every step forward has only been achieved after many hard-fought battles between the Lay and Professional sides'.[80]

Although Turner's personal authority stood high, he was also soon disillusioned by colonial bureaucracy. When he resigned he spoke out forcibly on the impossible situation in which he and Gregory were forced to work:

> The Health Department is undermanned. You can easily ascertain this by finding what proportion of the public documents come before either my Colleague or myself, I say public documents because our work is not confined to one Department. Undermanning is bad enough, but it is not nearly so troublesome as a bad system. The first one can fight against by overwork but against the latter the best experience, intelligence and assiduity is powerless. I put it to you sir, is it just that I should be made answerable for a failure which I have predicted as inevitable and which is due to a system against which I have protested.... I have never shirked the inconvenience and in some cases even more than inconvenience, which work away from Cape Town has entailed, because I felt that I was at least doing good and gaining experience, while in the office I was wasting my time and my temper.[81]

This frustrating situation, in which responsibility was divided between the Colonial Office, which administered local government and hospitals, and the Health Branch, was ended in 1906 after a bitter struggle on Gregory's part and as a result of rationalisation in the civil service precipitated by the depression. A sub-department was created which gave Gregory control over most sectors of public health and local government apart from hospitals and asylums.[82] Shortly after this he wrote to Pratt Yule giving a rare glimpse of his views of the role of the government medical officer of health. He was content that the Minister should have the final authority, he said:

> An autocracy, however benevolent, wise and just, will not survive a week in these democratic days. And after all, a conscientious officer

should be mainly filled with the desire to carry out his work to the best advantage rather than aspiring to an autocratic position.[83]

The 1897 Act gave shape to colonial health administration, instituting a medical bureaucracy which grew quite rapidly. By 1903 the government health department consisted of four doctors including Gregory and a clerical staff of twelve, mainly English-speaking. Gregory took on so much work that he failed to produce annual reports for several years.[84] There was little rivalry from the local authorities. In 1905, apart from Cape Town, only Kimberley and Port Elizabeth had appointed full-time health officers, and the latter town retrenched theirs after a few months. Forty-three local authorities employed medical officers in a consultative capacity.[85] Consequently, by 1910 Cape Town was sharply differentiated from the rest of the colony in its provisions for public health, since it had the colonial medical officer resident in the city and one of the few permanent health officers of its own.

Despite its obvious deficiencies, the creation of public health institutions gave Cape doctors a public presence and an authority which greatly enhanced their status by 1910. This situation was to be short-lived. When, following the British victory in the South African War of 1899 to 1910, the four British colonies of the Cape, Natal, the Orange Free State and the Transvaal, united in 1910 to form the Union of South Africa, conservative policies of the old Boer republics prevailed and medical concerns were subordinated to other interests. The Union had no public health department until the crisis following the 1918 influenza epidemic.[86] Health legislation took second place to the protection of mining interests against that of their labour, and public health was increasingly a tool of segregation.[87]

Race and gender in the Cape medical profession

Nothing speaks so loudly of the improved social position of the medical profession in the Cape Colony as the inclusivity of the 1891 Act. The 1891 Act made no attempt to exclude anyone from the practice of medicine on the grounds of race or gender. This was in keeping with the Cape's 'liberal' race-free franchise, but it is, nonetheless, worthy of comment. Undoubtedly the principal reason for this lacuna was the lack of anyone who might threaten the dominance of the white men in the profession. But it was also a token of respect to the Cape's only woman doctor, Jane Elizabeth Waterston, and perhaps also to the few black doctors at that time.

Andrew Christopher Jackson, who practised at the Cape from

1866 to 1906, was the first black man to be registered as a doctor at the Cape. The fact that Jackson was not a local African but a West Indian may have eased his way in racist South Africa. However, he did not find the same the acceptance in the Transvaal when he migrated north to try his fortune on the goldfields. Chastened, he returned to Cape Town where he became active in the emergent pan-African movement.[88]

Before 1910 there were only three colonial-born black doctors. William Anderson Soga was the son of Tiyo Soga, the first black ordained minister of the United Presbyterian Church in South Africa, and a Scottish mother. Tiyo Soga, a Xhosa missionary, had his son educated in Scotland to avoid the limitations his colour imposed on him at the Cape. Like his father, William Anderson Soga married a Scots woman, reinforcing a somewhat ambiguous position in the colony, for he was officially categorised as 'European'.[89] W.A. Soga became a medical missionary, founding the Miller Mission at Elliotdale in the Transkei. There his status was all that the missionaries could have wished, for he amassed a fair amount of property and lived, materially at least, in the style of a Victorian gentleman, dying on the local golf course.[90] As the only doctor for some distance, Soga's practice included whites as well as blacks. His obituary described him not only as popular, but as a man 'who impressed even on a slight acquaintance'. Soga's son followed in his footsteps, also qualifying as a doctor in Glasgow, and serving in the British forces during the First World War.[91]

The other two black doctors, Mohammed Omer Dollie and Abdullah Abdurahman, were both Muslims, so-called 'Malays', the descendants of slaves who had been urbanised almost from the foundation of the colony, and a few of whom had accumulated wealth since emancipation. Virtually nothing is known of Dollie. Jackson found some space in the interstices in Cape Town's social structures while Soga appears to have been contented with his isolated position in the depths of the Transkei. Jane Waterston and Abdullah Abdurahman, by contrast, found their place in the mainstream of Cape medical and political life.

Jane Elizabeth Waterston (1843-1932)

Jane Waterston came to the Cape as a missionary, the founder of the Girls' Institution at Lovedale, working under Dr James Stewart, formerly associate of David Livingstone.[92] Like Stewart, Waterston believed that medicine had an evangelical and moral purpose. A Scot from Inverness, the daughter of a bank manager, she had been recruited by Stewart in 1866 to start a girls' school at Lovedale. Although an effective teacher, Waterston was determined to work as a medical missionary in the north. In letters to Stewart she explained her views. An African mission, she considered, 'should be a *civilising*, and and *energising*, as well as a Christianizing Agent'. Her main goal was to help 'these poor wretches of women up country'. She felt she had a special understanding of their plight: 'I am a woman myself and it haunts me more than I can tell you, the thought of these poor wretches whose present life is misery, and their hereafter.'[93]

In 1874 Jane Waterston returned to Britain, where she was one of the first students at the London School of Medicine for Women. After qualifying in 1879, she went to the Livingstonia Mission in Nyasaland (Malawi) but she found the experience bitterly disillusioning and left after six months. Eventually she moved to Cape Town, where she practised as a doctor to the end of her long life in 1932. In Cape Town the same sense of mission motivated her. She expected to find a niche as a women's doctor but she soon acquired a larger practice, including black patients. 'They feel, I think, that I treat them like human beings and not *niggers* as the term is here.'[94] Her patients included African dock labourers, female prisoners, leprosy and mental patients on Robben Island, and the women of the slums. In 1888 she founded the Ladies' Branch of the Free Dispensary to improve maternity care.

In many respects Jane Waterston epitomizes the doctor as 'agent of empire'. As a committed imperialist and ardent supporter of Milner's expansionist policies, she would have been proud to bear that title.[95] Her concept of the imperial mission was multi-faceted, embracing political expansion and the imposition of Western values which were defined by education, hard work, the wearing of European dress, and the proper relation of men to women. Waterston was undoubtedly paternalist and class-bound but she rejected a racism which saw black people as inherently inferior. In the final analysis evangelical religion governed her thinking.

Although Waterston was a woman, uniquely she was also a member of the ruling establishment in Cape Town. She was accepted by the local medical fraternity, and from 1905 to 1906 she was president of the Western Cape branch of the BMA. She was never in full-time government employment but she was an official inspector to several institutions and frequently acted in an advisory capacity. Probably as a result of Milner's influence, she was also a member of the Committee of Ladies, led by Millicent Garrett Fawcett, which was set up by Britain to inquire into concentration camp conditions during the South African War.

Waterston's position in Cape Town society and her ability to assert such values were inseparable from her role as a doctor. It was also dependent on her manipulation of her gender. Her austere appearance and blunt manner led others to treat her more as a man than as a woman.[96] At the same time she was able to attract female patients and to treat Cape Town's poor precisely because that seemed appropriate to female behaviour.

A handful of women followed Waterston onto the Cape register before 1910. Others included an Anglican medical missionary, Edith Pellatt, whose career was cut short by the onset of blindness and she returned to Britain in 1896. The only colonial-born woman doctor at this time was Edith Gertrude Pycroft, the daugher of a pharmacist. None were as highly qualified as Waterston who later returned to Europe to obtain her M.D.

Abdullah Abdurahman (1872?-1940)

Abdullah Abdurahman is well known because of his leadership of the African Political (People's) Organisation (APO), one of the Cape's earliest black political organisations, founded in 1902. Abdurahman was the grandson of slaves and was, uniquely for a Muslim, educated at the South African College. He qualified in Glasgow and returned to Cape Town in 1895. While much has been written about him as a politician,[97] little has been said of his medical career. He was the first black member of the Cape Town municipal council on which, at least in his earlier years, health concerns were subordinated to political interests for he espoused the 'dirty party' cause of the small property owners and tenants who objected to expensive water schemes.

As a Muslim doctor, however, Abdurahman seems to have done much to reconcile Muslims to 'white' medicine. The Muslims had a rich medical tradition of their own, combined with a legacy of bitter resistance to vaccination and such sanitary measures as the closure of cemeteries.[98] In 1901, when a plague epidemic struck Cape Town, Abdurahman became an important intermediary between the Muslim community and the Cape government when rapid and arbitrary measures were introduced to control the disease. Muslim resistance to these sanitary controls crumbled, not only because the government was relatively sensitive to their traditions but because, in Abdurahman they had an intermediary whose status was on a par with the white élite.

Abdurahman died in 1940. Throughout his long political career he had remained the principal spokesman not only for Muslims but also for the rest of the Cape's coloured community. Like Waterston he was consulted by government on issues related to his community. His relative conservatism and non-confrontational manner undoubtedly eased his way but his status in Cape society was, above all, contingent upon his education as a doctor.

Conclusion

By 1910, when the Cape was incorporated into the Union of South Africa, the colony had a medical profession which was strongly entrenched in law and in society. The professionalisation of the practitioners took place within a legal framework which recognised the growing pre-eminence of the medical profession in the colony. A fully fledged public health system had been put in place, while the doctors themselves had established a society and journal which enabled them to share their experiences and voice their concerns. In doing so, they had a public voice as a pressure group which had been almost entirely absent thirty years before.

These advances ensured that the Cape entered Union with the most sophisticated health care system in South Africa. To some extent this advantage was maintained for the Western Cape has remained in the forefront of medicine. But the backwardness of the other colonies, combined with the dominance of Afrikaner culture in the post-Union years meant that some of these gains were lost. A Department of Public Health was only established after the crisis of the Spanish flu epidemic in 1918, while the provision of health care to the majority of the population was a low priority for most of the next century.

Notes

1. D. Dyason, 'The Medical Profession in Colonial Victoria, 1834-1901' in R. McLeod and M. Lewis (eds), *Disease, Empire and Medicine* (London: Routledge, 1988),194–216.
2. E.H. Burrows, *A History of Medicine in South Africa* (Cape Town: Balkema, 1958), 79, 92–3.
3. Resident Magistrate, East London to the Col. Sec. 8 November 1853, Resident Magistrate, Port Elizabeth to the Col. Sec. 5 December 1853, Resident Magistrate, Grahamstown to the Col. Sec. 8 December 1853, CA, CO 640.
4. Secretary, CMC to Mr C. Cornish, Surgeon, Aliwal North 25 February 1851, CA, CO 606.
5. Secretary, CMC to the Col. Sec. 10 February 1852, CA, CO 606;

see also President, CMC to the Col. Sec. 13 May 1853, CA, CO 627.

6. Secretary, CMC to the Col. Sec. 18 February 1870, CA, CO 927.
7. H. White, Surgeon to the Resident Magistrate, Swellendam 3 December 1853, CA, CO 640.
8. Secretary, CMC to the Col. Sec. 27 January 1854, CA, CO 640; Secretary, CMC to the Col. Sec. 1 July 1862, CA, CO 797.
9. SC 25-1883, *Report of the Select Committee on Medical Law Reform*, 1-3, Ebden's evidence; Acting UCS to the Secretary, CMC 18 March 1880, CA, MC 12; Secretary, CMC to the Col. Sec. 23 September 1881, CA, MC 30.
10. Secretary, CMC to the Col. Sec. 11 May 1888, CA, MC 30.
11. Secretary, CMC to the Col. Sec. 6 October 1871, CA, CO 940; Secretary, CMC to the Col. Sec. 31 December 1875, CA, CO 1008.
12. Quinn vs Harris, 8 May 1884, CA, MC 17.
13. Dr Matthews to the Secretary, CMC 13 May 1884, CA, MC 17.
14. F. Rutherfoord Harris to the Secretary, CMC, undated, CA, MC 17.
15. Secretary, CMC to F. Rutherfoord Harris, 16 May 1884, CA, MC 30.
16. Secretary, CMC to the Col. Sec. 16 May 1884, 21 June 1884, CA, MC 30.
17. Secretary, CMC to the Col. Sec. 5 September 1884, CA, MC 30.
18. SC 25-1883, 2, Ebden's evidence.
19. R.J. Reinecke to the Secretary, CMC 4 November 1883, CA, MC 17.
20. UCS to the President, CMC 11 February 1890, CA, MC 13; Secretary, CMC to the State Attorney, OFS, 6 March 1890, CA, MC 30.
21. Secretary, CMC to the Col. Sec. 19 June 1877, CA, CO 1045.
22. SC 25-1883, 2, Ebden's evidence.
23. Secretary, CMC to the Col. Sec. 12 June 1863, CA, CO 972; Secretary, CMC to the Col. Sec. *c.*1873, CA, CO 955; Secretary, CMC to the Col. Sec. 24 February 1872, CA, CO 814.
24. Cape of Good Hope, *House of Assembly Debates*, 1886, 217; 1888, 288.
25. Secretary, CMC to the Col. Sec. 3 August 1888, CA, MC 30.
26. Cape of Good Hope, *House of Assembly Debates*, 1889, 203.
27. M. Ryan, *A History of Organised Pharmacy in South Africa 1885-1950* (Cape Town: Society for the History of Pharmacy in South Africa, 1986), 43–6.
28. SC 6-1890, *Report of the Select Committee on the Medical Practitioners' Bill*, 37-8, Dr C.L. Herman's evidence.

29. SC 6-1890, 37, Dr C.L. Herman's evidence.
30. SC 6-1890, 39, Dr C.L. Herman's evidence.
31. C. Searle, *The History of the Development of Nursing in South Africa 1652-1960* (Cape Town: Struik, 1965), 102–3; Burrows, *op. cit.* (note 2), 332–3.
32. *SAMR,* vi, 15, 10 August 1908, 237–9.
33. President, CMC to the UCS 5 June 1893 and reply 10 July 1893, CA, CO 1527.
34. BMA annual reports, 1890-91, UCT, BC 328.
35. Burrows, *op. cit.* (note 2), 350–2; C. Blumberg, 'The Provision of Medical Literature and Information in the Cape, 1827-1973', (unpublished M.Bibl. thesis, University of South Africa, 1974), 30.
36. T.J. Johnson and M. Caygill, 'The British Medical Association and its Overseas Branches: A Short History', *Journal of Imperial and Commonwealth History,* i (1972-3), 303–29.
37. *Ibid.*, 304, 306.
38. *Ibid.*, 303.
39. *Ibid.*, 303–8.
40. *SAMJ,* ii, 9 (January 1895), 262–6.
41. *SAMJ,* ii, 11 (March 1895), 301.
42. The first branch was established in Griqualand West in 1888, followed by the Cape of Good Hope (1889), Grahamstown and Eastern Cape (1893), Natal (1896), Border (1907), Transvaal (1907), Rhodesia (1912), OFS (1913); Johnson and Caygill, *op. cit.* (note 36), 314.
43. *SAMJ,* i, 1 (May 1893), 1. A South African Medical Association was founded in 1897 but it had little influence in Cape Town; Burrows, *op. cit.* (note 2), 360.
44. Darley-Hartley had previously published a *South African Medical Journal* (1884-1889) in East London but this had failed.
45. *SAMJ,* i, 1 (May 1893), 2.
46. *SAMR,* vi, 2 (25 January 1908), 24; *SAMR,* vi, 4 (25 February 1908), 62; *SAMR,* vi, 7 (10 April 1908), 10; *SAMR,* viii, 5 (12 March 1910), 49.
47. *SAMJ,* ii, 6 (October 1894), 147–8.
48. V. Bickford-Smith, *Ethnic Pride and Racial Prejudice in Victorian Cape Town: Group Identity and Social Practice, 1875-1902* (Cambridge: Cambridge University Press, 1995), 11. Numbers have been rounded off.
49. C. Simkins and E. van Heyningen, 'Fertility, Mortality and Migration in the Cape Colony, 1891-1904', *International Journal of African Historical Studies,* xx, 1 (1989), 86–8. Bickford-Smith

estimated that there were about 70,000 immigrants of all races in the city of whom about 36,000 were white. Bickford-Smith, *op. cit.* (note 48), 44.

50. This increase arose partly from the inclusion in the Colony of African territories on the eastern border.

51. G 13-1888, *Report of the District Surgeons for 1887*, 9.

52. M.W. Swanson, 'The Sanitation Syndrome: Bubonic Plague and Urban Native Policy in the Cape Colony, 1900-1909' *JAH*, xvi, 3 (1977), 387–410.

53. M. Naude, 'The Role of the Free Dispensary in Public Health in Cape Town' (unpublished B.A. thesis, UCT, 1987), 17–26.

54. *Ibid.*, Chapter 3.

55. *The Epidemic in Cape Town*, 1867-68 (Cape Town: Juta, 1868). They were unable to identify the fever which did not appear to be typhoid or typhus and they concluded that it was some form of continued fever.

56. *Cape Argus*, 21 July 1868. These figures are only intermittently available, scattered through the archival files; *Cape Times*, 14 October 1886. Of the first 474 interments in the cemetery, 250–300 had not been certified.

57. Burrows, *op. cit.* (note 2), 86–8.

58. G 91-1883, *Reports by Civil Commissioners and Residents Magistrates and District Surgeons for 1882.*

59. See Chapter 7.

60. *DSAB*, iii, 212.

61. Cape of Good Hope, *Civil Service List*, 1910; Application for appointment as medical officer of health, 13 March 1895, CA, CO 8048; *Cape Argus*, 18 July 1927; *SAMJ*, i, 14 (23 July 1927), 377.

62. G 19-1894, *Report on Public Health for 1893*, iii; G 24-1895, *Report on Public Health for 1894.*

63. *Civil Service List*, 1910, 157; G19-1894, iii.

64. *Cape Monthly Magazine*, viii (March 1874), 165.

65. G 67-1884, *Report of the District Surgeons for 1883*, 3.

66. Deaths per thousand.

67. G 14-1893, xv–xviii, xl.

68. G 14-1893, iii; G 19-1894, iv.

69. G 15-1891, *Public health reports for 1890*, 6; G 14-1893, xl–xli.

70. G 5-1894, *Report of the Colonial Bacteriological Institute for 1893*, 18-19; *Cape Times*, 6 January 1894; A.J. Gregory to the Col. Sec., 24 August 1894, CA, CO 7019; Cape of Good Hope, *House of Assembly Debates*, 1894, 477.

71. *SAMR*, xiii, 6 (27 March 1915), 84; Files relating to the

appointment of the medical officer of health, 1893, CA, CO 8048.

72. AB 5-1894, *Bill to Amend and Add to the Law with Regard to Public Health, and to Consolidate, Extend and Define the Jurisdiction and Powers of Local Authorities, in Respect to Matters Relating to Public Health.*

73. House of Assembly, *Debates*, 1894, 34–6; SC 3-1894, *Report of the Select Committee on the Public Health Bill*, 31, 34.

74. SC 3-1894, 33, 73, 117.

75. House of Assembly, *Debates*, 1892, 264.

76. A 8-1895, *Report of Births and Deaths Registration*, January-March, 1895, 11.

77. G 74-1896, *Report of the Medical Officer of Health for 1895*, 7, 22. For a full analysis of vital statistics derived from this legislation see Simkins and van Heyningen, *op. cit.* (note 49). Simkins points out that there are difficulties with Turner's methodology. More correctly, in the principal towns of the colony the total number of white deaths per 1,000 was 21.53. Had the age specific mortality rates in England and Wales from 1871 to 1881 applied, the figure would have been 18.82.

78. Memorandum of T.W. Smartt on the position of the medical officer of health, 27 June 1898, CA, MOH 338-P119c; H. de Smidt to the UCS, 9 July 1898, CA, MOH 338-P119c.

79. A.J. Gregory to the Col. Sec., 13 September 1901, CA, MOH 338-P119c.

80. A.J. Gregory to G. Pratt Yule, 21 March 1905, CA, MOH 79-320; A.J. Gregory to G. Pratt Yule, 22 September 1906, CA, MOH 320-G117b.

81. Dr G. Turner to the Col. Sec., 31 August 1900, CA, CO 7266.

82. CA, GN 53-1907 and GN 54-1907.

83. A.J. Gregory to G. Pratt Yule, 26 May 1908, CA. MOH 415-P119a.

84. List of permanent staff, 11 March 1903, CA, MOH 79-320; A.J. Gregory to the UCS, 21 March 1904, CA, MOH 78-311.

85. Memorandum on the provisions of the new Public Health Act, n.d. (*c.* 1906), CA, MOH 328-L117l.

86. H. Phillips, '"Black October": The Impact of the Spanish Influenza Epidemic of 1918 on South Africa' *Archives Year Book for South African History*, i (1990), 203–6.

87. R.M. Packard, *White Plague, Black Labor: Tuberculosis and the Political Economy of Health and Disease in South Africa* (Berkeley: University of California Press, 1989); S. Marks, and N. Andersson, 'Typhus and Social Control: South Africa, 1917-50' in McLeod and Lewis, *op. cit.* (note 1), 219–41.

88. Bickford-Smith, *op. cit.* (note 48), 32, 86, 105, 192.

89. Death notice, CA, MOOC 6/9/828-1743.

90. D. Williams, *Umfundisi: A Biography of Tiyo Soga, 1829-1871*
(Lovedale: Lovedale Press, 1978), 87–8, 118, Liquidation of estate,
CA, MOOC 13/1/3856-133.

91. *SAMR*, xiv, 15 (12 August 1916), 232–3; Williams, *op. cit.*
(note 90), 87–8, 118; Liquidation of estate, CA, MOOC
13/1/3856-133.

92. J. Wells, *Stewart of Lovedale: The Life of James Stewart, D.D., M.D.*
(London: Hodder & Stoughton, 1908), 94–6; S.M. Brock, 'James
Stewart and Lovedale: A Reappraisal of Missionary Attitudes and
African Response in the Eastern Cape, South Africa, 1870-1895',
(unpublished Ph.D. thesis, University of Edinburgh, 1974).

93. L. Bean and E. van Heyningen (eds), *The Letters of Dr Jane Elizabeth
Waterston 1866-1905* (Cape Town: Van Riebeeck Society, 1983), 21,
22.

94. *Ibid.*, 196.

95. For Waterston's involvement in the Jameson Raid and her relations
with Sir Alfred Milner, South African High Commissioner,
see G. Shaw (ed.), *The Garrett Papers* (Cape Town: Van Riebeeck
Society, 1984).

96. Bean and van Heyningen, *op. cit.* (note 93), 39, 208.

97. *DSAB*, i, 1–4; G. Lewis, *Between the Wire and the Wall: A History of
South African 'Coloured' Politics* (Cape Town: David Philip, 1987),
27 ff.; R.E. van der Ross, *The Rise and Decline of Apartheid: A Study
of Political Movements Among the Coloured People of South Africa,
1880-1985* (Cape Town: Tafelberg, 1986), 28 ff.

98. E.B. van Heyningen, 'Public Health and Society in Cape Town,
1880-1910' (unpublished Ph.D. thesis, University of Cape Town,
1989), 167–225.

8

Mineral Wealth and Medical Opportunity

Harriet Deacon, Elizabeth van Heyningen,
Sally Swartz and Felicity Swanson

With the increase in population and in colonial revenues after the
discovery of diamonds and gold in the last quarter of the
nineteenth century, public and private hospitals proliferated,
particularly in larger centres such as Cape Town. The numbers of
practitioners engaged in public health also increased. Perhaps as
important, doctors were now accepted as skilled professionals
and remunerated accordingly. At the same time there was also a
greater demand for doctors in the employment of business and
industry, particularly the insurance industry and the railways.
These opportunities for salaried employment somewhat reduced
doctors' professional autonomy and occasionally encouraged
intra-professional squabbles. Yet they also provided a springboard
for general professional regulation, growing professional status in
specialisms like psychiatry, and a solid base for the economic
survival of country doctors.

Before the late 1860s the Cape had a relatively stagnant economy.
Although the colony had attained representative government in 1854
and responsible government in 1872, revenues remained too
restricted to attract either capital or immigrants in substantial
numbers. The change came with the discovery of diamonds on the
Cape-Orange Free State border in 1868, and the discovery of gold on
the Witwatersrand in 1886. The prosperity derived from diamonds
was limited but it provided a welcome avenue of employment for
colonists. Indeed, the flow of people to Kimberley was so great at one
stage that many of the official services, such as the underpaid police,
were denuded of staff.[1] Diamond mining, however, was an
economically unstable operation until Cecil John Rhodes and his De
Beers Company had established a monopoly by about 1880. Gold,
on the other hand, brought greater stability and prosperity. Although
the mines were on the Witwatersrand, in the South African Republic,

223

the Cape profited as well. For many years it was the base from which goods of all kinds were transported to the Rand, and the building of the railway in 1892 gave the colony a lead over alternative routes for some time. Gold also brought immigrants, many of whom found employment in the Cape, never reaching the Witwatersrand. Much mining profit was invested in the colony, mainly in property and financial institutions. Colonial revenues increased considerably, making money available to improve both public and private services, including health care.

With the increase in population and in colonial revenues, public and private hospitals proliferated, particularly in larger centres such as Cape Town. By 1900 Cape Town had a Lock Hospital (for the treatment of venereal diseases), the City Hospital (for infectious diseases), the Valkenberg Asylum, plans for the Alexandra Hospital and a number of suburban cottage hospitals and private sanatoria, in addition to the Old and New Somerset Hospitals and Robben Island institutions. Other centres showed the same proliferation of medical services.[2] Although in 1865 there were only 143 doctors recorded in the census, by 1891 there were nearly 550 doctors on the Cape register, with twenty doctors in Kimberley, thirteen in Port Elizabeth, twelve in Grahamstown and nearly forty in Cape Town.[3]

The numbers of practitioners engaged in public health also increased. By 1909 the central government employed four doctors in the Health Department while the Hospitals and Asylums section employed another thirteen doctors, as well as a number of nurses and a substantial lay staff. Most towns of any size in the colony appointed medical officers of health at least in an advisory capacity. Perhaps as important, doctors were now accepted as skilled professionals and remunerated accordingly. In 1900 George Turner, the colonial medical officer of health, was earning the substantial salary of £1,000 a year. Nine years later this had increased to £1,200.[4]

At the same time there was a greater demand for doctors in the employment of business and industry. The insurance industry, already one of the more flourishing sectors of business in the colony, grew apace with a consequent need for more medical personnel. Railway lines proliferated. Every centre had its own list of railway doctors. By 1899, for instance, the opening of railway workshops in Mafeking led to the engagement of two doctors, one of whom also acted as district surgeon. This tiny border settlement, which had virtually no medical facilities in 1891, boasted at least three doctors and a hospital by the time the South African War started in October 1899.[5] Along with the creation of the De Beers monopoly over diamond mining in Kimberley came the establishment of tightly enclosed compounds for black labourers. Both they and other De Beers employees had recourse only to practitioners on the company list. Colonial doctors were often closely associated with this economic expansion, lending middle-class respectability to processes which brutally incorporated indigenous societies into waged labour.

Cape doctors were not simply the handmaidens of colonial capital, although there were clear instances where doctors helped mining companies to justify and perpetuate the harsh treatment of mineworkers. In the relationship between doctors and commercial employers, the opportunities for salaried employment somewhat reduced doctors' professional autonomy and occasionally encouraged intra-professional squabbles. Yet these opportunities also provided a springboard for general professional regulation, growing professional status in specialisms like psychiatry and formed a solid base for the economic survival of country doctors.

Employment in commerce

From the beginning of the insurance business at the Cape in the early nineteenth century, life insurance companies provided part-time employment for some doctors. In the 1830s, the new Cape of Good Hope Fire and Life Assurance Company appointed Samuel Bailey as their doctor, and in the 1840s three new companies appointed Louis Liesching, Pappe, Fleck, Laing, Bickersteth and Chiappini as doctors.[6] These doctors also continued to practice privately in Cape Town. Bailey and Bickersteth held hospital posts; Bailey was surgeon of the Vaccine Institution and district surgeon of Cape Town (until 1840),[7] and Pappe was physician to the European Sick and Burial Society and the S.A. Private Widow's Fund.[8] In a confidential report on Bickersteth in 1843 or 1844, Governor Napier noted that Bickersteth was 'obliged to search for private practice' as his salary of £200 per annum as resident assistant surgeon to Bailey in the Old Somerset Hospital was too low to 'bind ["a skilful surgeon"] to constant unremitting attention and attendance within the walls of a hospital'.[9] Insurance, charity and hospital work were thus often combined with each other and with private practice to allow Cape doctors the income they needed as 'professional gentlemen'.

The records of Chiappini's medical practice from the mid-1840s[10] show how doctors worked for insurance companies at that time. In the first year of his work for the Mutual Life Assurance Company, from June 1845 to May 1846, Chiappini examined about 260 prospective clients. By the end of his records in December 1851, he had examined a total of 510 prospective clients for the company, an average of around eighty per annum. Both Chiappini and Bickersteth examined prospective clients, and sometimes disagreed about whether they should be insured by the company. On examining the young Lotz in 1845, for example, Chiappini wished to reject him because he suspected disease in Lotz's right lung, but Bickersteth disagreed and the man was accepted. Although we do not know how much he earned from examining insurance applicants, Chiappini may have found his insurance work useful in his private practice as he noted down for his own records not only the sum for which their lives were insured but also the Cape Town applicants' usual doctors. The latter information would have given him the opportunity to offer his services to those applicants who did not yet have a doctor for general purposes, or whose doctor had recently died or moved away. Insurance practice thus gave private practitioners free advertising and exposure to new clients.

The Mutual Life Assurance Society (Old Mutual) remained the mainstay of insurance work until 1883, for most of the other life insurance societies were relatively small and financially unstable. Between 1845 and 1910, however, the Old Mutual employed a total of only seven doctors, and in two cases the job passed from father to son. Antonio Lorenzo Chiappini succeeded Peter, while C.T. Anderson followed his father, G.E.C. Anderson, in 1902, after the latter retired with fifteen years service behind him.[11] In 1883 the Melbourne-based Colonial Mutual Life Assurance Society set up shop in South Africa. This initiative was almost certainly inspired by the discovery of diamonds in 1868 and the hope of better prospects in the colony.[12] By the end of the 1880s other companies were following. In some cases, as with Dr J.R Zeederberg of Paarl, doctors also acted as agents for the companies, recruiting business in a double capacity.[13] It was this proliferation of branches and the increase in the numbers of members which brought in additional employment for doctors.

Railway doctors

The economic and social transformation of South Africa as a result of the mineral revolution also opened up other employment opportunities to the medical profession. Although the first railway line, from Cape Town to Wellington, was opened in 1863, with a suburban service in the Peninsula following the next year, substantial expansion came well after the discovery of diamonds. This was partly because of the mountainous terrain through which lines had to be

Illustration 8.1a
Railway appointments

The expansion of the Cape Government Railways opened up new
opportunities for country doctors. Although salaries were often poor,
they provided at basic income which could usually be supplemented
through private practice. (SAMR, 27 August 1909)

AMENDED NOTICE.

EENDE KUIL—GRAAFWATER CONSTRUCTION.

MEDICAL APPOINTMENT.

Applications are invited for the position of Construction Medical Officer on the above Railway. The
successful applicant will be required to attend to
Construction employees and their families between
Eende Kuil and Graafwater, and to reside at any point
along the line most convenient for the work, which will
be at the discretion of the Department. Hut or tent
accommodation, riding horse, and medicines will be
provided by the Department. Private practice will not
be allowed. The salary attached to the office is
£20 per month. Applications, with copies of
references, should be forwarded in time to reach this
Office not later than 12 noon on the 1st September,
1909.

ALAN GRANT-DALTON,
Engineer-in-Chief.

Office of the Engineer-in-Chief,
Cape Government Railways,
Cape Town.
17th August, 1909.

laid. The first train only reached Kimberley in 1885 but the line to
the Rand was completed much more rapidly, arriving at the
goldfields in September 1892. By this time other lines had
proliferated through the colony, for the first time putting the Eastern
Cape in easy reach of the western regions, and integrating the more

Illustration 8.1b
Railway appointments continued

Cape Government Railways.

MEDICAL APPOINTMENT.

Applications are invited for the position of Railway Medical Officer for the District Huguenot (exclusive) to Porterville-road (inclusive) ; to reside in Wellington.

Salary, £75 per annum and £2 2s. for every Railway Midwifery case attended under the Regulations.

Applications, stating whether married or single, and accompanied by copies of testimonials, should be addressed to and reach the Undersigned before Noon on the 9th September, 1909.

The successful Candidate will be required to take up his duties on the 1st October, 1909.

Further particulars can be obtained on application to the Undersigned.

By order,
CHAS. DRUMMOND.
Secretary.

Railway Sick Fund Board Office,
Cape Town,
16th August, 1909.

isolated rural districts into the larger economy.[14]

These developments did not occur without injury and some loss of life, making the provision of medical care for the labourers desirable. Moreover, for much of the time immigrant European labour was used for building the railway, in contrast to road building which was performed largely by convict labour. This was probably another inducement to furnish adequate medical care, for such labour could not be attracted without facilities comparable to those available at home. By the end of the century the Cape Government Railways had become an institution which embraced the families of railway employees as well, making medical care available to wives and children. All these developments ensured that there was ample work for a number of doctors in the colony.

The Cape Government Railways medical service was, 'Omega' noted in 1895, 'the only body of anything like respectable dimensions under an organised system of administration.'[15] The system was a mix of club and departmental organisation. The Railway Sick Fund was intended to provide employees and their families with medical assistance and to make provision for sick pay for those unable to work. At the same time medical officers had administrative duties, supervising sanitary arrangements and examining candidates for employment. There were, in addition, five medical boards managing the Fund, and appointing the medical officers. But the latter had no distinct tenure of office, being essentially contract workers, the only vestige of status being the right to free rail passes. Emoluments varied greatly, some receiving houses or a housing allowance and in some cases a cart and horse allowance as well. The areas which they supervised also varied considerably in size and character, some including large country districts, others being purely urban.

Railway doctors were allowed to practise privately but the range of their duties often made this difficult; 'in fact, it is only the ever present fear of those extraordinary waves of depression which at times reduce private practice (or payment for it) to a vanishing point, that induces the good men to hold on to their railway billets.' Boards were not consistent in the way they made their appointments, some calling for tenders, others appointing their officers on fixed salaries; some granted privileges, others did not. (These medical boards were not headed by medical men – an object of criticism.) Their situation was not unlike that of the district surgeon, for they were paid a flat rate, apart from midwifery, and had 'to attack things requiring any amount of skill and time and quite out of the run of everyday work, without one penny of extra remuneration'. The tender system of appointment was particularly criticised, for it was argued that it was likely to attract the black sheep of the profession.[16]

Despite their complaints about the hardships of railway service, railway doctors could enjoy a comfortable position in their communities. In Mafeking the two brothers, doctors William and Tom Hayes, were prominent members of the small society. Each acted as district surgeon at various times and had a number of private patients in the town. During the long siege of October 1899 to May 1900 a number of patients remarked on their kindness and care. As both were virulently jingoistic, Boer patients received little of this sympathy. Dr William Hayes complained that Boer women were dirty and ungrateful.[17] An irascible man, he was frequently in conflict

Illustration 8.2
Staff, Victoria Hospital, Lovedale.

The Victoria Hospital (1908), attached to the Lovedale Mission Institution in the Eastern Cape, was one of the first in South Africa to train black health care workers, opening up new opportunities for educated black men and women. Here some of the staff is shown with Dr MacVicar (1871-1949), the medical superintendent at Lovedale from 1902 to 1939, renowned for his work on tuberculosis. (CMM: A 35)

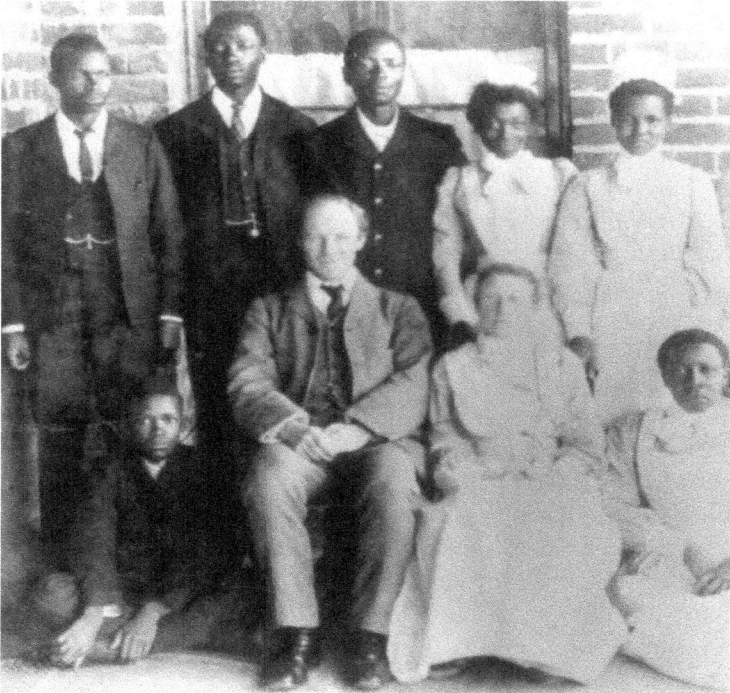

with other members of the small community and at least some of these quarrels arose from the tensions within the Railway Division.[18] His altercations with the volunteer nurses of the Victoria Hospital, on the other hand, were more probably related to the failure of the volunteers to accord him the deference which doctors of the day expected from the nursing staff.[19]

Kimberley and mining medicine

The discovery of diamonds in 1868 not only gave a boost to the Cape economy but also resulted in an influx of immigrants to a previously thinly populated area. Impoverished colonials and hopeful diggers from overseas swarmed to the diamond fields, along with blacks who traded their labour for guns and other goods. The most important diamond fields were located in a relatively arid area, some distance from the nearest water supply on the Vaal River.[20] Unregulated digging, the lack of water, poor sanitation and hastily erected dwellings, combined with the heat, led to a soaring mortality rate[21] and offered new opportunities for the medical profession. Within a short time Kimberley acquired one of the largest congregations of doctors in the Cape. Many of them, Burrows suggests, were a 'band of international adventurers who viewed their medical qualifications as no more than a comfortable "extra" to the more exciting task of living a full life.'[22]

The presence of this substantial wealth was a considerable attraction to the medical profession in Kimberley. A number of politically- and business-minded doctors congregated round Cecil John Rhodes, including his close associate, Dr Leander Starr Jameson,[23] and Hans Sauer,[24] Thomas Smartt[25] and Frederick Rutherford Harris.[26] The financial pickings were considerable and it was claimed that 'a doctor's assistant could earn £1,100 in seven months'.[27] The American Dr Prince's practice was reputed to be particularly prosperous and his partner, Dr Jameson, had an income of £5,000 a year.[28]

Jameson's career was fairly typical of these doctor-adventurers, if somewhat more inglorious. Born on 9 February 1853, the youngest son of an erratic and impecunious Scottish lawyer and journalist, Jameson grew up as one of the 'genteel poor'. After his father's death the family had sufficient resources to provide him with an unusually good medical education, which gave him an MD from London University, in addition to the more usual MRCS. Although he was well placed to achieve success in the competitive metropolitan medical world,[29] in 1878 Jameson abandoned this opportunity for the freer, more uncertain prospect of Africa.

Jameson seems to have been well adapted to colonial life. Despite his lively, dapper charm, which ensured his popularity with his patients, he had little taste for the conventions of middle-class Victorian life. Like Rhodes, Jameson preferred an austere bachelor existence – he admitted to his brother that he had little taste for marriage.[30] As a young man hunting, playing poker, travelling rough through the African veld, lording it over the local inhabitants and discussing 'big schemes' with Rhodes all had greater appeal.

By the time Jameson arrived in Kimberley the roughest days of the mining camp were over but mortality rates were still extremely high. There was plenty of work for an energetic young doctor. Jameson entered the lucrative practice of Dr James Perrot Prince, derived partly from treating mine labourers.[31] From the first, Jameson also treated the elite of the neighbourhood including, on one occasion, President Brand of the Orange Free State. Jameson apparently believed in the psychological ascendancy of the doctor over the patient. This included outward display for he drove 'a very smart victoria with two very fast black horses'.[32] There is a misogynist thread in Jameson's career, in his remarks in a sexual harassment case in which Jameson gave evidence, in his allusions to 'hysterical' women, to 'anxious ladies' with their 'imaginary' ailments, to a 'fanciful' patient recommended to rub a back pain with a brick. Skilled he may have been but style was crucial in establishing Jameson as the 'first doctor in Kimberley' – his cures were 'marvellous', his operations 'miraculous'.[33]

Although Jameson was clearly popular amongst the society doctors in Kimberley, he never became a member of the medical establishment of the colony, by contributing to the local medical journal or participating in the meetings of the local branches of the British Medical Association. He remained on the Cape register until 1911, but from 1890 he practised medicine only intermittently, mainly treating favoured patients like Rhodes. Exploration in Matabeleland (Zimbabwe) and politics became his chosen occupations. His poor judgement led him to undertake the Jameson Raid in early January 1896, leading a band of Rhodes's men over the Transvaal border to assist a rising of *Uitlanders* (mainly British immigrants) to overthrow the Kruger government. The failure of this incompetent enterprise severely damaged Rhodes's plans for expansion in Africa and he was forced to resign as prime minister of the Cape Colony. This did not entirely dampen Jameson's fortunes for he became prime minister himself in 1904, profiting from the disenfranchisement of the Cape rebels (colonial Boers who took up arms on behalf of the Boer republics) during the South African War of 1899-1902.[34]

The poor sanitary condition of Kimberley which gave Jameson his early opportunities also encouraged the establishment of hospitals. The first hospital in Kimberley, a rudimentary tent structure, was opened within a short time of the start of the diggings, followed by the Dry Diggings Hospital which was only slightly less primitive. In 1872 a somewhat more solid building, the Diggers Central Hospital, was erected in the town, catering for the poorest of the diggers, black and white. In 1874 the Provincial (Carnarvon) Hospital was established, soon staffed by the Anglican sisters of the Community of St Michael and All Angels.[35] In 1882 the two hospitals were amalgamated to form the Kimberley Hospital, double the size of the New Somerset Hospital, with a staff of almost fifty. Given the presence of a number of able doctors, the Kimberley Hospital earned the reputation of being the most advanced institution in the country and it was the first to make specialist appointments, in ophthalmology and pathology.[36] Erected during years of increasing racism, from the start the hospital was segregated racially and by class, with paying and non-paying patients in different wards.

Mine labourers did not benefit from the quality of the expertise at the Kimberley Hospital. Black mine labourers fared particularly badly, especially after De Beers Company had established a monopoly control over the Kimberley mines. In order to prevent the theft of diamonds, the mining industry introduced a compound system in which black workers were effectively incarcerated for the entire period of their employment contract. They were forced to submit to body searches to prevent them from hiding diamonds and, when they were ill, they were treated at hospitals in the compound.

Accidents were one source of health problems. By the 1890s there were six to seven fatalities per thousand employees and over twelve per thousand underground. The main cause of death amongst miners, however, was pneumonia, contributing to two-thirds of the fatalities in De Beers compound hospitals in the 1890s. A poor mining environment and overcrowded living conditions led to a situation in which company death rates were more than double those of the town.[37] Although doctors must have been aware of these conditions, self-interest as acolytes of Rhodes was often the first priority.

This self-interest was demonstrated most starkly in the infamous smallpox incident of 1883-1884. When smallpox broke out amongst black labourers travelling to Kimberley, the disease was diagnosed as 'a bulbous disease of the skin allied to pemphigus', infectious only to blacks. The victims were isolated on a local farm but, without proper checks, inevitably some trickled into the mine compounds. De Beers Company and the Town Council jointly took considerable effort to

Illustration 8.3
The Claremont Sanitarium

The luxurious Claremont Sanitarium was a striking example of the
opportunities opening up to medical entrepreneurs from the 1890s.
South Africa's bracing climate was regarded as particularly healthy
for tubercular patients – a feature which doctors were keen to
exploit. (NLSA: PHA, Cape Town, Claremont)

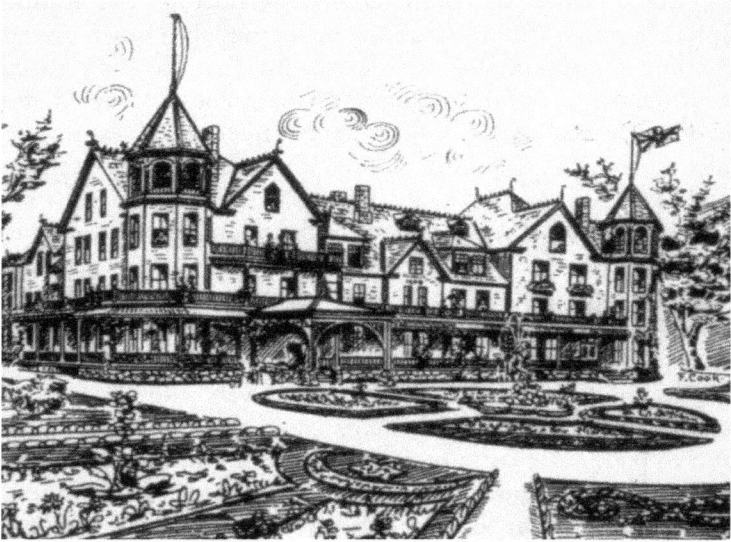

allay the fears of the mine owners and whites generally, that the
disease was smallpox, then prevalent in the country.[38] Mine officials
took no steps to quarantine the victims when the disease reached the
compounds and the epidemic spread rapidly. The local medical
officer of health, Dr Hans Sauer, was only able to introduce effective
controls after whites in the town began to fall ill. By the time the
epidemic had been defeated, over two thousand people had been
infected, with at least twenty-five per cent dying. To the last, mine
doctors continued to maintain their original diagnosis. Amongst
those most active in the cover-up was Jameson. Sister Henrietta
Stockdale, matron of the Kimberley Hospital, often revered as the
founder of nursing in South Africa, played her part by attempting to
exclude Sauer from inspecting the first patients in the hospital.[39]

The discovery of gold in the Transvaal soon attracted the medical

234

adventurers away from the Cape, leaving a small but significant core of career-minded doctors in Kimberley. Some were active in political life but, more important for the development of the Cape medical profession, they contributed to the evolution of the profession. With their enthusiasm the Griqualand West Medical Association was established in 1887, and the first South African Medical Congress was held in Kimberley in 1892.

It was also in Kimberley that another aspect of health care was introduced to South Africa – the hospital as luxury hotel. The Sanatorium in Belgravia, Kimberley's wealthiest suburb, was a handsome building, sponsored by De Beers Mining Company and initiated by Rhodes. The latter explained:

> The Sanatorium is a bit of a hobby of mine. I have always thought that Kimberley would be an admirable place for people with chest complaints from Home, if only there were sufficient and proper accommodation. The experience of many has been that this climate has been very successful in such complaints, and doctors all agree that Kimberley is a good place for a Sanatorium.[40]

In Kimberley, then, could be found the extreme ends of the scale of health care in the Cape in the late-nineteenth century. On the one hand black mine workers had one of the highest death rates in the country; on the other the wealthy could obtain the best and most luxurious care available. The medical profession was an integral part of this structure. While company doctors were more concerned with the interests of their employers than with those of the labourers, the medical profession of the town shared substantially in the profits to be made from mining. The status of the profession was improved as a result of practitioners' participation in the development of Kimberley, for many of the doctors moved in the same circles as the mining magnates, but neither the town nor the black labourers benefited much. This was a pattern which was to be further entrenched in the twentieth century throughout South Africa.

Professional specialisation

The mineral revolution, which brought immigrants and capital to South Africa, enabled a handful of doctors to specialise in particular branches of medicine. Ophthalmology was one of the first to emerge. We have seen that Dr FitzGerald at the Grey Hospital in King William's Town built his reputation partly on his skill as an eye surgeon. In Cape Town towards the end of the century Dr Andrew

Christopher Jackson also had standing as an ophthalmologist. He had need of this regard for he was a man of two worlds, a black man delicately maintaining his status in a racist, predominantly white medical world. Born in the West Indies, Jackson had trained in Britain and immigrated to the Cape in 1880. For a brief time he flirted with a career in Johannesburg, but the extremes of racism in the Transvaal drove him back to Cape Town. Here he lived in prosperous Buitenkant Street, on the fringes of the poor inner city area of District Six, a location which symbolised his own social position. In his private life he was active in promoting nascent black consciousness, working closely with the Trinidadian attorney, Henry Sylvester Williams. The latter was the first black man to practise law in South Africa, and he was one of the founders of the Pan-African movement. Despite such activities, which would have been anathema to the majority of the medical fraternity, Jackson retained the respect of the profession as his obituary in the *SAMJ* indicates.[41]

The private sanatorium

Kimberley was not the only town to acquire a private sanatorium. From the 1890s a number sprang up in different parts of the colony, designed to attract the more affluent middle classes or tubercular immigrants. Cape Town possessed several such places, including the Hygeia Sanitarium in the Gardens district of the town. The Hygeia offered modern treatment using electrical therapy of various kinds, as well as massage, 'medical gymnastics' and 'physical culture'. Rates were relatively modest at £3 13s 6d a week inclusive.[42]

Better known was the Claremont Medical and Surgical Sanitarium in Cape Town. This substantial institution was opened in 1897, funded largely by the Wessels family of Cape Town, but backed by the Medical and Missionary Benevolent Association of Michigan, United States of America. This philanthropic support was somewhat at odds with the custom which the sanatorium was seeking, for it advertised widely, emphasising that it was 'a well equipped scientific medical establishment', with both lady and gentlemen physicians on the premises.[43] This was not a 'mere health resort', another advertisement explained, but was a 'restful, homelike place for those who do not consider themselves sick, but who are in need of rest'.[44] The Claremont Sanitarium lasted a mere three years, for it was taken over by the British military authorities during the South African War and never recovered its initial popularity. Eventually it went bankrupt and the building was destroyed by fire in 1905.

During the course of the 1890s similar institutions sprang up in a number of the country towns. Dr G.A. Heberden started The Home in Barkly West, offering 'air dry and bracing', while The Poplars in Middelburg promoted itself as a 'private home for phthisical patients.'[45] The various hot springs in the Western Cape were yet another source of revenue to the medical entrepreneur.

Psychiatry as a medical specialty

Apart from surgery, psychiatry was the first specialty to be supported from public funds. The history of psychiatry in nineteenth-century British colonies has now begun to receive some attention from social historians.[46] The Cape is no exception. Recent work by Moyle, Deacon, Swanson, Foster and Swartz has traced the development of a racialised psychiatry in the Cape during the course of the nineteenth century, challenging the picture drawn by Minde and others of a progressive and scientific psychiatry.[47] However the development of a racist psychiatry is not the only interesting feature of the psychiatric specialism within the Cape medical profession of the nineteenth century. In this section we explore how Cape doctors used asylum appointments to carve out a position for themselves as specialist psychiatrists.

The Robben Island asylum[48] was the most prominent psychiatric institution at the Cape. It had been established as part of a trio of hospitals on the island in 1846 under the direction of a doctor, John Birtwhistle, who had no previous experience of tending the insane and an old-fashioned punitive approach to therapeutics. In 1862, after much parliamentary concern over the way Birtwhistle and his successor, Minto, managed the asylum, Dr William Edmunds was appointed as Surgeon Superintendent. He was an ex-military surgeon who, like his predecessor, had been working in the Eastern Cape before his appointment. He had no formal training in asylum management, but he was a knowledgeable and well-read man who sought to apply the latest British principles of asylum management to the establishment on Robben Island – then the only Cape asylum. This was in marked contrast to the attitude of most other doctors appointed to the island asylum during the nineteenth century. But it is interesting in that it prefigured the approach of Dodds and other asylum doctors to the treatment of white patients in the 1890s and after. These 'progressive' approaches towards the treatment of insanity, which all emphasised cure, were firmly entwined with the ambitious professional aims of a group – those now known as psychiatrists. While these men sought professional recognition as specialists, they were often looked down upon by the medical profession as a whole – then and perhaps even today.

Edmunds used his position as Surgeon Superintendent of the Island Infirmary to promote the use of the 'moral management' system in the asylum – a system which emphasised psychological treatment and the possibility of cure for the insane. This was in line with the demands of the colonial parliament (constituted in 1854) and the imperial government in London. The popularity of asylum reform was tied up with a general attempt to emphasize the humanitarian nature of colonial rule and colonial institutions, and specifically to demonstrate the modernity and political maturity of colonies like the Cape. The colonial government at the Cape thus willingly allocated Edmunds the funds to apply to the asylum some of the principles of moral management, which depended on the use of seclusion cells rather than straitjackets, high staff–patient ratios and the creation of an attractive garden environment. It was a great blow to both the colonial office in Cape Town and to Edmunds himself when, in 1863, London's inspection of the asylum, part of an imperial inspection tour, found evidence that these reforms had not been sufficient to remove physical punishment and to alleviate poor conditions of care in the asylum. This setback caused Edmunds and the colonial office to redouble their efforts to make the island asylum a model of humanitarian reform.

Because of the island situation, Edmunds had no opportunity to pursue his private practice while in the asylum post. He was responsible for the chronic sick and leper hospitals on the island as well, which must have taken up much of the time he was free from his duties at the asylum. His salary was thus higher than that of a district surgeon but his income may not have been. The importance of the asylum position for a man like Edmunds, therefore, lay less in the financial opportunities it might have offered, than in the chance to show that colonial asylum management could be modelled on modernity – the British humanitarian template. This was important for the colony's self-image but also for the professional image of the Cape doctor. Military doctors held no high status in Britain, and doctors who emigrated to colonial territories in particular were often thought to be the worst of the professional crop. By showing that Cape medical institutions could be run by the British book, Edmunds was able not only to improve the image of the asylum within the colony (thus attracting more wealthy patients) but also, if briefly, to improve the image of the Cape medical profession as modern and humane. His colleagues at Robben Island were much less successful at these goals, when indeed they shared them. Some, like Minto in the 1850s, used their position on the Island to start up private businesses like fish-curing, and others, like the asylum doctors of the early twentieth century, saw the (then largely black) asylum as a stepping stone to more prestigious posts in mainland asylums for white patients.

After Edmunds' death in 1872, the island asylum continued for some years to attract middle-class white patients and to treat them with the care thought to be necessary in the moral management model. By the late 1870s, however, the mood among Cape asylum doctors - and now there was another Cape asylum, at Grahamstown - was changing. Increasingly, the cure of the black insane was thought to rest, not on psychological treatment through 'moral management', but on physical restraint. This racist argument for the reduction of curative facilities for black 'lunatics' - who were increasingly held on the Island rather than in mainland asylums - resulted in a gradual decrease in the attention paid to Robben Island asylum and the status of its asylum doctors after 1880. For professional recognition, Cape doctors had to seek posts in mainly white asylums.

Valkenberg and the modernisation of psychiatric care

Sally Swartz has documented an important change in Cape government policy on the care of the insane from 1889.[49] This year marked the appointment of an Inspector of Asylums, and ushered in a period of legislative reform and the rapid expansion of asylum accommodation. Increased financial provision, improved legislation, better staff and institutional management of Cape asylums now made it easier for asylums to attract and retain good staff and improved the professional standing of asylum doctors. The difficulty of actually curing the insane remained a stumbling block, however, and this kept the status of medical jobs in asylums fairly low, relative to other medical institutions.

The first Inspector of Asylums, appointed in 1889, was a man named William John Dodds. Before his appointment to this post, and to the superintendency of the planned new Valkenberg Asylum, he had been Deputy Superintendent at Montrose Royal Asylum in Scotland. He was highly qualified academically, having M.B., C.M., M.D. and D.Sc. degrees behind his name, and was a meticulous and energetic administrator. His arrival at the Cape, together with the passing of the 1891 and 1897 Lunacy Acts, began the process of giving professional status to asylum medicine and provided the framework for reform. Dodds' asylum reports, providing a detailed

239

Illustration 8.4
Medical Superintendent and male nurses,
Fort Beaufort Hospital, 1894

The mental institution at Fort Beaufort was designed entirely for black patients, but the staff were all white. The distinctive uniforms worn by the nurses, bearing a close resemblance to police or military uniforms, suggest the coercive nature of control at the asylum. (CMM: N 20)

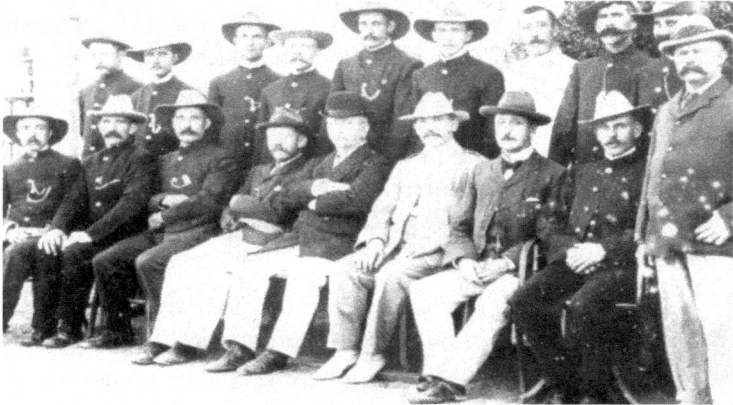

and lengthy record of asylum inspections and recommending improvements to asylum conditions, set the stage for a decade of vigorous reform of the colony's institutional provision for the insane. He made it clear from the beginning that, while lip-service was being paid to the tenets of 'moral management', existing asylums were predominantly custodial rather than curative and that they were also overcrowded, unhygienic and under-funded. The reforms that he put into motion helped not only to improve asylum conditions (albeit mainly for white patients) but also to establish a Cape psychiatric profession around a discourse of scientific classification and cure of the insane.

The creation of a psychiatric profession at the Cape was enabled not only by improved asylum conditions, but also by a revised legal framework for the care of the insane and a growing community of asylum doctors at the Cape who engaged in academic and managerial debates among themselves and with asylum doctors abroad. The 1891 and 1897 Lunacy Acts brought the colony into line with legal and medical practices around the treatment of insanity in Britain, although they did not provide for the accommodation of the insane on such a large scale. Dodds campaigned for changes to the 1891 legislation which would allow for temporary release of patients, urgent admissions and the admission of voluntary patients. Dodds's lobbying, and the tenor of the legislation, spelt out what had been a feature of Cape lunacy policy from the beginning – the centrality of medical doctors in the state-sponsored care of the insane. It also highlighted what was now felt to be the important position of doctors as specialists in the treatment of the insane, the difficult working conditions they faced and the need for appropriate legal and medical spaces within which they could perform their work. By assuming in his lobbying activities that his audience would respect specialized medical knowledge in this way, Dodds was making a political claim for a professional identity in relation to asylum medical practice.

One of the places in which Dodds and other doctors were able to cement this claim was in the new asylum at Valkenberg, opened in Cape Town in 1891. Valkenberg was the country's first whites-only asylum, and the first building specially designed to accommodate the insane. (Fort Beaufort, the first asylum solely for the black insane, was opened in an old barracks in 1894.) In 1910 the *Cape Town Guide* wrote of Valkenberg's 'picturesque position on the summit of a gentle eminence overlooking a landscape that, except for the mighty mass of Table Mountain overshadowing it, might well be an English one.' The buildings, setting, recreational activities (including garden parties and cricket matches) and the exclusively white patient body established Valkenberg as a colonial showpiece of the British model of treating the insane. It was particularly important for the psychiatric profession at the Cape that Valkenberg was deliberately associated with curing the insane, which aided the construction of asylum medical practice as skilled work, rather than custodial gaol-keeping. Those patients who did not fit into the category of early or curable cases were simply transferred to other asylums, particularly to Robben Island.

The rise of a professional psychiatry at the Cape was also helped by the growth of a professional discourse about the insane, centering around diagnostic and aetiological classifications of insanity. This helped to distinguish psychiatrists from general practitioners, and also to establish connections between Cape psychiatrists and those in higher-status places like British asylums. This professional discourse was used in Dodds' asylum reports, which contained numerous statistical tables recording the types of insanity, in academic meetings of the local British Medical Association branch and in academic journals such as the *British Journal of Mental Science* and the local *South African Medical Record* and *South African Medical Journal.* The sharing of asylum reports between Britain, America and Australia helped to construct international connections which boosted local doctors' status as professional specialists. And Dodds' regular tours of inspection through the Cape asylums helped to maintain a local community of asylum doctors who exchanged patients, case notes and personnel. This contributed to the establishment of a more uniform institutional culture with respect to the management of the insane.

Psychiatry in the Eastern Cape

In the Eastern Cape psychiatry developed on similar lines, particularly in the differing provisions for white and black patients. Fort England Asylum had been established in Grahamstown in 1875; it was the oldest Eastern Cape asylum and the second oldest Cape asylum after Robben Island (excluding the Old Somerset Hospital). Thomas Greenlees, a British-born doctor who sought better professional opportunities in the colonies, became medical superintendent of Fort England in 1890. His position as both asylum doctor and private practitioner in Grahamstown, and later as government pensioner, illustrates the opportunities available to doctors in the growing psychiatric profession at the Cape by the late nineteenth and early twentieth centuries.

Under Dodds' direction, the Eastern Cape asylum network was extended, with the establishment of Port Alfred Asylum in 1889 (for chronic, senile and pauper cases) and Fort Beaufort Asylum in 1894 (for chronic black male patients). A separate asylum for black female patients opened in Fort Beaufort in 1897, although it was administered by staff from the male asylum. Within this network, Fort England evolved into a high-status hospital, similar in function and ethos to Valkenberg, where medical treatment became focussed around the needs of white, paying patients. New patients were admitted into Fort England for specialist assessment and, if they were too dark-skinned or too poor to remain in the asylum, they were referred to other institutions. Port Alfred and Fort Beaufort were little more than custodial institutions, poorly resourced and staffed only by part-time visiting medical officers (the local district surgeons) until 1897, when a full-time doctor was appointed to Fort Beaufort.[50]

Greenlees' position within the asylum fraternity of the Eastern

Cape was, therefore, a powerful one. In 1890, he was paid £510 per annum: £410 as medical superintendent of Fort England and £100 as visiting medical officer of the chronic-sick hospital.[51] Greenlees also had to assist the police and general practitioners where a diagnosis of mental competency was required.[52] Three years later he was given a further £50 p.a. to attend the Institute for Imbecile (white) Children which had been established in the grounds of the asylum.[53] He earned a substantial commission on the income from private patients and on the recovery of bad debts (which topped £6,800 in 1905).[54] He was provided with free furnished accommodation in the asylum grounds and a horse and carriage (worth £30 per annum). His rations were drawn from the asylum account and he received fresh produce from the patients' farming activities. Convalescent patients were employed in his house as domestic servants, gardeners, grooms and stablehands.[55]

Greenlees fought for the right to establish a private practice in addition to his public duties. The Colonial Office was initially reluctant to allow this, as they anticipated a clash of interests between his private and public duties.[56] But Greenlees prevailed, and soon developed a private clientele whom he treated in his own home or admitted into the asylum.[57] The overlap between his private and public work enhanced both the image of the asylum and his standing as a private doctor. It augmented the intake of wealthier patients into the asylum, reducing the running costs of the asylum and earning Greenlees an increased commission. The combination of public duties and private practice thus benefited both Greenlees and his asylum.

With Dodds, Greenlees was an important player in negotiations with the colonial government for better working conditions and pension rights for his profession. These claims helped to represent asylum doctors to government as a skilled and powerful group within the medical profession. Dodds assisted Greenlees in negotiating six months' leave in Britain and America, with 68 days full pay and the remainder on half pay. They argued that Medical Superintendents of asylums did not have weekends or public holidays off duty and that the work was stressful and burdened with considerable responsibilities.[58] In 1907 Dodds and the Eastern Cape superintendents made a joint application to government for fourteen days special leave annually to compensate for their irregular working hours. A similar discourse, representing psychiatry as a difficult and demanding specialty, was used to justify calls for better retirement benefits. Greenlees claimed that asylum work was accompanied by 'more risks to life and limb than many of the other employments under government'.[59] He criticised the 'miserable pittance' provided by the government pension scales for asylum doctors in 1903 and, five years later, negotiated an early retirement with no loss of pension, on the argument that the job had been demanding and required extensive training which raised the starting age.[60]

By the late nineteenth century, therefore, psychiatry had been established as a solid, if often undervalued, specialism within the medical fraternity. It is not perhaps a coincidence that dentistry and psychiatry, which emerged from lower-status sections of the medical profession, were the first to try and establish themselves as medical specialties at the Cape.

Conclusion

As the Cape Colony entered the industrial era it gained new prosperity through the mineral discoveries. Fresh opportunities opened up for the medical profession. These existed on a number of fronts. The creation of a Health Department in the Colonial Office gave public health a professional status it had lacked before. Not only did the department itself expand in the 1890s, but it was able to pressure other local authorities into employing professional public health officials. Government hospitals increased in number and offered a wider range of health care, sometimes providing a rationale for controlling dissidents amongst the indigenous population. Semi-government organisations such as the railways also began to provide their own medical care, as did the diamond mining companies in Kimberley. As with government asylums a major consideration was often control rather than care for labourers, establishing a pattern which was to carry over into the twentieth century.

As the status of doctors and of hospitals improved, the medical profession was also able to tap into a more affluent market which demanded high-quality health care. C.J. Rhodes was the outstanding example of a valetudinarian who befriended doctors, made them part of his inner circle, drew them into his schemes for imperial aggrandisement and demanded their constant medical attention. Transvaal mining magnates, regular visitors to the Cape, also expected luxurious hospitals and specialist health care, creating a valuable market for the few who could respond to this demand.

By the end of the nineteenth century, then, the position of the Cape medical profession had become more similar to that of the metropolitan or the settlement colonies of Australia, New Zealand and Canada. Diamonds, gold and war all put South Africa on the map medically, but the resultant flow of doctors had its disadvantages as well, for some within the medical profession, but even more for black patients.

Notes

1. N. Worden, E. van Heyningen and V. Bickford-Smith, *Cape Town. The Making of a City* (Cape Town: David Philip, 1998), 211–7.
2. See Chapter 9.
3. Cape of Good Hope, *Government Gazette*, 2 January 1891.
4. Cape of Good Hope, *Civil Service List*, 1900, 1910.
5. I. Smith (ed.), *The Siege of Mafeking* (Johannesburg: The Brenthurst Press, 2001).
6. E. Burrows, *A History of Medicine in South Africa* (Cape Town: Balkema, 1958), 138.
7. *Ibid.*, 108.
8. See Chapter 5.
9. Confidential Reports on Civil Servants, 1843-45, CA, CO 8551.
10. Account book of Dr Peter Chiappini 1842-46, UCT Medical School Library, Cape Town, 'Names of Persons who Underwent an Examination'.
11. P. Simon, *Old Mutual 1845-1995* (Cape Town: Human & Rousseau, 1995), 122. C.T. Anderson remained in his post until 1938.
12. *Ibid.*, 64–5.
13. *Ibid.*, 51.
14. For a general account of these developments see J. Burman, *Early Railways at the Cape* (Cape Town: Human & Rousseau, 1984).
15. *SAMJ*, ii, 12 (April 1895), 333.
16. *Ibid.*, 333–9.
17. J. Bottomley, 'The Siege of Mafeking and the Imperial Mindset as Revealed in the Diaries of T.W.P. (Tom) Hayes and W.P. (William) Hayes, District Surgeons', *New Contree*, 41, (September 1997), 47.
18. Diary of Dr William Hayes, 31–137, CA, A 723.
19. E.B. van Heyningen, 'Women Under Siege' in Smith, *op. cit.* (note 5).
20. The diamond fields included the river diggings on the Vaal River including New Rush, and the dry diggings at Du Toit's Pan, Bultfontein, De Beers and Alexandersfontein (Kimberley and Beaconsfield).
21. B. Roberts, *Kimberley: Turbulent City* (Cape Town: David Philip, 1976), 71–6; S. Marks, *Divided Sisterhood: Race, Class and Gender in the South African Nursing Profession* (London: Macmillan, 1994), 24, 28.

22. Burrows, *op. cit.* (note 6), 257.
23. E. van Heyningen, 'Leander Starr Jameson' in J. Carruthers (ed.), *The Jameson Raid: A Centennial Retrospective* (Johannesburg: The Brenthurst Press, 1996), 181–91; *DSAB*, iii, 458.
24. *DSAB*, ii, 623; H. Sauer, *Ex Africa* (London: 1937).
25. *DSAB*, i, 725.
26. *DSAB*, iv, 210; R. Rotberg, *The Founder: Cecil Rhodes and the Pursuit of Power* (Oxford: Oxford University Press, 1988).
27. P.W. Laidler and M. Gelfand, *South Africa: Its Medical History* (Cape Town: Struik, 1971), 403.
28. I. Colvin, *The Life of Jameson* (London: T.C. and E. Jack, 1923), i, 26.
29. *Ibid.*, 9–10.
30. *Ibid.*, 38.
31. Rotberg, *op. cit.* (note 26), 127.
32. *Ibid.*, 27.
33. *Ibid.*, 26–7.
34. Van Heyningen, *op. cit.* (note 23), 181–191.
35. Sister Henrietta Stockdale is best known for her role in the initiation of nursing training. For opposing views on Sister Henrietta see Marks, *op. cit.* (note 21), 22–44 and C. Searle, *The History of the Development of Nursing in South Africa 1652-1960* (Cape Town: Struik, 1965), 137–45.
36. Burrows, *op. cit.* (note 6), 262–5; Laidler and Gelfand, *op. cit.* (note 27), 405.
37. W.H. Worger, *South Africa's City of Diamonds: Mine Workers and Monopoly Capitalism in Kimberley 1867-1895* (New Haven: Yale University Press, 1987), 64–5. See also 100, where Worger gives comparative death rates – in the 1870s Calcutta: 52/1,000, London: 23/1,000 and Kimberley: 80/1,000.
38. Burrows, *op. cit.* (note 6), 259–62; Laidler and Gelfand, *op. cit.* (note 27), 400–2.
39. Roberts, *op. cit.* (note 21), 218–27; Marks, *op. cit.* (note 21), 7–40; Worger, *op. cit.* (note 37), 103–4.
40. Roberts, *op. cit.* (note 21), 308.
41. See also Chapter 7.
42. *SAMR*, v (10 May 1907).
43. BOS 18/5
44. *SAMJ*, vii (Ocober 1899).
45. *SAMJ*, iii (December 1895).
46. W. Ernst, 'Lunatic Asylums in British India, 1800-1858', *Society for the Social History of Medicine Bulletin*, xxxix (1986), 27–31;

W. Ernst, 'The European Insane in British India 1800-1858: A Case Study in Psychiatry and Colonial Rule' in D. Arnold (ed.) *Imperial Medicine and Indigenous Societies* (Manchester: Manchester University Press, 1988); W. Ernst, *Mad Tales from the Raj: The European Insane in British India, 1800–1858* (London: Routledge, 1991); W. Mitchinson, 'The Toronto and Gladesville Asylums: Humane Alternatives for the Insane in Canada and Australia?', *Bulletin of the History of Medicine*, lxiii (1989), 52–72; M. Lewis, *Managing Madness: Psychiatry and Society in Australia 1788–1980* (Canberra: AGPS, 1988); M. Vaughan, 'Idioms of Madness: Zomba Lunatic Asylum, Nyasaland, in the Colonial Period', *JSAS*, ix, 2 (1983), 218–38; M. Vaughan, *Curing Their Ills: Colonial Power and African Illness* (Cambridge: Polity Press, 1991); J. McCulloch, *Colonial Psychiatry and 'The African Mind'* (Cambridge: Cambridge University Press, 1995).

47. S. Swartz, 'Colonialism and the Production of Psychiatric Knowledge in the Cape, 1891–1920' (unpublished Ph.D. thesis, UCT, 1996); F. Swanson, 'Colonial Madness: The Construction of Gender in the Grahamstown Lunatic Asylum, 1875–1905' (unpublished B.A. thesis, UCT, 1994); M. Minde, 'History of Mental Health Services in South Africa', in fourteen parts, *SAMJ* (1974-77); D. Moyle, 'Drawing the Line: the Early History of Lunacy in South Africa' (unpublished paper, Psychology Department, UCT), 1987); D. Moyle, 'Laying Down the Line: the Emergence of a Racial Psychiatric Practice in the Cape Colony during the Nineteenth Century' (unpublished paper, Psychology Department, UCT, 1988); D. Foster, 'Introduction' in S. Lea and D. Foster (eds) *Perspectives on Mental Handicap in South Africa* (Durban: Butterworths, 1990). See also R.C. Warwick, 'Mental Health Care at Valkenberg Asylum 1891–1909' (unpublished B.A. thesis, UCT, 1989); S. Dubow, 'Mental Testing and the Understanding of Race in Twentieth Century South Africa' in T. Meade and M. Walker (eds), *Science, Medicine and Cultural Imperialism* (Basingstoke: Macmillan, 1991).

48. H.J. Deacon, 'A History of the Medical Institutions on Robben Island, 1846-1910' (unpublished Ph.D. thesis, University of Cambridge, 1994), chapters 3 and 5; H.J. Deacon, 'Madness, Race and Moral Treatment on Robben Island Lunatic Asylum, Cape Colony, 1846-1890', *History of Psychiatry*, vii (1996), 87–297.

49. Swartz, *op. cit.* (note 47).

50. Swanson, *op. cit.* (note 47).

51. CA, CO 1458, n.d.

52. CA, CO 1458, 18 November 1890.
53. *Annual Report, Grahamstown Lunatic Asylum* 1893, G24-1894.
54. *Annual Report, Grahamstown Lunatic Asylum* 1905, G32-1906.
55. Swanson, *op. cit.* (note 47).
56. CA, CO 1458, 21 October 1890.
57. CA, CO 1570, 16 January 1893.
58. CA, CO 7161, 13 March 1894.
59. T.D. Greenlees, 'Remarks on Lunacy Legislation in the Cape Colony', *SAMJ*, v, 9 (January 1898).
60. T.D. Greenlees, 'Lunacy Administration in Cape Colony', *Journal of Mental Science*, lxi (1910), 269–70 and Burrows, *op. cit.* (note 6), 343.

9

Making a Medical Living:
The Economics of Medical Practice in the Cape
c.1860-1910[1]

Anne Digby

The economics of colonial medicine have been largely neglected. This chapter shall seek first to give an overview of the medical market in the Cape during the late nineteenth and early twentieth centuries, before turning to a fuller exploration of the nature of private and public practice, and their inter-relationship. The chapter will end with a case study of Dr William Darley-Hartley whose life exemplified some typical features of life in the Cape medical profession at this time.

The medical market and private practice

The Cape medical market was characterised by a comparatively early regulation of medicine, by economically mixed practices with frequent dependence on public appointments to eke out a modest income from private practice, and by what was perceived to be an increasingly crowded profession in relation to effective demand, which led in turn to conspicuous mobility amongst practitioners.

In forty years from 1864 to 1904 the Cape population tripled, but the number of doctors quadrupled.[2] One reason for the increase was immigration by British doctors. From the 1880s until the National Health Insurance Act of 1911, the very large increase in the supply of graduates of British medical schools had not been matched by an expansion of medical opportunities at home.[3] The Cape was seen as a promising opportunity for those without capital to set up a new practice, often with the help of an official appointment such as that of district surgeon.[4] Among Cape medical practitioners registered between 1880 and 1910, Elizabeth van Heyningen has found that British-born and British-trained doctors were overwhelmingly preponderant, with only a small cohort of doctors with German medical qualifications, and with weak Dutch representation.[5] Chapter 4 has indicated that over the century as a whole only one in seven of the Cape's doctors had been trained in Holland or Germany. And, in the absence of medical degrees in South Africa until the 1920s, only a very small minority of those who had had a British training had actually been born in the Cape. Chapter 4 has indicated that only one in ten nineteenth-century Cape doctors had actually been born in the colony.

Following the South African War (1899-1902), numbers of doctors were further swollen because British doctors sought to convert a temporary military position into a permanent civilian one.[6] But a severe trade depression then restricted practice opportunities, incomes declined and, by 1906, medical departures outweighed new recruits.[7] A medical exodus from the Cape to the Transvaal's gold fields, as well as to Rhodesia and New Zealand, resulted and helped to relieve perceived medical overcrowding.[8] A profession of 617 registered Cape practitioners in 1904 had, by 1911, shrunk to 562.

According to the census categories, the registered profession remained almost entirely a white, male one; in 1911 there were only four white or European female practitioners, and seven coloured or African or Malay male practitioners.[9] However, the character of the practitioner did not necessarily restrict the profile of patients. Dr Jane Waterston, the first registered medical woman at the Cape, wrote with satisfaction that 'I have had two gentlemen patients today and I am getting more of them. I shall not refuse any without good cause. I am also getting more black patients.'[10] And the Scottish doctor, James Mackenzie, who from 1906 developed a practice in the working-class community of Salt River in Cape Town, recruited 'a cross-section of the less affluent members of the South African community. White and brown lived side by side, English speakers and Afrikaans speakers were near neighbours.'[11]

Until the 1880s practice prospects in this huge territory were quite good for aspiring doctors. Doctors were at first geographically concentrated in major settlements and along the coast, but more of them gradually moved into rural areas as well, a catalyst being the diamond mining rush of the 1870s when a substantial railway infrastructure was created.[12] Even in 1911, however, the census indicated that nine out of ten Cape medics were located in larger towns,[13] an even greater urban concentration than in the Union as a whole. Here six out of seven were urban practitioners; the 'Garden Colony' of Natal being exceptional in having as many as two out of five doctors in country areas. But in these rural areas it was difficult to establish a permanent practice, even with the help of an official appointment as district surgeon. Drought and depressed farm prices could lead to the swift collapse of a practice, since cheaper alternatives to the doctor existed such as the household medicine chest, itinerant unlicensed practitioners, local chemists, or missionary medicine.[14]

Mobility was thus endemic within the South African medical profession: its peripatetic nature being influenced by the volatility of the economy, by the lure of practice or speculation associated with mining developments, by a moving frontier of settlement, and also by the character of immigrant doctors attracted by the adventure of practice in a 'new' land. First the sparkle of diamonds in Kimberley and then, from 1886 to 1889, the glitter of gold in Johannesburg, stimulated migration. In the 'medical El Dorado'[15] of the Witwatersrand an influx of colonial and immigrant doctors soon outpaced restricted openings for practice. This was overwhelmingly a male mining settlement, yet practice opportunities were generally acknowledged to be more plentiful with women and children. 'Despite the attempts of the Sanitary Board to keep the town in as foul a condition as possible, there are not enough patients', the profession wryly concluded.[16]

For the unfortunate cohorts of young doctors who graduated from the swollen British medical schools of the 1880s to 1900s, the absence of sufficient openings at home applied a stick to professional mobility, to add to the carrot of imagined colonial opportunities.[17] But, unknown to British emigrants, practice in nineteenth-century and early-twentieth-century South Africa involved higher risks than in Britain. Few Cape medical practices became sufficiently well-established for transfer to another practitioner so that the market for the sale of good practices remained a small one (see Illustrations 9.1a and 9.1b, pp.270–1). A more pronounced economic orientation than was found in Britain resulted from difficulties of practising in South Africa. Medical journals devoted far more space to practitioners' finances and their business anxieties, whilst regulatory fee tariffs appeared earlier and developed into more complicated tables than were found elsewhere. Doctors also appear to have been less reticent about the economic basis of practice. An extreme example was the action of the Transvaal Medical Union in compiling a blacklist of patients in 1907, when its members declared that they would not treat such patients without cash in advance.[18]

During the decade before Union in 1910, Cape practitioners indicated the extent of the financial pressures they felt themselves to be experiencing by their extraordinary sensitivity to, and intolerance of, doctors who gained competitive advantage through unprofessional advertising. Practices which were tolerated in other countries, such as giving a public notification that a doctor was setting up a practice, or had moved his or her office, were viewed as unethical. In Cape Town, membership of the local professional association was denied to new colleagues held to have breached this rule, whilst established members who had transgressed this custom might be expelled. In vain did one culprit plead that such procedures were seen as unexceptional in Australia or Johannesburg where he had practised previously![19]

The early registration of doctors in the Cape in 1807, through a single or double qualification in medicine and/or surgery, should have ensured that registered practitioners had a privileged monopolistic position in the medical market, since unlicensed practice was prohibited. Only registered doctors could sue for fees in a court of law, sign medical certificates or hold an official medical appointment (see Chapter 3).[20] In reality those registered found that their certificate gave them only very limited protection against competition by many rivals. Contemporary medical journals were full of complaints about opposition from unlicensed practitioners, whether missionaries, chemists or itinerants, all offering cheaper medical services. And in the early 1890s doctors protested against, and attempted to amend, the licensing of doctors who, although not meeting the stringent regulations for formal qualifications, were enabled under the Medical and Pharmacy Act of 1891 to be placed upon the roll of medical practitioners if they had had long experience of medical practice.[21]

Amongst the registered there was also fierce contention for the finite supply of paying private patients. An important factor in creating this situation was that enterprising doctors found it possible to set up new practices as 'squatters', rather than buying an established practice. Admission to the medical market was thus facilitated by the low entry costs of doing so, and overcrowding was common in desirable locations. This tended to subvert the very conditions which had attracted doctors initially, by producing very competitive practice conditions. Despite almost continuous efforts, it proved impossible for medical associations to enforce collective restrictive practices such as formalised schedules of minimum fees, since there was every incentive for individual doctors to acquire a competitive advantage by recruiting their patients through undercutting a colleague's charges.

Recruiting patients was also often easier than extracting payment from them. A rural practice often involved long journeys with several days on horseback. As a result the cost of treatment was multiplied several times by high mileage charges. In the towns doctors might even employ an accountant/collector to make out and get in the bills, as did Dr Chiappini in Cape Town, or Dr Te Water in Graaff Reinet.[22] Alternatively, as did Dr J.R. Mackenzie in Salt River, the doctor could either resort to payment by instalments or substitute for monetary payment a job of work by a grateful working-class patient.[23] In country districts patients might resort to payment in kind. A few practitioners resorted to legal action against some of their patients, but could be faced with counterclaims from assertive patients claiming that malpractice had occurred, and hence that they were justified in the non-payment of the doctor's bill![24]

Public appointments

Given the difficulties of earning private fees, Cape doctors were eager for the additional income brought in from public appointments. The most common of these was that of government district surgeons, but there were also a variety of public positions offered by voluntary bodies, notably by friendly societies. In comparison with fees from private practice, these appointments offered certain advantages such as security of income and freedom from bad debts. However, a price might be paid for this in terms of lay control, low remuneration or even tendering for appointment. Lay control could mean that unqualified people might be appointed in preference to the regular practitioner, and in 1856 Eastern Cape practitioners complained that the Cape government was itself illicitly employing unqualified men.[25] Tendering was always deprecated by the medical profession, whether this was adopted by small clubs[26] or by the Cape government. The South African Medical Association complained to the Cape government in 1886 that tendering was being employed on the railways, arguing that 'the Public Service would be well and economically managed if appointments were offered at fixed salaries, and made upon a basis of competency, rather than upon the purely *Trade Principles* of Tender.'[27] This 'respectful protest' produced an unrepentant response, in that it was asserted that tendering in the public service had 'brought about a considerable saving of public expenditure, without loss of professional efficiency.'[28]

Government appointments were the most important component of Cape doctors' income that did not come from private practice fees. The post of district surgeon was the most accessible public post because it was the most numerous and thus the most geographically

Table 9.1
Numbers and remuneration of district surgeons in
the Cape, 1811-1909

Date	Number	Fees / Salary Range (£)	Standard Part-Time Salary p.a. (£)
1811	6	-	-
1826	11	125-150*	-
1844	-	Fee schedule	-
1856	33	75-150	75
1866	48	75-200	75
1876	62	75-200	75
1886	91	75-400	75
1896	96	50-400	75
1909	141 part-time** [5 full-time]	40-350 part-time [465-810 full-time]	75

Source: see note 22
* Rules in 1828 laid down that £150 would be paid for posts without house, or £120 with a house provided (Cape Archives, MC 24.)
** The increase in numbers had arisen mainly from the creation of additional district surgeoncies in frontier areas where divisions were very large.

widespread. By the end of the period rather more than one in four Cape doctors drew part of their income from this office. The Cape administration found that this post gave (and still gives today) a flexible and economical medical service. In consequence, the number of such appointments grew from six in 1811 to 141 part-time appointments as well as five more recently established full-time ones by 1910 (see Table 9.1).[29] Salaries were at first standardised but later became more differentiated, varying both according to the weight of the duties and whether it was thought likely that a private practice could be built up. Fees for certain duties were also payable in addition (for instance, for giving evidence in court), as well as a travelling allowance per mile. Both the amount and the variability of these caused continual resentment, but protest only resulted when additional duties were given without recompense, as in 1895-6.[30]

Duties were first laid down in 1823, and a surviving copy of the Instructions for District Surgeons of 1828 reveals the minute detail in which these were specified. Article 3 made clear that 'The Surgeon shall be fully at liberty to carry on the Private Practice of his profession, provided the same do not interfere with his Official Duties.'[31] Duties might include certifying the insane, attending government officers such as members of the police and gaol officials and their families, being present during the physical punishment of prisoners, attending executions, conducting examinations or post-mortems where the cause of death was uncertain, visiting sick prisoners in gaol, giving expert medical testimony in the circuit court, providing medical attendance to paupers (i.e. those unable to pay), and providing free vaccinations. By the end of the colonial period additional duties in the realm of public health were specified in some detail: the district surgeon had to write an annual report on the state of the water supply and sanitation, slaughter houses, wash houses and native locations, as well as charting the incidence of infectious diseases and the measures taken against them.[32]

In spite of the litany of allegations in the medical press about the manifold disadvantages of the post, practitioners continued to apply for it. Young doctors – particularly immigrant ones – found the position of district surgeon to be a useful one. Rather like a Poor Law position in England and Wales, it gave a status and thus an introduction to a district, together with a nucleus of secure income, on which it was hoped later private practice could be added to achieve a viable medical living. More established practitioners may well have taken or retained such a post, despite its low remuneration, since not to do so would have given an opening for a new competitor. The government consequently found no difficulty in filling posts, and – in the absence of inflationary pressures – saw no reason to raise the official remuneration.[33] Table 9.1, column four indicates that, in the absence of any significant inflation, the typical salary of the district surgeon remained static between 1856 and 1909.

In favourable locations the aggregation of public and private income was satisfactory, although it produced a dual standard of medical care in which 'passable knowledge' sufficed in the former, whilst a more up-to-date clinical knowledge was requisite in the latter.[34] In other less auspicious places, private practice was thought insufficient to compensate for uncomfortable conditions and high living expenses, including the cost of replacement horses for those succumbing to long, waterless rides. For posts in Herschel and Garies (salaries of £150), Williston (salary of £100), and Britstown (salary of £75) the editor of the *South African Medical Record*, Dr W. Darley-Hartley, tried to discourage applications through unfavourable comment on the lack of potential. For Britstown, in the Fraserburg Division, he commented, 'We do not advise application for this. The village is a most miserable one, and the district sparsely populated and poor. Total income from all sources would little, if at all, exceed £300 p.a.'[35] In this kind of situation the government might pay larger sums to surgeons in selected districts than were justified by the duties, in order that a 'camouflaged subsidy' would attract them into areas so unappealing for private practice that otherwise they would have remained without a registered doctor.[36]

The combination of public service and private practice was not always easy because the freedom which the doctor saw as his right in private practice might conflict with the lay authority exercised by the civil commissioner, later resident magistrate (RM), over his public duties.[37] Indeed, it is instructive to compare the earlier (1828) and later (1896) nineteenth-century rules for district surgeons, which reveal a growth both in the bureaucratic detail with which the duties and fees of the district surgeon were specified and, in tandem with this, a more obtrusive imposition of lay authority.[38] Such tensions might be exacerbated because of the requirement that the district surgeon reside in the town where the resident magistracy was located. The profession thus felt that the magistracy was attempting to be 'lord and master of the District Surgeon.'[39].

Correspondence between Dr W.G. Atherstone and the Cape administration reveals some of the financial pitfalls of district surgeoncies. Having succeeded his father in the post of District Surgeon of Albany, Atherstone found the administration reluctant to continue paying the same emoluments. They now wanted to pay only £150 for the post, and not the additional £50 for running the Vaccine Establishment for the Eastern District, which had previously been associated with the post. This economical attitude towards public expenditure had been evident from 1844, when a fixed fee schedule had temporarily replaced salaried appointments, in the mistaken hope that this would be cheaper. But when salaries were reinstated their amount had been reduced, by as much as a quarter in the case of Albany.[40]

The long-term result of this refusal to pay what doctors perceived to be an adequate sum for the requisite medical services could be serious. By the 1880s, a district surgeon such as Charles Gorman in Knysna was reluctant to exert himself for services like vaccination for which the Cape administration no longer gave additional fees. No smallpox vaccinations had been performed in Knysna for five years, and Gorman stated that 'if District Surgeons were given a yearly allowance for vaccination this state of affairs would cease to exist.'[41] It was not only salaries but other allowances too that doctors complained did not form adequate recompense, with allegedly miserly travelling allowances being an especially contentious subject.[42]

The adequacy of the service that the district surgeon could perform was also increasingly thrown into doubt. The inhabitants of Namaqualand petitioned in 1872 that one district surgeon for 25,000 square miles and 10,000 inhabitants was insufficient, more especially since journeys to the circuit town of Clanwilliam, might involve the surgeon in a round trip of 800 miles:

> That in consequence of the frequent and necessary attendance of the only available medical man in the division, your petitioners are frequently debarred from medical privileges, and that fatal results have [resulted from]... the serious absences of fourteen or sixteen days of the district surgeon.[43]

A later case of an aggrieved patient indicated the human costs that such a situation could involve. In 1903 the Chief Constable of Clanwilliam accused the District Surgeon, Dr Hayes, of lack of attention both to his infant daughter, who died of bronchitis, and to his wife during a confinement. The doctor defended himself against the first accusation by stating that no amount of care could have altered the outcome, and against the second by stating that he had had a more serious case to deal with nearly forty miles away. Significantly, the Resident Magistrate sided with the District Surgeon.[44]

As outlying areas became settled, so the pressure on a district surgeon built up because of the long journeys. Accompanying private practice was also disadvantaged because extensive travel resulted in large bills and frequently in large debts. In the fullness of time, the Cape government might ease the situation by making an additional appointment, as in the King William's Town Division at Keiskama Hoek in 1887.[45] However, the life of the district surgeon continued to be a hard one and practitioners needed to be physically robust to sustain the life. The obituary of young Dr P.D. Frick, who was appointed to Caledon in 1893, and died five years later at the age of twenty-eight, was salutary: 'No doubt the incessant long rough cart journeys in a large scattered country district had unhappily in a measure hastened his end.'[46]

Apart from the post of district surgeon, there were public appointments as medical officers of health, as well as a range of others, including medical posts in the army, police force, prisons, asylums, hospitals and railways. Within the confined space of this chapter it is only possible to deal with these selectively and briefly.

The growth in the number of hospitals during the second half of the nineteenth century gave expanding opportunities for public positions, in which there was a trend to supplement an earlier pattern of visiting, honorary positions held by senior doctors through paid, resident appointments held by junior colleagues. For example, at the Kimberley Hospital (founded in 1882), there were five visiting surgeons in 1889 who gave their services freely, as well as a Senior House Surgeon.[47] A few years later the hospital advertised two posts: the Senior House Surgeon at £650 with quarters for a single man and, in addition, a Junior House Surgeon at £300, with board and lodging. Each was envisaged as a full-time post so that private practice was prohibited.[48] By 1910 there were thirteen such resident medical officer posts in Cape hospitals.[49] Hospitals varied both in the medical hierarchies they created and in the payment made. In 1884 at the Frere Hospital in East London, for example, there was one honorary surgeon together with two active surgeons who were each paid an honorarium of £75 per annum.[50] (The latter was a post later held by William Darley-Hartley, the subject of a case study below.[51])

Opportunities for full-time medical positions grew with the expansion of responsibilities undertaken by the Cape government. In this context it is interesting to contrast the four medical posts (other than district surgeons) financed in 1866 with the range of posts nearly half a century later, listed in Table 9.2.[52] The range of remuneration offered in 1909 was in line with that of the Cape medical profession more generally, with top salaries of £1,000 or more, and lowest ones at less than £300. However, for the fortunate minority who gained these public positions, the distribution of income within these twenty-seven posts was markedly better than in the profession more generally. Only eleven per cent were in the lowest income category of less than £300, and seven per cent had more than £1,000 per annum.[53]

Government service also offered part-time appointments and the income from these was a useful supplement to that from private practice. Apart from the 140 district surgeoncies, there were another sixteen appointments which included eight posts as port health officers (remuneration from £25 to £225); a post as vaccination

Source for Table 9.2:
G26-1909 and G48-1909, *Estimates of Expenditure of Year Ending 30 June 1910.*
*Includes allowances for board and lodging.

Table 9.2
Full-time government medical appointments in the Cape, 1909-10

Appointment	Salary, p.a. (£)
Asylums	
Valkenberg, Inspector of Asylums and Medical Superintendent	1000*
Assistant MO	500*
Grahamstown, Medical Superintendent	550*
Assistant MO	300
Port Alfred, Medical Superintendent	746*
Fort Beaufort, Medical Superintendent	575*
Assistant MO	275
Hospitals	
Old Somerset, Cape Town, Surgeon in Charge	350
Grahamstown Chronic Sick Hospital, Medical Superintendent	240*
Robben Island, Senior MO	700
Assistant MO	400
Assistant MO	275
Leprosy Research MO	450
Emjanyana Leper Asylum, MO in Charge	450
Penal Establishments	
Tokai Convict Station, MO	440*
Cape Town Convict Station and Prison, MO	810*
Porter Reformatory, Resident MO	440
Colonial forces and volunteers	
Colonial Forces, Principal MO	700
Cape Mounted Rifleman, Surgeon Lieutenant	444
Public health	
Cape Colony, MOH	1200
Assistant MOH	850
Additional MOH	650
District Surgeons	
Cape Town, District Surgeon	810*
Additional District Surgeon	465*
Wynberg	650*
Port Elizabeth	700*
East London	600*

officer to the Cape District at £150; three posts as visiting medical officers to convict stations (at £50 to £100); and allowances to two visiting medical officers at African townships ('native locations') at £110 and £150.[54]

By the end of the colonial period, one in three Cape doctors might have had access to a full-time or part-time public appointment. This underlines the extent to which a liberal administration was attempting to extend the reach of Western medicine in the colony, not least because Western medicine was seen as being an important part of the civilising mission of imperialism. The medical practitioner was at the same time both financial beneficiary and loser by this arrangement, since by spreading the finite money so thinly, many benefited to some extent, but few gained what they themselves perceived to be an adequate recompense for their professional work. The same was also true of the voluntary sector where many appointments were offered by friendly societies but where only modest remuneration was proffered.

The voluntary sector

An official report of 1899-1900 indicated that there were 128 friendly societies in the Cape, of which more than half were in Cape Town and the surrounding semi-urban area. The number of societies in 1900 was comparable to that in the census of 1891, which suggests that the number of societies that could remain solvent was fairly static so that doctors' income from this source was not buoyant.[55] Nevertheless, friendly societies employed large numbers of medical practitioners, the post of surgeon to a friendly society being second only to that of district surgeon in its frequency. But, whereas the latter were found in rural as well as urban areas, the former were almost exclusively urban. In urban areas a practitioner might be both district surgeon and hold multiple appointments with friendly or medical aid societies, as did James Mackenzie in Salt River. He was appointed District Surgeon in Woodstock and also did paid surgical work for the Loyal St. George, the Ancient Order of Forester, the Nil Desperandum, and the Independent Order of Oddfellows. In addition he received some remuneration from a timber yard, and from the South African Railways and Harbours.[56]

Methods of payment by societies and clubs were diverse. The highly variable sums paid to doctors indicates that many societies paid a doctor as, and when, he was required for a sick member. However, some societies paid an inclusive sum per member per head; in 1890, for example, the Jubilee Benefit Society in Paarl paid seven shillings and sixpence per head, and the St Francis Church Friendly Society, Simon's Town, six shillings.[57] A decade later the English Church paid its doctors £150 per annum in Cape Town, and £40 in Claremont.[58] The branches of the large affiliated orders such as the Foresters or Oddfellows were also more likely to pay an annual salary than capitation fees; for example, the Foresters' South Africa Hope Lodge (in Cape Town) paid £72 per annum to their surgeon, Dr E.V. von Landsley.[59]

How adequate was the medical remuneration? In 1900 the Loyal South African Bud of Hope Lodge of the Independent Order of Oddfellows, then with 453 members, offered a salary of £120 per annum.[60] This appears a substantial sum but worked out at five shillings and three pence per member per year. Taking the sums for medical attendance from the official report of 1899-1900, where membership numbers were also given for a minority of societies, enables an estimate to be made of the kind of remuneration that a doctor might expect to receive. There was an effective range of payment from three shillings and ten pence to six shillings and ten pence, with the average payment amounting to five shillings and four pence per member per year. Yet five shillings per member per year was alleged by the colonial medical profession to be exploitation.[61] In Australia, too, where the profession was even more dependent on friendly society income, there were bitter struggles.[62] Like the British Medical Association in Britain, professional associations in South Africa attempted to restrain their members from accepting what they perceived to be low-paid 'club' practice.[63] Predictably, this was unsuccessful, not least because – in reality – the remuneration did not compare particularly badly with other sources of income.[64] The economic failure of those Cape friendly societies which offered higher rates, should have been a salutary lesson to the medical profession in suggesting the inadvisability of attempting to raise remuneration significantly. For instance, in the town of George the St Mark's Benefit Society for Working Men paid their medical officer fifteen shillings per member per annum. They were warned by the Government Actuary that this was actuarially unsound since this took up eighty-four per cent of contributions. The society accepted the advice but then entirely discontinued the services of the doctor.[65]

Cape doctors complained of 'the slavery of medical men to the Friendly Societies.'[66] Only occasionally did the local medical profession succeed in taking effective action against medical aid schemes which they found objectionable. In 1906 the BMA Cape of Good Hope (Western) branch managed to end the African Homes

Trust's new sick benefit scheme because it denied subscribers the right to be reimbursed for their bills after consultation with their own doctors, as distinct from the medical practitioners chosen by the trust.[67] According to the editor of the *South African Medical Record*, William Darley-Hartley, the profession was unable to take efficient collective action because:

> We are at present helplessly open to such sweating, simply because the man who wants to build up a practice by the dubious method of squatting will take clubs at any rate... as will also to some extent, the established man who, from professional inability to hold his own, is getting left behind in private practice.[68]

This was only a partial explanation. Given the volatility of the medical market in the Cape, such an appointment would provide a relatively secure bedrock of income. And, whatever the state of the private practice, an individual doctor would assume that such an appointment would involve only a minimal addition to expenses, and therefore see it as an attractive income-generating option.[69]

The medical profession's attitude towards appointments with friendly societies was influenced by the tension between the advantage of income and the disadvantage of lay control. The friendly society with the largest medical expenditures in the Cape was the De Beers Consolidated Mines Ltd Benefit Society, Kimberley.[70] Professional sensitivities seem to have been heeded in this society, and an enthusiastic editorial in the *South African Medical Record* wrote approvingly of it avoiding 'most of the abuses which have rendered the club system so degrading and oppressive to the medical profession.' The scheme was unusual in allowing prospective patients to choose from a panel of doctors, and in providing adequate remuneration for the medical work performed.[71] Elsewhere, friendly societies specified the duties for medical practitioners and monitored their performance carefully. A Forester's Lodge Surgeon had to visit those sick members in the town whose 'pence card' was left at the consulting rooms, certify them as sick or healthy, and provide a fortnightly report to the branch meeting. Doctors had to examine applicants for membership to determine their state of health.[72]

Professional pride was at stake, given the assumption by lay people that they could censure the doctor for inadequate service. Dr Chiappini was paid £80 per annum as Lodge Surgeon by the Loyal South African Bud of Hope Lodge of the Independent Order of Oddfellows during the late seventies and early eighties. Chiappini was then 'the most skilful surgeon of his day', and a leading member of the Cape profession who served on the Colonial Medical Committee.[73] Despite this, he was censured by the Lodge because it was considered that 'in many cases he has not attended to the brothers of the Lodge as he should have done.'[74] Equally irksome to the profession was the fact that doctors who were not paid a salary were not allowed to charge their customary private fees, but were remunerated by fees for visiting. The Foresters supplemented the work of the Cape Town surgeon by appointing additional doctors to visit in the suburbs, but would only authorise these doctors to charge two shillings and sixpence per visit, rather than the three shillings and sixpence or five shillings that the medic thought appropriate.[75] However, if the doctor managed to keep on the right side of the brethren then there might be an occasional bonus, as was the case with the Forester's Court of South African Hope who voted a testimonial to the doctor of £25.[76]

Rewards of public and private practice

Given the risks of South African medicine, and the conspicuous economic orientation this produced in practice, what kind of medical living was achieved by Cape doctors? Individual medical incomes were far more buoyant than 'Jeremiahs' in the medical press would have led the unsuspecting reader to expect. Unexpectedly, when viewed from the perspective of this earlier journalism, it was discovered that doctors had the highest average net income of any occupation in 1908-9! However, their reference group – the lawyers – had proportionately more high earners of over £1,000 per annum than did doctors, although there were fewer struggling doctors earning less than £300 per annum than lawyers (see Table 9.3). A significant reason for the relative paucity of high medical earners compared to lawyers was the slow development of consultancy work in the Cape medical profession. In Johannesburg, where consultancy developed earlier, there was a higher proportion of 'thousand a year' medics. However, during the early years of the Union doctors in the Cape were second only to those in the Transvaal in their high earning power, and much ahead of those in both the Orange Free State and in Natal (see Table 9.4).

These returns of medical incomes are intriguing not least in relation to the constant whingeing by doctors about their poorly remunerated labours. Further work is required on the economic history of medicine to fully elucidate some of the issues raised. For example, the reliability of these figures in terms of providing a

Table 9.3
Structure of Cape medical and other taxable incomes in the Cape,
1908-9 (%)

Profession	Under £50	£51-£300	£301-£1000	Over £1000
Medical	0	25.7	63.2	11.1
Legal	0	30.3	53.2	16.5
Other professions	0	74.1	23.9	2.0
All taxpayers	0	91.9	7.3	0.8

Source: Report of Cape of Good Hope Commissioner of Taxes, 1908-9

representative cross sample of the profession needs to be ascertained. So too does the extent to which the moving northern frontier removed many of the economic failures from the Cape profession, as those with an unviable practice migrated to the Transvaal or to Rhodesia, and thus raised average medical incomes. Offsetting monetary gains, however, were the continuing high costs of practice in South Africa. The very high cost of living in South Africa was one of the first things to strike the immigrant. One new arrival in Cape Town wrote in 1882, 'The price of everything is nearly double that in England. Rent is exorbitantly high.'[77] In real, as distinct from monetary terms, medical incomes might therefore not compare so very well with those in the home country.[78]

Patients

The range of a doctor's patients expanded both directly and indirectly because of appointments, notably through rural posts as district surgeons or through posts with urban friendly societies. That club practice or social insurance was being extended to groups who could well afford to pay the doctor independently was an international professional preoccupation. But evidence is lacking to support such an argument for Cape Town's friendly societies (as even the alarmist rhetoric of the editor of the *South African Medical Record* conceded) because the majority of each friendly society's members was poor.[79] Cape friendly societies therefore tended to extend the practitioner's practice to new social groups, whether in terms of race, class, age or gender. For example, the Saint Francis's Church Friendly Society at Simon's Town had a membership mainly of poor coloured people; the South African Hope Female Friendly Benefit Society provided a limited attendance for women at the time of their confinement;

Table 9.4
Distribution of individual taxable incomes in South Africa exceeding
£1,000, 1914-5 (%)

Profession	Cape	Natal	Transvaal	Orange Free State
Medical	35.6	11.2	44.2	9.0
Legal	39.8	11.2	36.6	12.4

Source: UG24/1917, Report of Commissioner of Inland Revenue and Taxes, 1915-6

while Oddfellows and Foresters often had juvenile branches, such as the Loyal Kaffrarian Oddfellows Lodge at King William's Town. Over 14,000 Cape people obtained medical assistance from doctors through this kind of collective provision. Despite the graduated income-related fee scales for patients operated by some doctors (for example, Dr Chiappini operated first, second and third-class rates), it is possible that without such collective provision, many sufferers would not have been able to pay for medical treatment. Since, for the doctor, the alternative even to the low payments of friendly societies, could be entirely unremunerated *pro Deo* work, this kind of practice was also advantageous

In rural or frontier districts the district surgeon might provide the only service by a registered practitioner. The first encounter with Western medicine for many Africans was likely to have been that of being vaccinated against smallpox by a district surgeon. In Albany in 1857, for example, 1,950 'Kafirs [Africans from the Transkei], who had recently come into the colony' were vaccinated, because 'none of them had previously been vaccinated.'[80] But it was the doctor who needed to take the initiative, as the district surgeon for the Transkei commented thirty years later: 'Natives [Africans] do not present themselves for vaccination unless smallpox is prevalent.'[81] Or, as another colleague commented, 'the natives have become indifferent to its [smallpox's] presence, but when a death occurs, panic results and there is a rush for vaccination.'[82] Apart from smallpox vaccination, there was also treatment by the district surgeon for syphilis.[83]

Africans were both cautious and discriminating in their attitudes to Western medicine. A new district surgeon needed to win personal trust and also show that Western medicine was effective. Newly appointed district surgeons might not be aware that this was a slow process and thus write of 'hostility', and of 'natives' being 'peculiarly averse to medical treatment.'[84] In areas where a district surgeon had been appointed for the first time, and where Western medicine was probably unknown to Africans, the process of gaining African patients was even slower. Thus the first district surgeon to be appointed in East Griqualand wrote in 1889 that, during his first year of appointment when his 'practice so far has been almost entirely confined to Europeans, that the few native cases which have come under my supervision so far have been of a trivial nature.'[85] Africans were more unfamiliar with Western ideas of preventive, than curative, medicine and therefore tended to seek vaccination when smallpox was already in the area, rather than before. Once smallpox was present, however, they showed some faith in vaccination, saying, 'We don't want to get the pox, so we have come to be vaccinated.'[86] But it was perhaps personal trust in the healing power of an individual, and the doctor's patience and honesty, rather than a more general belief in the power of Western medicine that was most evident in African attitudes. Long journeys would be undertaken to consult such a healer, more especially for acute conditions.[87] Extensive travel was also thought worthwhile to receive treatment in a hospital.[88] And, in areas where there had been long-standing missions, such as Lovedale or Healdtown, Africans had been exposed to Western medicine for decades, were familiar with its strengths and hence in these localities would seek its benefits.

With good reason, however, Africans might show a generalised distrust towards white doctors, who were usually district surgeons in the 'native territories', and so were members of an official white bureaucracy which had the power *inter alia* to remove them forcibly to a leper colony or lunatic asylum. In this context it is instructive to read in the *Report of the Tuberculosis Commission* of 1914 that:

> [So] suspicious are natives of official interference that medical men practising among them found it detrimental to their practices and to the confidence which the native placed in them, to associate themselves publicly with the proceedings of the Commission.... When we remember how disinclined the native is to seek European medical treatment, the large number coming under the notice of medical practitioners must connote a very considerable amount of the disease in the general population, with a pretty widespread infection.[89]

Doctors were aware that TB (a notifiable disease since 1904) had spread from mining to rural areas with migratory labour,[90] and reported that TB was increasing, with rates of from three to fifty per cent of their 'native' patients. They acknowledged that only a small percentage of cases sought their care; significantly these were acute cases, those that were chronic being self-treated with patent medicines.[91] Ironically, such famed patent medicines as 'pink pills for pale people' were available in the 'native territories', along with advertisements that targeted the African patient by including expressions of gratitude written in Xhosa.[92]

Some Western-trained doctors in rural areas built up extensive private practice amongst Africans, once familiarity had established social confidence and efficacious treatment had then created medical trust. The District Surgeon of Xalanga observed:

> I find an increasing desire among the natives of this district to accept and adopt our European method of medical treatment; they purchase our medicines freely, and the witch doctor's occupation among the natives hereabouts is reduced to a minimum.[93]

There was an element of wish-fulfilment here, as well as a view of Western medicine as a civilising agent pushing back frontiers of ignorance symbolised by the 'witch doctor.' Nevertheless, areas where an individual had become well-known through acting as a District Surgeon for a long period were those where a substantial private practice could be created amongst Africans. Dr Welsh, the District Surgeon for Umtata for twenty years, saw around 1,500 new patients annually in his 'native private practice.' And practising in 1914 in a district that was 'one of the oldest to come into contact with civilisation', Dr C.P. Bligh-Wall, the District Surgeon at Butterworth, stated that he had seen 2,661 individual 'native' patients in 1908 which had risen to over nearly 4,000 by 1911, when the increase in numbers meant that he could take on a junior partner. Within a year the practice's African clientele had grown by a further one-third.[94] The growth of practice amongst Africans continued, such that in 1918 it was stated complacently that 'recourse to European medical practitioners is very common, and not a few practitioners regard the Native work as one of the most satisfactory departments of their practice.'[95]

The Cape Medical Officer of Health characteristically wrote in 1908 of 'a Native and Coloured population, with its ignorance, and its insanitary and uncivilised habits.'[96] District surgeons followed this lead in writing of 'the Kafir location' as a 'menace to the health of the

Illustration 9.1a
Advertisements for medical practitioners

The economic value of medical practices was carefully evaluated in the *SAMR*. Many of these appointments, however, were closed to immigrant doctors with no knowledge of Dutch. Dr Darley-Hartley's medical agency ran in association with the columns of the *SAMR*. (*SAMR*, 10 February 1907)

48   SOUTH AFRICAN MEDICAL RECORD.   FEBRUARY 10.

S.A. MEDICAL RECORD AGENCY DEPARTMENT.

Sale or purchase of practices and partnerships negotiated. Locum tenencies arranged. Medical arbitrations and valuations undertaken. Advice given as regards settling in practice, and appointments. Agencies in England, Australia, and New Zealand.

A. 101. Sound practice on railway near Cape Town, with lucrative appointment for disposal with or without preliminary partnership. Only suitable for Africander.

A. 133. Good O.R.C. practice. Income £800, including appointment about £350.

A. 134. Well-established practice, bringing in over £1,000 a year, in large town on railway, within easy reach of Cape Town. Rich agricultural district.

A. 138. For immediate disposal, unopposed practice in good Karoo district. Cash premium £100, to include good stock of drugs.

A. 139. Compact well established and light practice of £600 per annum, in district town on Karoo. Premium very low. Suitable for gentleman in delicate health.

A. 142. Well-established practice, first-class, Cape Town, residential suburb. Income £1,200. Excellent house, at reasonable rental. Purchaser must be prepared to invest some capital.

A. 146. Very old established practice, divisional town, Midland Districts, Cape. Receipts last year £1,130. Large house. Knowledge of Dutch necessary.

A. 151. Small but light practice with appointment of £150 in good Karoo town; opposition slight. Nominal premium to include drugs.

A. 156. For disposal well established practice of £1,300 in large coast town Cape Colony, two appointments. Premium £800.

A. 157. For disposal. Well-established practice in small town on railway, near Cape Town. Income about £780. Knowledge of Dutch necessary. An Afrikander could expand this practice rapidly.

A. 159. For disposal. Well-established practice in an important town on railway in northern part of Cape Colony. Opposition slight. Present income £800, but expansible. Premium low to a prompt purchaser, as vendor has to leave South Africa through pressing family reasons.

A. 161 and 162. For disposal, two good unopposed Karoo practices, one with appointment, at nominal premiums.

A. 163. For disposal, medium country practice in Midlands, Cape.

A. 164. For disposal, well established practice of £700, in good divisional town in Cape Midlands.

A. 168. For disposal, an old established and very cheaply worked practice in good mining town in Transvaal. Income keeps steady at £800, for last four years.

B. 102. Elderly practitioner, experienced, open to purchase good practice on railway, in Western Province, Cape Colony. Income not less than £1,200.

B. 113. Well qualified practitioner, with ample South African experience and well up in Surgery, desires partnership or practice in good town in inland district. Could invest up to £1,000.

B. 117. Highly qualified gentleman, married, about 30, with extensive experience in surgery, is open to purchase good partnership or practice in a large town, Cape Peninsula preferred.

C. 127. Wanted, for six months, locum tenens House Surgeon for good Hospital. Inland.

C. 131. Wanted a locum for six months for a Railway M.O. Terms liberal, but applicant must be well up in surgery.

C. 132. Wanted, assistant for six months, for practice on Witwatersrand.

C. 133. Wanted a Dutch speaking locum, for about six months, in a good practice in a particularly pleasant town on railway, C.C. Dispenser kept, all found. Must be a thoroughly competent man, with fair knowledge of gynæcology and surgery.

C. 137. Wanted, assistant, indoor, for O.R.C. town.

D. 108. Thoroughly experienced and reliable married practitioner, speaking Dutch fluently, requires good assistancy, preferably out door.

D. 109. Married practitioner, no children, ample South African experience, thoroughly reliable, and speaking some Dutch, requires long locum tenency or out door assistancy.

D. 115. Married gentleman, Dutch speaking colonial, requires good assistancy outdoor, highly recommended.

No connection with any other Agency in South Africa.

town' or of it being 'useless issuing written instructions in Kafir owing to the ignorance of the most elementary principles of sanitation.'[97] District surgeons perceived themselves to be a front line not just in the fight against disease, but thereby also in the advance of imperial civilisation.

Illustration 9.1b

A. 134. Well-established practice, bringing in over £1,000 a year, in large town on railway, within easy reach of Cape Town. Rich agricultural district.

A. 138. For immediate disposal, unopposed practice in good Karoo district. Cash premium £100, to include good stock of drugs.

A. 139. Compact well established and light practice of £600 per annum, in district town on Karoo. Premium very low. Suitable for gentleman in delicate health.

A. 142. Well-established practice, first-class, Cape Town, residential suburb. Income £1,200. Excellent house, at reasonable rental. Purchaser must be prepared to invest some capital.

A. 146. Very old established practice, divisional town, Midland Districts, Cape. Receipts last year £1,130. Large house. Knowledge of Dutch necesary.

A. 151. Small but light practice with appointment of £150 in good Karoo town ; opposition slight. Nominal premium to include drugs.

A. 156. For disposal well established practice of £1,300 in large coast town Cape Colony, two appointments. Premium £800.

A. 157. For disposal. Well-established practice in small town on railway, near Cape Town. Income about £750. Knowledge of Dutch necessary. An Afrikander could expand this practice rapidly.

A. 159. For disposal. Well-established practice in an important town on railway in northern part of Cape Colony. Opposition slight. Present income £800, but expansible. Premium low to a prompt purchaser, as vendor has to leave South Africa through pressing family reasons.

Imperialist, peripatetic practioner and editor: A case study of Dr W. Darley-Hartley

The opportunities that the imperial relationship of the late nineteenth and early twentieth centuries provided are demonstrated in the career of William Darley-Hartley (1854-1934). Despite unusual drive and ambition, his early career in South Africa exemplified many of the economic problems that individual doctors faced in attempting to make a medical living in the volatile economy and politics of the colonial Cape. He practised privately but also held public appointments. He endured hardship but ultimately succeeded in making a successful career – not least through his flexibility in making the best use of the openings which were presented to him.

William Darley-Hartley came out from Britain to the Cape, probably influenced by the surge of imperialistic activity between 1872 and 1878 under Disraeli's premiership.[98] At this time the majority of Cape doctors were British-born practitioners who had been trained in either London or Edinburgh.[99] Darley-Hartley was born in England, trained at Guy's, London, and qualified MRCS (England) in 1878, later obtaining further qualifications (LRCP, Edinburgh, 1879; MRCP, London, 1898; MD, Durham, 1898.)[100] A keen imperialist, he came out to South Africa immediately after qualifying. Like so many doctors in the Cape, his civilian practice was pursued in tandem with military service. He served as surgeon-captain to the Cape Mounted Rifleman in the Ninth Frontier War in 1878, and in the 24th regiment (the South Wales Borderers) in the Anglo-Zulu Wars in 1879, where he ran a field hospital. Fortunately he was invalided home with sunstroke before his regiment was annihilated at Isandhlwana. Later, in 1897, he undertook service as a surgeon-captain in the Kaffrarian Rifles during the Langeberg campaign in the Bechuanaland War; he was a civil surgeon at Woodstock Military Hospital during the second South African War of 1899-1902 and, in 1917, at the age of 63, he acted as a temporary major in the South African Medical Corps.

His military service was likely to have been primarily motivated by imperialist sentiment, but an economic rationale (in finding a post) and a medical justification (in extending skills), may also have been present. A fellow surgeon who served in the Anglo-Zulu War wrote of the 'opportunity to test my surgical skill on a fair scale' and of the satisfaction of giving service.[101] Darley-Hartley echoed this thought in 1918 when he wrote that the medical profession 'has "played the game" in the way of patriotism' during the First World War, impelled through duty to make self-sacrifices, including the loss of practice.[102] A fervent imperialist, in sympathy with Rhodes, he had been the first President of the South African League in 1896, which aimed to support, and provide a justification for, the British government's policies. In professional matters also, he was an enthusiast for close ties with the British Medical Association, which he referred to as 'the great Association',[103] and he served during the second Anglo-Boer War as a correspondent for its journal – the *British Medical Journal*

To the four disjunctures in his civilian practice resulting from war, were others caused by economic difficulty. In the diverse and migratory pattern of his early professional life he was typical of his colleagues. Darley-Hartley's reasons for beginning practice by 'squatting' in East London in 1879 are unknown. They may have sprung from mixed motives in an imperialist desire to serve on the moving frontier of empire, as well as in a financial calculation that the medical market of the Eastern Cape offered better opportunities than in areas settled earlier in the Western Cape. East London was a frontier town with British and German settlers, which had been founded in 1848 for military reasons, only becoming a municipality in 1873. Darley-Hartley was said to have built up a large practice in the area, but the fact that economic depression literally drove him out of private practice in the town for several years, suggests that, like many others in South Africa, the practice was not secure enough to withstand economic fluctuations. These years from 1880 to 1886 have been called the 'blackest period' in South Africa's colonial history because of economic depression and drought.[104] Darley-Hartley was forced to move to Cathcart in 1885 where he kept body and soul together by holding the post of district surgeon for three years. However, the good health of the area may not have resulted in much private practice,[105] so that years later Darley-Harley recollected a passage of weeks when he did not earn anything beyond his district surgeon's salary.[106] At this time he also acted as a surgeon in the Frontier Armed and Mounted Police. The importance of medical personnel in bodies such as this is suggested by the fact that, whereas only one surgeon served in this force before 1877, thirty-six were involved by 1880, and then – after the cessation of hostilities – this again dwindled to only three.[107]

Always a staunch upholder of professional solidarity he was active in the foundation of the Frontier Medical Association at Queenstown in 1886, which aimed to promote scientific and social contact amongst practitioners as well as to advance the interests of the medical profession. Given the large area that the association covered, it was agreed to rotate meetings amongst four towns, one of them being East London.[108] In 1889 William Darley-Hartley moved from Cathcart back to East London, having first taken the precaution of obtaining the security of a regular salary as a railway medical officer, and a part-time post as Medical Officer of Health. As has been mentioned earlier, he also received a modest honorarium as a medical officer to the Frere Hospital – a small institution that had been established in the town in 1881. In addition he became medical officer to the East London Medical Aid Society, and held the same position with the local Oddfellows. With income from these varied appointments to supplement his fees from private practice Darley-Hartley was doing well enough to stay in the town for over a decade. His clinical experience in the town is illuminated by an article he wrote on 'Case-Taking in General Practice', which indicated his awareness of the need to gain his patient's confidence, as well as indicating a methodical approach to diagnosis and treatment.[109]

It was during this period in the Eastern Cape that he resumed the medical journalism earlier begun as a student when he had edited *Guy's Hospital Gazette*. In 1884 Darley-Hartley founded the *South African Medical Journal* as a private venture, probably motivated as much by the hope of creating a successful business venture as of aspiring to shape the South African medical profession through editorial input. The journal survived for only five years, and even this short period had a short intermission because of pecuniary losses. Later, Darley-Hartley referred to the 'weary struggle of the last five years', and to his accumulating financial deficit on this venture, commenting wryly that 'the individual efforts of one man can be of but little avail when met by the apathy of the great mass of one's confreres.'[110] It is a testimony to his resilience that in 1903 he was prepared to start another medical journal – the *South African Medical Record* – to which was attached a medical agency for the sale of practices. This journalistic enterprise was mostly 'stress and struggle', making for the most part a 'meagre income' until the 1920s, when it finally became 'a really satisfactory proposition.'[111] But this was a more serious business venture than had been the earlier *Journal* since, at the age of 52, Darley-Hartley gave up full-time medical practice to concentrate on the *Record*.[112]

By this time he was in Cape Town, having moved to the colony's capital and major economic centre eight years previously in 1898. No doubt he had been attracted to the enhanced opportunities there, not only for professional practice and collegial contact but also for medical politics.[113] His active involvement as a medical politician had taken off with his appointment to the Colonial Medical Council in 1904. In his later writings, however, it is apparent that it was earlier experience in the Eastern Cape that had already decisively shaped his outlook. His liberal stance towards African medical practice, together with his interest in the pharmacological possibilities of Cape plants, seem likely to have been formed during his time as district surgeon for Cathcart.[114] Throughout a long life his medical journalism was dominated by economic anxieties about the state of the medical market and the ethical problems that resulted from this, in terms of unprofessional behaviour such as undercutting colleagues or doctors' advertising their services. These concerns were most fully developed in a long paper delivered to the Fourth South African Medical Congress, where Darley-Harley spoke feelingly about the difficulties of achieving medically ethical behaviour in the South African context, and thus of the need for a South African Medical Association.[115]

It was not until 1926 that an association whose membership truly lived up to this title was achieved, and the gulf between the Afrikaner and English members of the medical profession was bridged. More than any other, Darley-Hartley had worked towards this end, especially as a medical journalist where he was the foremost opinion-former and mouthpiece of the Cape profession. Having been editor of the *South African Medical Record* from its inception, he became joint editor when it was subsumed in 1926 into the *Journal of the Medical Association of South Africa*, but served in that capacity for only a year. Darley-Hartley also served as the last president of the old Colonial Medical Council during 1927 to 1928, and topped the poll for membership of the new South African Medical Council, which replaced it. A year later he was awarded the first Gold Medal of the Medical Association of South Africa (BMA) for distinguished service to the profession in South Africa. 'By sheer force of character, from being a general practitioner in the Eastern Province, he came to be the trusted adviser in things medical to the whole profession in South Africa.'[116]

That Darley-Hartley was enabled to give this effective leadership to Cape doctors in his later years stemmed from the knowledge that earlier stages of his career had given him, when he had suffered the insecure earnings, and peripatetic medical practice which were all too evident amongst the rank and file members of the Cape profession. These early years illustrated vividly private medical practice's vulnerability to economic and political change, and hence the importance of public practice to supplement it. The continual preoccupation with money that these insecurities forged in Darley-Hartley's mind was typical of the South African doctor. Many of the general character traits that underpinned clinical ability in a Cape general practitioner were also displayed by Darley-Hartley: a physical resilience, capacity for hard work and ability to network professionally. The experiences of this doctor therefore exemplified many of the difficulties of the Cape medical profession, where an individual's personality, social connection and ability increased the chances of making a viable medical living within a volatile colonial context.

Notes

1. The financial assistance of the Wellcome Trust for this research is gratefully acknowledged.
2. G20-1866, G6-1892, G19-1905, *Cape censuses.*
3. A. Digby, *Making a Medical Living: Doctors and Patients in the English Market for Medicine, 1720-1911* (Cambridge: Cambridge University Press, 1994) 14, 112 144–55, 168–9; A. Digby, *The Evolution of British General Practice, 1850-1948* (Oxford: Oxford University Press, 1999), chapters two and three, *passim.*
4. *South African Medical Journal* (hereafter *SAMJ*), v (1897), 36; *South African Medical Record* (hereafter *SAMR*), iv (1906), 156–8; D. Dyason, 'The medical profession in Colonial Victoria, 1834-1901' in R. MacLeod and M. Lewis (eds), *Medicine and Empire: Perspectives on Western Medicine and the Experience of European Expansion* (London: Routledge, 1988), 197–9.
5. E. van Heyningen, 'Public Health and Society in Cape Town, 1880-1910' (unpublished PhD thesis, University of Cape Town, 1989), 71-2, 74; 'Agents of Empire: The Medical Profession in the Cape Colony, 1880-1910', *Medical History*, xxx (1986), 452–3.
6. *SAMR*, i (1903), 25; iii (1905), 230–2.
7. C.G.W. Schumann, *Structural Change and Business Cycles in South Africa, 1806-1936* (London: P.S. King, 1938), 112; *SAMR*, ii (1904), 193; iv (1906), 337. The editor, W. Darley-Hartley, (see case study at the end of the chapter) ran a medical agency and was in an excellent position to judge the ebb and flow of medical personnel.
8. *SAMR*, v (1907), 46; vii (1909), 169; viii (1910), 166.
9. A. Digby, '"A Medical El Dorado"? Colonial Medical Incomes and Practice at the Cape', *Social History of Medicine*, viii (1995), table 1, 474
10. Jane Waterston to Dr Stewart, 18 March 1884, UCT, Department of Manuscripts and Archives, BC 700.
11. B. Mackenzie, *Salt River Doctor* (Cape Town: Faircape Books, 1981), 36.
12. E H. Burrows, *A History of Medicine in South Africa* (Cape Town: Balkema, 1958), 179.
13. South Africa, UG 32-1912, *Census, 1911, Part V, Occupations*, 706-7.

14. *SAMJ*, ii (1887) 119; iii (1887), 13-14.
15. *SAMR*, iv (1906), 62; *SAMJ*, iii (1888), 189.
16. *SAMJ*, iv (1889), 169; iii (1888), 208.
17. Digby, *op. cit.* (note 3b), chapters two and three. The National Health Insurance Act of 1911 obviated this pressure by providing insurance for poorer manual workers on which 'panel practices' could be created.
18. P.W. Laidler and M. Gelfand, *South Africa: Its Medical History, 1652-1898* (Cape Town: Struik, 1971), 187; *Transvaal Medical Journal*, iii (1907), 93.
19. Dr Durham to Dr Alston and Dr Richardson, 9 April 1903, 4 June 1904, UCT, Department of Manuscripts and Archives, BC 328.
20. Digby, *op. cit.* (note 9), 468.
21. Petition of BMA Cape of Good Hope branch against the 1891 bill, UCT, Department of Manuscripts and Archives, BC 328.
22. UCT Medical School, MS Africana collection; Visit and cash books of Dr Thomas N.G. Te Water, CA, A467/86.
23. Mackenzie, *op. cit.* (note 11), 36-7.
24. *SAMJ*, ii (1887), 69.
25. Memorial of Members of the Medical Profession Practising at Port Elizabeth and Uitenhage, April 1856, CA, HA 8-56.
26. *SAMJ*, iii (1888), 161; *SAMR*, i (1903), 114.
27. Minutes of the South African Medical Association (SAMA), 1883-8, letter from Dr J.H.M. Beck to C.B. Elliott, General Manager of Railways, 20 January 1886, UCT, Medical School Africana Collection.
28. Minutes of SAMA, letter from A. Difford, Secretary to the Manager of the Railways, to Dr J.H.M. Beck, 31 March 1886, UCT, Medical School Africana collection.
29. Laidler and Gelfand, *op. cit.* (note 18), 107–8, 224–5, 230; Unnumbered government paper, *Estimates of Revenue and Expenditure of Cape of Good Hope, 1856*; G22-1866, G41-1876, G29-1885, G22-1895, G48-1909, *Estimates of Expenditure*, 1866, 1876, 1886, 1896, 1909 for year ending 30 June, except for 1866, when the calendar year was used.
30. *SAMJ*, iii (1895-6), 80; IV (1896-7), 221-3.
31. Accounts for Medical Attendance etc., 1806-96, CA, MC 24, Cape Medical Committee.
32. See for example, G43-1909, *Report of MOH for Colony on Public Health, 1908*, where the summaries of district surgeons' reports on public health are given.
33. *SAMJ*, iii (1895-6), 194; *SAMR*, ii (1904), 91.

34. *SAMR*, vii (1909), 40–1
35. *SAMR*, ii (1904), 78, 139; v (1907), 36.
36. *SAMR*, xxiv (1926), 146.
37. A.J.T. Roux, 'The Relationship Between the Government and the Medical Profession in South Africa', *SAMR*, xxiv (1926), 250–2.
38. Instructions for District Surgeons, 1828, CA, MC 24; *Regulations for the Instruction of District Surgeons in the Performance of Their Duties* (Cape Town: 1896); *SAMR*, ii (1904), 76–8.
39. *SAMJ*, ii (1894-5), 13.
40. A98-1861, *Correspondence Between District Surgeon of Albany and the Government.*
41. G4-1889, *Reports of District Surgeons, 1889*, 73–4.
42. *SAMJ*, iii (1895-6), 195; *SAMR*, ii (1904), 90–2.
43. A11-1872, *Petition of Merchants, Miners, Farmers and Others Residing in the Division of Namaqualand, 1872.*
44. F. Kilpatrick, 'The Contagious Diseases Act of 1885 and the Dynamics of the Clanwilliam District, 1880-1910' (unpublished UCT BA Honours dissertation, 1998), 34–7.
45. *SAMJ*, ii (1887), 73.
46. *SAMJ*, iii (1895-6), 177.
47. G29-90, *Report on Hospitals and Asylums, 1889.*
48. *SAMJ*, i (1893-4), 146, 167; *SAMR*, i (1903), 100.
49. *SAMR*, viii (1910), 246.
50. *SAMJ*, i (1884), 13.
51. G29-1890, *Report* from Frere Hospital, East London, by J. Hewitt Paley and W. Darley-Hartley, 43–4.
52. G26-1866, *Estimates of Expenditure for the Year 1866.*
53. Digby, *op. cit.* (note 9), 479.
54. G26-1909 and G48-1909, *Estimates of Expenditure of Year Ending 30 June 1910.*
55. G64-1901, *Report on Friendly Societies for the Years 1899 and 1900*, 8–10. It should be noted that 32 societies had recently been dissolved.
56. Mackenzie, *op. cit.* (note 11), 40.
57. G5-1891, *Report by the Government Actuary upon Friendly Societies, 1890*, 21, 41.
58. G64-1901, *Report*, 18.
59. Minutes of Lodge of Court South Africa Hope Number 5236 of Ancient Order of Foresters, Minute Book, 1907-17, CA, A2011/1.
60. G64-1901, *Report on Friendly Societies*, 11.
61. *SAMR*, ii, 1904, 212.
62. T.A. Pensabene, *The Rise of the Medical Profession in Victoria*

(Canberra: Australian National University, 1980).

63. For example, *SAMR*, iii (1905), 128; iv (1906), 341, 371–2.

64. *SAMR*, v (1907), 8–10.

65. G5-1891, *Report by the Government Actuary upon Friendly Societies*, 43–4.

66. *SAMR*, ix (1911), 123.

67. Secretary to the African Homes Trust to Secretary of Colonial Medical Council, 2 June 1906, UCT, Department of Manuscripts and Archives, BC 328.

68. W. Darley-Hartley, 'Medical Economics: The Expenditure Side', *SAMR*, xxiv (1926), 353–4.

69. *Ibid.*, 353–4.

70. G64-1901 *Report on Friendly Societies for the Years 1899-1900*, 22.

71. *SAMR*, ix (1911), 289–91.

72. Minutes of Court South Africa Hope Number 5236 of Ancient Order of Foresters, Minutes, 1907-17, CA, A2011/1.

73. 'Antonio Lorenzo Chiappini (1841-1883)', *DSAB*, iii (1981), 148.

74. Minutes, 20 January and 17 February 1880, CA, A 1967/1/1/3.

75. Minutes 9 December 1907, 17 February 1908, CA, A 2011/1.

76. G64-1901, *Report on Friendly Societies, 1899-1900*, 11.

77. Diary of Rev. A.J. Gould of the London Missionary Society, Entry 24 August 1882, CA, A 1999.

78. Digby, *op. cit.* (note 9), 479.

79. *SAMR*, v (1907), 8–10.

80. A98-1861, *Correspondence Between District Surgeon of Albany and the Government.*

81. G4-1889, *Reports of District Surgeons*, 130.

82. G43-1909, *Report of MOH for Colony on Public Health, 1908*, Comment by District Surgeon for Idutywa, Dr C. Armstrong Lumley.

83. For example, G28-1910, *Blue Book on Native Affairs.*

84. G4-1889, *Report of District Surgeon*, for Cathcart, then in post for only four months.

85. G4-1889, *Reports of District Surgeons*, 125.

86. G13-1888, *Reports of District Surgeons*, on Xalanga, 56.

87. Obituary of J.W. Weir, *Journal of the Medical Association of South Africa*, iii (1929), 86; *SAMR*, xvi (1918), 103

88. G29-1890 *Report on Grey Hospital, King William's Town*, 1889.

89. South Africa, UG 34/1914, *Report of the Tuberculosis Commission*, 77, para 144, 82, para 158.

90. R.M. Packard, 'Industrialization, Rural Poverty and Tuberculosis in South Africa, 1850-1950' in S. Feierman and J.M. Janzen (eds), *The*

Social Basis of Healing in Africa (Berkeley: University of California Press, 1992), 113–4, 121–3.

91. South Africa, UG 34/1914, *Report of the Tuberculosis Commission,* comment of Dr F.H. Walker, the District Surgeon of Nqanduli for seventeen years.

92. G. Callaway, *Sketches of Kafir Life* (Oxford: Mowbray, 1905), 93. In this case patent medicines had been sent for by post.

93. G13-1888, *Reports of District Surgeon* for Xalanga, 53.

94. South Africa, UG34/1914, *Report of the Tuberculosis Commission,* evidence of district surgeons.

95. W. Darley-Hartley, 'A Native Medical Service', *SAMR,* xvi (1918), 162.

96. G43-1909, *Report of MOH, 1908,* xviii.

97. G43-1909, *Report of MOH, 1908,* reports by Dr H.H. Joubert on Willowmere and by Dr T L Craister on Xalanga.

98. A.Thomas, *Rhodes* (London: BBC Books, 1996), 107.

99. H. Deacon, 'Cape Town and "Country Doctors" in the Cape Colony during the First Half of the Nineteenth Century', *Social History of Medicine,* x (1997), 33.

100. The principal sources used for the narrative of his life are entries in medical directories, the entry in the *DSAB,* iv (Pretoria: Human Sciences Research Council, 1981), 101–2; obituaries in *SAMR,* viii (1934), 119–23; Burrows, *op. cit.* (note 12), 363–5 and plate xxxii. Other sources are cited below.

101. D. Blair Brown, *Surgical Experiences in the Zulu and Transvaal Wars 1879 and 1881* (Edinburgh: Oliver & Boyd, 1883), 7–9, 92.

102. Editorial, *SAMR,* xvi (1918), 333–5.

103. *SAMR,* xxiv (1926), 9 January 1926.

104. C.W. de Kiewet, *A History of South Africa, Social and Economic* (Oxford: Oxford University Press, 1941), 109.

105. G13-1888, *Report of District Surgeon for 1887,* Cathcart, 14.

106. Editorial, *SAMR,* xxiv (1926), 27 March 1926.

107. *SAMJ,* i (1884), 155–6.

108. C. Blumberg, 'The Provision of Medical Literature and Information in the Cape, 1827-1973 (unpublished M.Bibl. thesis, University of South Africa, 1974).

109. *SAMR,* iv (1905), 51–3.

110. *SAMJ,* September 1889, editorial. Circulation must have been small as surviving sets of the journal are rare.

111. Last editorial by W. Darley-Hartley as editor of *SAMR,* xxiv (1926), 37–8.

112. He was still prepared to serve in a consulting capacity, as he later did

as consulting physician to the Cape Town Free Dispensary.

113. See Deacon, *op. cit.* (note 99), for discussion of this point for an earlier period.

114. *SAMR*, ii (1904), 26; xvi (1918), 161–3, 209–11.

115. *SAMJ*, v (1897), 34–9.

116. Obituary note by E. Barnard Fuller in *SAMR*, viii (1934).

10

The Cape Doctor 1807-1910:
Perspectives

Howard Phillips

This chapter contrasts the Cape doctor in 1807 and in 1910, and finds that, in a whole variety of ways, the differences between the two were not of degree but of kind. Underlying this sea-change was the germ revolution of the late Victorian era, which transformed the Cape doctor out of all recognition, thereby laying important foundations for the development of the twentieth-century South African doctor.

Thinking back over half a century to his student years in London in the 1850s, Dr F. Ensor of Port Elizabeth recalled with a smile:

> [the days] when there was no temperature chart above the patient's bed, when Rontgen [sic] Rays, and the ubiquitous microbe were unknown... [and] unrecognized till the genius of Pasteur and of Lister gave them their true interpretation, involving quite a new aspect and theory of disease.[1]

Echoing these sentiments, another Cape doctor of similar vintage wrote:

> [I was] struck with astonishment at the vast improvement which has taken place, both in the better knowledge of the nature and causation of many diseases, the improvement in the means of diagnosis with the certainty which later science has rendered possible, in the improved modes of treatment, and the addition of many new and valuable remedies which chemical science has provided us with.[2]

What both of these veteran doctors were expressing was their sense that the practice of medicine had changed out of all recognition just during own careers since the 1850s, let alone since the beginning of the nineteenth century. With such an overarching judgement no historian today will disagree, despite the persistence into the twentieth century of some pre-1850 features like the one-doctor practice and a dependence on clubs and insurance companies for custom.

Like biomedicine all over the world, the nature of biomedicine practised at the Cape in 1910 – even by the most conservative of its doctors – was a world away from that practised there a century earlier. Already by 1910, science in all its diverse nineteenth century technical and intellectual forms had transformed biomedicine sufficiently for it to be identifiably 'modern', even when seen from the year 2004, and in so doing had profoundly altered its contents, modus operandi, self-perception and the form and social relations of its distinctive consultation and examination processes. Among the more obvious public manifestations of this at the Cape were the appearance of specialists within the profession, the creation of two medical laboratories for pathological analysis, and the transformation of hospitals into sites par excellence for the practice of state-of-the-art clinical medicine in the interests of the community as a whole, a change most clearly illustrated by the difference in intention between the Old Somerset Hospital and Lunatic Asylum, opened in 1818 'for the reception of Merchant Seamen, and the Slave Population',[3] and the Nightingale-inspired New Somerset Hospital opened as Cape Town's first general hospital in 1862. As Bynum has made clear, 'modern medicine... was the product of nineteenth-century society... Modern medicine has been built on the foundations that were firmly established before World War I.'[4]

Nor was it just the kind of medicine practised by Cape doctors which changed comprehensively during the 'long' nineteenth century. Taking advantage of the prestige conferred by these accumulating breakthroughs in the later decades of the century and their own numerical growth as a result of the mineral revolution, Cape doctors were gradually able to enhance their standing in a society itself undergoing major social, economic and demographic modernisation, so that by 1910 they were well on their way to becoming the uniformly trained, homogeneous, well-organised, influential and financially secure profession which dominated healthcare discourse in South Africa for the rest of the century. Following the example of their counterparts in Britain and its settler colonies, they sought to make their profession part of what has been called 'the most powerful trade union in the British Empire'.[5] In pursuit of this in the larger Union of South Africa, they and their aggrandising Transvaal *confreres* led the way towards making medicine the epitome of applied modern science, consequently enjoying what Paul Starr has described as a 'dominant... position in... [the] new world of rationality and power.'[6]

Alongside them, the motley array within the ranks of those practising biomedicine a century before – including military surgeons, apprenticeship-trained apothecaries and Continental MDs – were barely recognisable as members of the same group: in training, ethos, self-confidence and outlook they now shared a uniformity undreamt of in 1807. Within biomedicine in 1910, like doctors elsewhere in the British Empire, they stood unchallenged at the summit of the healthcare hierarchy, commanding deference from nurses, midwives and pharmacists; among Cape healthcare practitioners more broadly conceived, they alone had the ear of the political, religious and cultural establishment and so, paradoxically, enjoyed an influence in conceptualising the body, disease and its treatment far in excess of the extent of their actual biomedical practice among the colony's population at large, surely a key element in any definition of a colonial medical profession. African traditional healers who, in 1807, had been unchallenged in their *weltantschauung* and ministrations were, a century later, probably still treating a majority of the Cape's population, but were now doing so under increasing pressure from a burgeoning biomedicine which would have no truck with any other form of healing. Particularly in urban areas of the colony, Muslim and Dutch folk medicine were already in retreat in the face of this advancing 'biomedicalisation' of Cape society. In these confrontations with other medical systems biomedicine was most obviously at the cutting edge of Europe's colonial enterprise.

Those who stood at the forefront of this biomedical advance in 1910 were still overwhelmingly white men born and trained in Europe. Yet, in this regard, the situation in 1910 apparently did not represent the shape of things to come in the new century, but rather the acme of a trend which stretched back to 1807 and beyond. Within fifteen years of 1910, male and female doctors trained wholly in South Africa were starting to enter practice in the country, the forerunners of thousands more similarly trained practitioners in subsequent decades, while from the 1940s they began to be joined by a trickle of their black peers, also locally trained. In 2004 South Africa's doctors span a far wider ethnic and gender spectrum than was conceivable in 1910, but whether the kind of medicine most of them were taught to practise differs significantly from that taught in the old colonial metropoles is a moot point.

Yet, although the Cape doctor, as characterised in the preceding chapters, no longer exists, the social, economic, cultural, scientific and imperial forces which made him and (in a few cases) her in the watershed half-century after 1860 left their mark indelibly on their successors. The South African doctor who emerged in the following decades inherited a number of distinctive traits from the Cape doctor, which became part and parcel of his/her new identity – an intellectual dependence on and deference to metropolitan biomedicine (tellingly, until 1946 the doctors' 'trade union', the Medical Association of South Africa, retained the colonial signifier, 'British Medical Association', as part of its official title); a sense of cultural superiority vis-à-vis all other types of healing and a belief in the role of biomedicine in spreading Western civilisation; a willingness to pathologise the 'other' race/gender/class all too readily; a belief in the need for sovereignty, effective self-control and lobbying as a united profession; a concern not to alienate the political powers-that-be unduly; a self-conscious sensitivity about and striving for social status, respectability and just financial rewards; a preference for a curative, hospital-based medicine which utilised cutting-edge technology in all spheres of practice and which was concentrated in the cities; and a relationship with others in the healthcare professions which was decidedly top-down.

Though in the year 2004 a number of these historical traits are on the wane, many still occupy a fundamental place in the character of the South African medical profession today, part of the longlasting bequest of the nineteenth-century Cape doctor to the South African doctor of the twentieth, and even the twenty-first century.

Notes

1. F. Ensor, 'Typhoid Fever from a Student's Note-book 50 Years Ago', *South African Medical Record [SAMR]* (15 July 1903), 69, 71.
2. H. Lawrence, 'Some Reminiscences of Medical Practice', *SAMR* (24 August 1912), 345.
3. *Cape Town Gazette* (18 July 1818).
4. W.F. Bynum, *Science and the Practice of Medicine in the Nineteenth Century* (Cambridge: Cambridge University Press, 1994), xi.
5. Cited in J.A. Gillespie, *The Price of Health: Australian Governments and Medical Politics 1910-1960* (Cambridge: Cambridge University Press, 1991), x.
6. P. Starr, *The Social Transformation of American Medicine* (New York: Basic Books, 1982), 4.

Select Bibliography

'Hollandse Medisijne', *SAMJ*, xxvii, 25 (20 June 1953), 532–33.

'South African Snake-Bites', *Chambers's Journal*, (29 March 1890), 208.

A.M.L.R., 'An American Girl at the Cape in 1834', *QBSAL*, xxiii, 3 (March 1969), 83–96.

B. Abel Smith, *The Hospitals 1800-1948: A Study in Social Administration in England and Wales* (London: Heinemann, 1964).

J.E. Alexander, *Expedition of Discovery into the Interior of Africa* (London: Colburn, 1838).

D. Arnold (ed.), *Imperial Medicine and Indigenous Societies* (Manchester: Manchester University Press, 1988).

E.C. Atwater, 'The Medical Profession in a New Society, Rochester New York (1811-60)', *Bulletin of the History of Medicine*, lxvii, 3 (1973), 221–35.

J. Backhouse, *Extracts from the Journal of James Backhouse* (London: Hamilton Adams, 1840).

A. Bank, 'Of "Native Skulls" and "Noble Caucasians": Phrenology in Colonial South Africa', *JSAS*, xx, 3 (September 1996), 387–403.

J. Barrow, *Travels into the Interior of Southern Africa*, Vol.1 (London: T. Cadell & Davies, 1806).

L. Bean and E.B. van Heyningen (eds), *The Letters of Dr Jane Elizabeth Waterston 1866-1905* (Cape Town: Van Riebeeck Society, 1983).

W. Beinart and S. Dubow (eds), *Segregation and Apartheid in Twentieth-Century South Africa* (London: Routledge, 1995).

E. Bergh, 'Memorie over de Kaap de Goede Hoop' (1801) in G.M. Theal (ed.), *Important Historical Documents*, iii (Cape Town: 1911), 13–120.

M. Bevan (comp.), *Dr James Barry 1795-1865: Inspector-General of Military Hospitals: A Bibliography* (Johannesburg: Public Library. 1966).

J.V. Bickford-Smith, *Ethnic Pride and Racial Prejudice in Victorian Cape Town* (Cambridge: Cambridge University Press, 1995).

J.V. Bickford-Smith, E. Van Heyningen and N. Worden, *Cape Town in the Twentieth Century* (Cape Town: David Philip, 1999).

C. Blumberg, 'The provision of medical literature and information in the Cape, 1827-1973' (unpublished M.Bibl. thesis, University of South Africa, 1974).

C. Blumberg, 'The South African Medical Society and its Library', *Cabo*, ii, 4 (1978), 18–25.

BMA meeting report, 'Notes on the Pharmacology of Some South African Drugs', *SAMJ*, vii (October 1899), 123–28.

T.F. Bonner, *Becoming a Physician – Medical Education in Britain, France, Germany and the United States 1750-1945* (New York: Oxford University Press, 1995).

J. Bottomley, 'The Siege of Mafeking and the Imperial Mindset as Revealed in the Diaries of T.W.P. (Tom) Hayes and W.P. (William) Hayes, District Surgeons', *New Contree*, lxi, (September 1997), 25–161.

M. Boucher and N. Penn (eds), *Britain at the Cape, 1795-1803* (Johannesburg: The Brenthurst Press, 1992).

J. Bradley, A. Crowther and M. Dupree, 'Mobility and Selection in Scottish University Medical Education, 1858-1886', *Medical History*, lx (1996), 1–24.

E. Bradlow, '"The Oldest Charitable Society in South Africa": One Hundred Years and More of the Ladies' Benevolent Society at the Cape of Good Hope', *South African Historical Journal*, xxv (November 1991), 77–104.

J. Branford, *A Dictionary of South African English* (Oxford: Oxford University Press, 1978).

S.M. Brock, 'James Stewart and Lovedale: a Reappraisal of Missionary Attitudes and African Response in the Eastern Cape, South Africa, 1870-1895', (unpublished Ph.D. thesis, University of Edinburgh, 1974).

D. Blair, Brown, *Surgical Experiences in the Zulu and Transvaal Wars 1879 and 1881* (Edinburgh: Oliver & Boyd, 1883).

J. Brown, 'Some Reminiscences of Practice in the Cape Half a Century Ago', *SAMR*, xiv (1916), 216–18, 248–50, 321–23, 384–86.

P.S. Brown, 'The Providers of Medical Treatment in Mid-Nineteenth Century Bristol', *Medical History*, xxiv (1980), 297–314.

D. Bunn, 'Of Poison and Painting "The Brown Serpent of the Rocks": Bushman Arrow Toxins in the Dutch and British Imagination, 1735-1850', Appropriations conference papers, Centre for African Studies, University of Cape Town, September 1993.

J. Burman, *Early Railways at the Cape* (Cape Town: Human & Rousseau, 1984).

C. Burns, 'Louisa Mvemve: A Woman's Advice to the Public on the Cure of Various Diseases', *Kronos: Journal of Cape History*, xxiii (1996), 108–134.

E. Burrows, *A History of Medicine in South Africa* (Cape Town: Balkema, 1958).

E.H. Burrows, 'The Leyden Tradition in South African Medicine', *SAMJ* xxx, 11, (17 March 1956).

W.F. Bynum and R. Porter (eds), *Companion Encyclopedia of the History of Medicine*, vols 1 & 2 (London and New York: Routledge, 1993).

W.F. Bynum, *Science and the Practice of Medicine in the Nineteenth Century* (Cambridge: Cambridge University Press, 1994).

G. Callaway, *Sketches of Kafir Life* (Oxford: Mowbray, 1905).

J. Campbell, *Travels in South Africa Undertaken at the Request of the Missionary Society* (London: Black and Parry, 1815).

A.J. Christopher, *Southern Africa* (Folkestone: Dawson, 1976).

I. Colvin, *The Life of Jameson*, 2 vols (London: T.C. and E. Jack, 1923).

J. Connor, 'A Sort of Felo-de-se: Eclecticism, Related Medical Sects and Their Decline in Victorian Ontario', *Bulletin of the History of Medicine*, lxv (1991), 503–527.

P.J. Corfield, *Power and the Professions in Britain, 1700-1850* (London: Routledge, 1995).

L.G. Couch, *A Short Medical History of Grahamstown* (Grahamstown: Grocott & Sherry, 1976).

C.H. Creswell, *The Royal College of Surgeons of Edinburgh – Historical Notes from 1510 to 1905* (Edinburgh: The College, 1926).

P. Curtin, *The Image of Africa. British Ideas and British Action, 1780-1850* (London: Macmillan, 1965).

W. Darley-Hartley, 'Medical Economics: The Expenditure Side', *SAMR*, xxiv (1926).

W. Darley-Hartley, 'A Native Medical Service', *SAMR*, xvi (1918), 210–1.

C. De Jong, *Reizen naar de Kaap de Goede Hoop* (Haarlem: Francois Bohm, 1802).

C.W. De Kiewiet, *A History of South Africa, Social and Economic* (Oxford: Oxford University Press, 1941).

V. De Kock, *Those in Bondage* (Pretoria: Allen & Unwin, 1963).

H.J. Deacon, 'A History of the Medical Institutions on Robben Island, 1846-1910' (unpublished Ph.D. thesis, University of Cambridge, 1994).

H.J. Deacon, 'Leprosy and Racism at Robben Island' in E. van Heyningen (ed.) *Studies in the History of Cape Town*, vii (Cape Town, 1994), 45–83.

H.J. Deacon, 'Madness, Race and Moral Treatment at Robben Island Lunatic Asylum, 1846-1910', *History of Psychiatry*, vii (1996), 287–97.

H.J. Deacon, 'Midwives and Medical Men in the Cape Colony, 1800-1860', *JSAS*, xxxix (1998), 271–92.

H.J. Deacon, 'Cape Town and Country Doctors in the Cape Colony During the First Half of the Nineteenth Century', *Social History of Medicine*, x, 1 (1997), 25–52.

H.J. Deacon, 'Racial Segregation and Medical Discourse in Nineteenth-Century Cape Town', *JSAS*, xx, 2 (1996), 287–308.

A. Digby, *The Evolution of British General Practice, 1850-1948* (Oxford: Oxford University Press, 1999).

A. Digby, *Making a Medical Living: Doctors and Patients in the English Market for Medicine, 1720-1911* (Cambridge: Cambridge University Press, 1994).

A. Digby, 'A Medical El Dorado?: Colonial Medical Incomes and Practice at the Cape', *Social History of Medicine*, vii, 3 (1995), 473–9.

J. Dixon (ed.), *Social welfare in Africa* (London: Croom Helm, 1987), 184–217.

R.S. Downie and B. Charlton, *The Making of a Doctor – Medical Education in Theory and Practice* (New York: Oxford Univeristy Press, 1992).

D. Dyason, 'The Medical Profession in Colonial Victoria, 1834-1901' in R. MacLeod and M. Lewis (eds), *Disease, Medicine and Empire* (London: Routledge, 1988), 194–216.

S.N. Eaton, 'A Housewife at the Cape in 1818', *QBSAL*, viii, 2 (December 1953), 45–9.

R. Edgecome, 'The Letters of Hannah Dennison, 1820 Settler, 1822-1847' (unpublished M.A. thesis, Rhodes University, 1968).

R. Elphick, and H. Giliomee (eds), *The Shaping of South African Society*, 1652-1840, 2nd ed. (Cape Town: Maskew Miller Longman, 1989), 521–66.

N. Erlank, 'Letters Home: The Experiences and Perceptions of Middle-class British Women at the Cape, 1820-1850' (unpublished M.A. thesis, UCT, 1995).

W. Ernst, 'Lunatic Asylums in British India, 1800-1858', *Society for the Social History of Medicine Bulletin*, xxxix (1986).

W. Ernst, *Mad Tales from the Raj: the European Insane in British India, 1800-1858* (London: Routledge, 1991).

S. Feierman and J.M. Janzen (eds), *The Social Basis of Healing in Africa* (Berkeley: University of California Press, 1992), 104–130.

G.H. Findlay, *Dr Robert Broom, F.R.S., Palaeontologist and Physician, 1855-1951* (Cape Town: Balkema, 1972).

J.P. FitzGerald, *A Short History of the Native Hospital and Permanent Canvas Marquees* (King William's Town: S.E. Rowles, 1885).

D. Foster, 'Introduction' in D. Lea and D. Foster (eds), *Perspectives on Mental Handicap in South Africa* (Durban: Butterworths, 1990).

D. Fox, *Health Policies, Health Politics: The British and American Experience 1911-1965* (Princeton: Princeton University Press, 1986).

C. Friedman-Spits, *The Fraenkel Saga* (Pinelands: South African Medical Association, 1998).

E. Friedson, *Profession of Medicine: A Study of the Sociology of Applied Knowledge,* 2nd edn (New York: Harper & Row, 1988).

W. Frijhoff, '"Non Satis Dignitatis": Over de Maatchappelijke Status van Geneeskundigen tijdens de Republiek', *Nederlandsche Tijdschrift voor Geschiedenis,* lcvi (1983), 379–406.

B. Gandevia, 'A History of General Practice in Australia', *Medical Journal of Australia,* ii (12 August 1972), 381–385.

T. Gelfand, *Professionalising Modern Medicine: Paris Surgeons and Medical Science and Institutions in the Eighteenth Century* (London: Greenwood Press, 1980).

R.D. Gidney and W. Millar, *Professional Gentlemen: The Professions in Nineteenth Century Ontario* (Toronto: University of Toronto Press, 1994).

J.A. Gillespie, *The Price of Health: Australian Governments and Medical Politics 1910-1960* (Cambridge: Cambridge University Press, 1991).

C.J. Glacken, *Traces on the Rhodian Shore: Nature and Culture in Western Thought from Ancient Times to the End of the Eighteenth Century* (Berkeley: University of California Press, 1967).

J. Goldswain, *The Chronicle of Jeremiah Goldswain,* 2 vols (Cape Town: Van Riebeeck Society, 1946-1949).

B. Good, *Medicine, Rationality and Experience: An Anthropological Perspective* (Cambridge: Cambridge University Press, 1994).

D. Gordon, 'From Rituals of Rapture to Dependence: The Political Economy of Khoikhoi Narcotic Consumption, c.1487-1870', *SAHJ*, xxxv (November 1996), 62–88.

D. Gordon, 'Science, Superstition and Colonialism: Disease and Therapy at Kingwilliamstown, Xhosaland, 1847-91' (unpublished paper, SSHM Simmer Conference, Medicine and the Colonies, July 1996).

L. Granshaw & R. Porter (eds), *The Hospital in History*, (London: Routledge, 1989).

D.G. Green, *Working Class Patients and the Medical Establishment: Self-help in Britain from the Mid Nineteenth Century to 1948* (New York: St Martin's Press, 1985).

T.D. Greenlees, 'Lunacy Administration in Cape Colony', *Journal of Mental Science*, lix (1910), 269–70.

T.D. Greenlees, 'Remarks on Lunacy Legislation in the Cape Colony', *SAMJ*, v, 9 (Jan. 1898), 228–34.

P.W. Grobbelaar, C.W. Hudson and H. Van der Merwe (eds), *Die Afrikaner en sy Kultuur, deel VI: Boerewysheid* (Cape Town: Tafelberg, 1977).

D. Hammond-Tooke, *Rituals and Medicines: Indigenous Healing in South Africa* (Johannesburg: A.D. Donker, 1989).

C.A. Harrison, 'The King of Native Customs: SPD Madiehe and the Ambiguities of African Traditional Healers' Associations, 1928-1948' (unpublished Honours thesis, University of the Witwatersrand, 1993).

M. Harrison, *Public Health in British India* (Cambridge: Cambridge University Press, 1994).

D.V. Hart, 'Bisayan Filipino and Malayan Humoral Pathologies: Folk Medicine and Ethnohistory in South East Asia', Data Paper 76, SE Asia Program, Dept. of Asian Studies, Cornell University, Ithaca, New York, Nov. 1969.

C.F. Hofman, *Korte Beschreijving van de Caab de Goede Hoop* (University of Natal facsimile reproduction, 1967 [n.d. on original]).

G.H. Hofmeyr, 'King William's Town and the Xhosa, 1854-1861. The Role of a Frontier Capital During the High Commissionership of Sir George Grey' (unpublished M.A. thesis, University of Cape Town, 1981).

H. Hoving, 'Thunberg en die Kaapse inwoners' (unpublished MA, University of Stellenbosch, 1939).

M. Hunter, *Reaction to Conquest: Effects of Contact with Europeans on the Pondo of South Africa* (London: Oxford University Press, 1936).

G.A. Hutton, *Reminiscences in the Life of Surgeon-Major George A. Hutton* (London: 1907).

J. Iliffe, *The African Poor* (Cambridge: Cambridge University Press, 1987).

T. James, 'Sieketroost: Dr. James Barry's contribution to Materia Medica', *SAMJ*, lx (15 July 1972), 1013–16.

T.J. Johnson and M. Caygill, 'The British Medical Association and its Overseas Branches: A Short History', *Journal of Imperial and Commonwealth History*, i, (1972-3), 303–29.

H. Juta, *Reports of Cases in the Supreme Court*, 6 (Cape Town: Juta, 1890).

S. Kalff, 'Batavische Doctoren uit de 17e eeuw', *Staatkundig, Economisch en Letterkundig Tijdschrift*, xxxii (1910), 1136–292.

F. Kilpatrick, 'The Contagious Diseases Act of 1885 and the Dynamics of the Clanwilliam District, 1880-1910' (unpublished UCT BA Honours dissertation, 1998).

P.R. Kirby (ed.), *Andrew Smith and Natal. Documents Relating to the Early History of that Province* (Cape Town: Van Riebeeck Society, 1955).

P.R. Kirby, *Sir Andrew Smith: His Life, Letters and Work* (Cape Town: Balkema, 1965).

C. Koeman (ed.) *Tabulae Geographicae: Eighteenth-century Cartography of the Cape Colony* (Amsterdam: Hollandsch-afrikaansche Uitgewers, 1952).

P. Kolbe, *The Present State of the Cape of Good Hope*, 2 vols (London: W. Innys, 1731).

S. Koolhof and R. Ross, 'Upas, September and the Bugis at the Cape of Good Hope: The Context of a Slave's Letter', *SARI: A Journal of Malay Studies*, (forthcoming).

C.F. Krige, *To Cure Sometimes – A Doctor's Autobiography* (Johannesburg: n.d.)

B. Kruger, *The Pear Tree Blossoms: A History of the Moravian Mission Stations in South Africa 1737-1869* (Genadendal: The Provincial Board of the Moravian Church of South Africa, 1966).

P. Laidler and M. Gelfand, *South Africa: Its Medical History* (Cape Town: Struik, 1971).

M. Last, and G.L. Chavunduka (eds), *The Professionalisation of African Medicine* (Manchester: Manchester University Press, 1986).

E. Lastovica, 'Sequah, a Quack in Nineteenth Century Cape Town', *Cabo*, iv, 2 (1987), 10–18.

P. Le Feuvre, 'Cultural and Theological Factors affecting Relationships Between the Nederduitse-Gereformeerde Kerk and the Anglican Church of the Province of South Africa in the Cape Colony 1806-1910' (unpublished Ph.D. thesis, UCT, 1980).

M. Lewis, *Managing Madness: Psychiatry and Society in Australia 1788-1980* (Canberra: 1988).

M. Lichtenstein, *Foundation of the Cape*, O.H. Spohr (ed.), (Cape Town: Balkema, 1973).

M. Lichtenstein, *Travels in Southern Africa*, 2 vols (Cape Town: Van Riebeeck Society, 1928-30).

T.O. Lloyd, *The British Empire 1558-1883* (Oxford: Oxford University Press, 1984).

U. Long, *An Index to Authors of Unofficial, Privately-Owned Manuscripts Relating to the History of South Africa 1812-1920* (London: n.p., 1947).

I. Loudon, 'Medical Practitioners 1750-1850 and the Period of Medical Reform in Britain' in A. Wear (ed.), *Medicine in Society* (Cambridge: Cambridge University Press, 1992), 219–47.

J.H. Louw, *In the Shadow of Table Mountain – A History of the University of Cape Town Medical School and its Associated Teaching Hospitals up to 1940* (Cape Town: Struik, 1969).

T.J. Lucas, *Camp Life and Sport in South Africa* (Johannesburg: Africana Book Society, 1975).

J. Maberley, 'South African Pharmacology', *Transvaal Medical Journal*, i, 4 (1 November 1905), 99–104.

B. Mackenzie, *Salt River Doctor* (Cape Town: Faircape Books, 1981).

R. MacLeod and M. Lewis, *Disease, Medicine and Empire* (London: Routledge, 1988),

F. and W. Malherbe, *H.A.J.B. Hammerschmidt: Medical Practitioner in Stellenbosch 1858-1860* (Stellenbosch: Stellenbosch Museum, 1999).

S. Marks, 'What is Colonial About Colonial Medicine? And What Has Happened to Imperialism and Health?', *Social History of Medicine*, x, 2 (1997), 205–19.

S. Marks, *Divided Sisterhood: Class and Gender in the South African Nursing Profession* (London: Macmillan, 1994).

N. Mathie, *Man of Many Facets: Atherstone, Dr. W.G.* 3 vols (Grahamstown: Grocott & Sherry, 1997-8).

J. McCulloch, *Colonial Psychiatry and 'The African Mind'* (Cambridge: Cambridge University Press, 1995).

P. McMagh, *The Three Lieschings: Their Times and Contribution to Cape Medicine 1800-1843* (Cape Town: The Society for the History of Pharmacy in South Africa, 1992).

T. Meade and M. Walker (eds), *Science, Medicine and Cultural Imperialism* (Basingstoke: Macmillan, 1991).

H.S.N. Menko, *Contributions of the Netherlands to the Development of South African Medicine (1652-1902)* (Amsterdam: De Bussy, 1954).

W. Menzies, *Cases Decided in the Supreme Court of the Cape of Good Hope* (Cape Town: Juta, 1903).

F.C. Metrowich, *Assegai over the Hills* (Cape Town: Timmins, 1953).

M. Minde, 'History of Mental Health Services in South Africa', in fourteen parts, *SAMJ* (1974-77).

A. Mitchell, 'The Function and Malfunction of Mutual Aid Societies in Nineteenth-Century France' in J. Barry and C. Jones (eds) *Medicine and Charity before the Welfare State* (London: Routledge, 1991).

W. Mitchinson, 'The Toronto and Gladesville Asylums: Humane Alternatives for the Insane in Canada and Australia?', *Bulletin of the History of Medicine*, lxiii (1989), 52–72.

S.M. Mitra, *The Life and Letters of Sir John Hall* (London: Longmans, Green and Co., 1911).

E.C.G Molsbergen (ed.), *Reizen in Zuid-Afrika in de Hollandse Tijd* iv ('s-Gravenhage: Martinus Nijhoff, 1932).

J.W.D. Moodie, *Ten Years in South Africa* (London: Richard Bentley, 1835).

D. Moyle, 'Drawing the Line: The Early History of Lunacy in South Africa' (unpublished paper, Psychology Department, UCT, 1987).

D. Moyle, 'Laying Down the Line: the Emergence of a Racial Psychiatric Practice in the Cape Colony During the Nineteenth Century' (unpublished paper, Psychology Department, UCT, 1988).

J. Murray (ed.) *Mrs Dale's Diary 1857-72* (Cape Town: Balkema, 1966).

M. Naude, 'The Role of the Free Dispensary in Public Health in Cape Town' (unpublished B.A. thesis, UCT, 1987).

C. Newman, *The Evolution of Medical Education in the Nineteenth Century* (New York: Oxford University Press, 1957).

H. Ngubane, *Body and Mind in Zulu Medicine* (London: New York Academic Press, 1977).

J. Noble (ed.) *The Cape and its People, and Other Essays* (Cape Town: Juta, 1869).

J.M. Orpen, *Reminiscences of Life in South Africa from 1846 to the Present Day* (Cape Town: Struik, 1964).

R.M. Packard, *White Plague, Black Labor: Tuberculosis and the Political Economy of Health and Disease in South Africa* (Berkeley: University of California Press, 1989).

L. Pappe, 'A List of South African Indigenous Plants used as Remedies by the Colonists', *Cape Town Medical Gazette*, i, 2 & 4 (April, October 1847).

J.B. Peires, *The Dead Will Arise: Nongqawuse and the Great Xhosa Cattle-Killing Movement Of 1856-7* (Johannesburg: Ravan, 1989).

J.B. Peires, *The House of Phalo: A History of the Xhosa People in the Days of their Independence* (Johannesburg: Ravan, 1981).

A.N. Pelzer, *Geskiedenis van die Suid-Afrikaanse Republiek*, 3 vols (Cape Town: Balkema. 1950).

T.S. Pensabene, *The Rise of the Medical Practitioner in Victoria* (Canberra: Australian National University, 1980).

R. Percival, *An Account of the Cape of Good Hope* (London: Baldwin, 1804).

H. Phillips, '"Black October": The Impact of the Spanish Influenza epidemic of 1918 on South Africa,' *Archives Year Book for South African History*, i (1990).

E. Pretorius, 'Alternative (Complementary?) Medicine in South Africa', *SA Sociological Journal*, xxiv, 1 (1993), 13–17.

C.H. Price, 'Diary of Dr. Mackrill', *Africana Notes and News*, xiii, 8 (Dec. 1959), 314–16.

C.H. Price, 'J.T. Pocock – Pioneer – Pharmacist Part II', *South African Pharmaceutical Journal*, xxvii, 6 (February 1961), 15–21.

W.H.J. Punt, *Louis Trichardt se Laaste Skof* (Pretoria: Van Schaik, 1953).

S.R. Quah, 'The Social Position and Organisation of the Medical Profession in the Third World: The Case of Singapore', *Journal of Health and Social Behaviour*, xxx (1989), 450–66.

I. Rae, *The Strange Story of Dr James Barry* (London: Longmans Green, 1958).

B.M. Randles, *A History of the Kaffrarian Museum* (King William's Town: The Museum, 1984).

B. Roberts, *Kimberley: Turbulent City* (Cape Town: David Philip, 1976).

C.G. Roland (ed.) *Health, Disease and Medicine: Essays in Canadian history* (Toronto: Hannah Institute 1984), 65–95.

T.M. Romano, 'Professional Identity and the Nineteenth Century Ontario Medical Profession', *Social History*, xxviii, 55 (May 1995).

J. Rose, *The Perfect Gentleman: The Remarkable Life of Dr James Miranda Barry* (London: 1977).

C.E. Rosenberg, *The Care of Strangers: The Rise of America's Hospital System* (Baltimore: Johns Hopkins University Press, 1987).

L. Rosner, *Medical Education in the Age of Improvement – Edinburgh Students and Apprentices 1760-1826* (Edinburgh: Edinburgh University Press, 1994).

J. Ross, *A Few Chapters on Public Health, Adapted for South Africa*, (King William's Town: Hay, 1887).

R. Ross, 'The anthropology of the Germanic-speaking Peoples of Southern Africa', paper presented at the Conference on History and Anthropology, University of Manchester, 1980, *JSAS* 8, 1, (1981).

R. Rotberg, *The Founder: Cecil Rhodes and the Pursuit of Power* (Oxford: Southern Book Publishers, 1988).

A.J.T. Roux, 'The Relationship Between the Government and the Medical Profession in South Africa', *SAMR*, xxiv (1926).

M. Ryan, *A History of Organised Pharmacy in South Africa 1885-1950* (Cape Town: The Society for the History of Pharmacy in South Africa, 1986).

E.M. Sandler (ed.), *Dear Dr Bolus – Letters... by C. Louis Leipoldt to Harry Bolus... 1897 to 1911* (Cape Town: Balkema, 1979).

E.M. Sandler, 'The First Caesarean Section at the Cape of Good Hope', *South African Journal of Obstetrics and Gynaecology* (17 June 1967).

E.M. Sandler, 'Lichtenstein's Vaccination Tour – 1805', Supplement to *SAMJ*, lxviii (1974).

H. Sauer, *Ex Africa* (London: Geoffrey Bles, 1937).

C. Saunders, 'The Creation of Ndabeni: Urban Segregation and African Resistance in Cape Town', *Studies in the History of Cape Town*, i (Cape Town, 1984), 165-193

C.G.W. Schumann, *Structural Change and Business Cycles in South Africa, 1806-1946* (London: P.S. King, 1938).

C. Searle, *A History of the Development of Nursing in South Africa 1652-1960* (Cape Town: Struik, 1965).

M.W. Searle (ed.) *Cases Decided in the Supreme Court, 1857-1860,* vol.3 (Cape Town: Juta, 1888).

S.E. Shortt (ed.) *Medicine in Canadian Society* (Montreal: McGill-Queen's University Press, 1981).

S.E.D. Shortt, 'Physicians, Science and Status: Issues in the Professionalisation of Anglo-American Medicine in the 19th Century', *Medical History* xxvii (1983), 51–68.

C. Simkins and E. Van Heyningen, 'Fertility, Mortality and Migration in the Cape Colony, 1891-1904', *International Journal of African Historical Studies*, xx, 1 (1989), 79–111.

P. Simon, *Old Mutual 1845-1995* (Cape Town: Human & Rousseau, 1995).

A.R. Skelley, *The Victorian Army at Home: The Recruitment and Terms and Conditions of the British Regular, 1859-1988* (London: Croom Helm, 1977).

A. Smith, *A Contribution to South African Materia Medica Chiefly from Plants in Use among the Natives* (Lovedale: Lovedale Press, 1888).

I. Smith (ed.), *The Siege of Mafeking* (Johannesburg: The Brenthurst Press, 2001).

A. Sparrman, *A Voyage to the Cape of Good Hope* (London: G.G.J. & J. Robinson, 1786).

P. Starr, *The Social Transformation of American Medicine* (New York: Basic Books, 1982).

E.S. Stevenson, *The Adventures of a Medical Man* (Cape Town: Juta, 1925).

A.L. Stoler and F. Cooper, 'Between Metropole and Colony' in F. Cooper and A.L. Stoler (eds) *Tensions of Empire: Colonial Cultures in a Bourgeois World* (Berkeley: University of California Press, 1997), 1–56.

F. Swanson, 'Colonial Madness: The Construction of Gender in the Grahamstown Lunatic Asylum, 1875-1905' (unpublished B.A. thesis, UCT, 1994)

M.W. Swanson, 'The Sanitation Syndrome: Bubonic Plague and Urban Native Policy in the Cape Colony, 1900-1909,' *JAH*, xvi 3, (1977).

S. Swartz, '"Work of Mercy and Necessity": British Rule and Psychiatric Practice in the Cape Colony 1891-1910', *International Journal of Mental Health*, xxviii, 2 (Summer 1999), 72–90.

S. Swartz, 'Colonialism and the Production of Psychiatric Knowledge in the Cape, 1891-1920' (unpublished Ph.D. thesis, UCT, 1996).

A. Thomas, *Rhodes* (London: BBC Books, 1996).

R. Thornton and T.E. Fuller, *The Epidemic in Cape Town, 1867-68* (Cape Town: Juta, 1868).

C.P. Thunberg, *Travels at the Cape of Good Hope 1772-1775*, V.S. Forbes (ed.), (Cape Town: Van Riebeeck Society, 1986).

J.H. Treble, *Urban poverty in Britain 1830-1914* (London: Batsford Academic Press, 1979).

E.B. van Heyningen, 'Agents of Empire: The Medical Profession in the Cape Colony, 1880-1910', *Medical History*, xxx (1989), 450–71.

E.B. van Heyningen, 'Cape Town and the Plague of 1901', *Studies in the History of Cape Town*, iv (Cape Town: UCT History Workshop, 1984), 66–107.

E.B. van Heyningen, 'Leander Starr Jameson' in J. Carruthers (ed.), *The Jameson Raid. A Centennial Retrospective* (Johannesburg: The Brenthurst Press, 1996), 181–91.

E.B. van Heyningen, 'Medicine and Empire: The Transmission of Ideas and Disease Between India, Australia, New Zealand and the Cape Colony in the Nineteenth Century', paper presented at the Ninth Historical Geography Conference, Perth, 1995.

E.B. van Heyningen, 'Poverty, Self-Help and Community: The Survival of the Poor in Cape Town, 1880-1910', *SAHJ*, xxiv (1991), 128–43.

E.B. van Heyningen, 'Public Health and Society in Cape Town, 1880-1910' (unpublished Ph.D. thesis, University of Cape Town, 1989).

E.B.. van Heyningen, 'The Social Evil in the Cape Colony 1868-1902: Prostitution and the Contagious Diseases Acts', *JSAS*, x, 2 (April 1984), 170–97.

E.B. van Heyningen, 'Women and Disease: The Clash of Medical Cultures in the Concentration Camps' in University of South Africa Library, *Rethinking the South African War* (forthcoming).

E.B. van Heyningen, 'Women Under Siege' in I. Smith (ed.), *The Siege of Mafeking* (Johannesburg: The Brenthurst Press, 2001).

M.J. van Lieburg and H. Marland, 'Midwife Regulation, Education, and Practice in the Netherlands during the Nineteenth Century', *Medical History*, xxxiii (1989), 296–317.

M. Vaughan, *Curing Their Ills: Colonial Power and African Illness* (Cambridge: Cambridge University Press, 1991).

M. Vaughan, 'Idioms of Madness: Zomba Lunatic Asylum, Nyasaland, in the Colonial Period', *JSAS*, ix, 2 (1983), 218–38.

R. Viljoen, 'Disease and Society: VOC Cape Town, its People and the Smallpox Epidemics of 1713, 1755 and 1767', *Kleio*, xxvii (1995), 22–45.

R. Viljoen, 'Diseases and Doctoring: Khoikhoi, Diseases and Medicine at the Cape of Good Hope', unpublished paper presented at the SSHM Summer Conference, Medicine and the Colonies, Oxford, July 1996.

J. Walton, B.B. Beeson and R.B. Scott (eds), *Oxford Companion to Medicine*, 2 vols (Oxford and New York: Oxford University Press, 1986).

H. Ward, *Five Years in Kaffirland*, 2 vols (London: Colburn, 1948)

J.H. Warner, *The Therapeutic Perspective: Medical Practice, Knowledge and Identity in America, 1820-1885* (Princeton: Princeton University Press, 1986).

R.C. Warwick, 'Mental Health Care at Valkenberg Asylum 1891-1909' (unpublished B.A. thesis, UCT, 1989).

D. Warren, 'Merchants, Commissioners and Wardmasters: Municipal Politics in Cape Town 1840-1854' (unpublished M.A. thesis, UCT, 1986).

J.M. Watt, 'The History of Pharmacology in South Africa', *Journal of the Medical Association of South Africa*, i (22 October 1927), 528–34.

J.M. Watt and M.G. Breyer-Brandwijk, *The Medicinal and Poisonous Plants of Southern Africa* (Edinburgh: Livingstone, 1932).

J. Wells, *Stewart of Lovedale: the life of James Stewart, D.D., M.D.* (London: Hodder & Stoughton, 1908).

J.D.H. Widdess, *The Royal College of Surgeons in Ireland and its Medical School 1784-1966*, 2nd edn (Edinburgh and London: E. & S. Livingstone, 1967).

D. Williams, *Umfundisi. A Biography of Tiyo Soga, 1829-1871* (Lovedale: Lovedale Press, 1978).

M. Wilson, and L. Thompson (eds), *The Oxford History of South Africa*, Vol. I – *South Africa to 1870* (Oxford: Oxford University Press, 1969).

N.Worden, E. Van Heyningen, and J.V. Bickford-Smith, *Cape Town: The Making of a City* (Cape Town: David Philip, 1998).

W.H. Worger, *South Africa's City of Diamonds: Mine Workers and Monopoly Capitalism in Kimberley 1867-1895* (New Haven: Yale University Press, 1987).

A.J. Youngson, *The Scientific Revolution in Victorian Medicine* (London: Croom Helm, 1979).

Index

303

INTERNATIONAL JOURNAL OF HEALTH SERVICES
Editor-in-Chief: Vicente Navarro

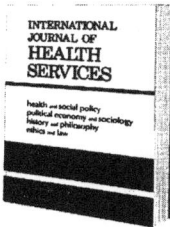

The *International Journal of Health Services* is one of the best known refereed quarterlies that covers health and social policy, political economy and sociology, history and philosophy, ethics and law, focusing on issues of health, social well being, and quality of life, with analyses of the socioeconomic and political interventions that affect them. Recent topics include studies on social inequalities and the impact of globalization on health and social policies. The *International Journal of Health Services* has been called one of the most stimulating and exciting journals in the health and social policy field.

RECENTLY PUBLISHED ARTICLES

Special Report on the Political and Social Contexts of Health:

Part 1——Introduction: Objectives and Purposes of the Study • *Vicente Navarro*

The Importance of the Political and the Social in Explaining Mortality Differentials among the Countries of the OECD, 1950-1998
Vicente Navarro, Carme Borrell, Joan Benach, Carles Muntaner, Agueda Quiroga, Maica Rodriguez-Sanz, Nuria Vergés, Jordi Gumá, and M. Isabel Pasarin

Do Social Policies and Political Context Matter for Health in the United Kingdom? • *Tim Doran and Margaret Whitehead*

An Analysis of the Role of Health Care in Reducing Socioeconomic Inequalities in Health: The Case of the Netherlands • *Johan P. Mackenbach*

The Health of Peoples: Predicaments Facing a Reasoned Utopia • *Richard Horton*

Sex and Gender: The Challenges for Epidemiologists • *Lesley Doyal*

Globalization and the Pharmaceutical Industry Revisited • *Joan Busfield*

Uneven Health Outcomes and Political Resistance under Residual Neoliberalism in Africa • *Patrick Bond and George Dor*

Complimentary sample issue available upon request

Subscription Information: ISSN: 0020-7314, Price per volume (4 issues yearly)
$252.00 Institutional;$64.00 Individual
Postage and handling: $10.00 U.S. and Canada; $18.00 elsewhere

BAYWOOD PUBLISHING COMPANY, INC.
26 Austin Avenue, PO Box 337, Amityville, NY 11701
phone (631) 691-1270 • fax (631) 691-1770 • toll-free orderline (800) 638-7819
e-mail: baywood@baywood.com • web site: http://baywood.com

Africa and Its Significant Others.
Forty Years of Intercultural Entanglement.

Edited by Isabel Hoving, Frans-Willem Korsten and Ernst van Alphen.

Amsterdam/New York, NY 2003. 208 pp.
(Thamyris Intersecting Place, Sex and Race 11)
ISBN: 90-420-1029-0   € 40,/US$ 50.-

When did the intimate dialogue between Africa, Europe, and the Americas begin? Looking back, it seems as if these three continents have always been each other's significant others. Europe created its own modern identity by using Africa as a mirror, but Africans traveled to Europe and America long before the European age of discovery, and African cultures can be said to lie at the root of European culture. This intertwining has become ever more visible: Nowadays Africa emerges as a highly visible presence in the Americas, and African American styles capture Europe's youth, many of whom are of (North-) African descent. This entanglement, however, remains both productive and destructive. The continental economies are intertwined in ways disastrous for Africa, and African knowledge is all too often exported and translated for US and European scholarly aims, which increases the intercontinental knowledge gap.

This volume proposes a fresh look at the vigorous and painful, but inescapable, relationships between these significant others. It does so as a gesture of gratitude and respect to one of the pioneering figures in this field. Dutch Africanist and literary scholar Mineke Schipper, who is taking her leave from her chair in Intercultural Literary Studies at the University of Leiden. Where have the past four decades of African studies brought us? What is the present-day state of this intercontinental dialogue?

USA/Canada: One Rockefeller Plaza, Ste. 1420, New York, NY 10020,
Tel. (212) 265-6360, Call toll-free (U.S. only) 1-800-225-3998,
Fax (212) 265-6402
All other countries: Tijnmuiden 7, 1046 AK Amsterdam, The Netherlands.
Tel. ++ 31 (0)20 611 48 21, Fax ++ 31 (0)20 447 29 79
Orders-queries@rodopi.nl   **www.rodopi.nl**
Please note that the exchange rate is subject to fluctuations

Africa's Quest for a Philosophy of Decolonization.

Messay Kebede

Amsterdam/New York, NY 2004. XIII, 256 pp.
(Value Inquiry Book Series 153)
ISBN: 90-420-0810-5   € 52,-/ US$ 68.-

This book discovers freedom in the colonial idea of African primitiveness. As human transcendence, freedom escapes the drawbacks of otherness, as defended by ethnophilosophy, while exposing the idiosyncratic inspiration of Eurocentric universalism. Decolonization calls for the reconnection with freedom, that is, with myth-making understood as the inaugural act of cultural pluralism. The cultural condition of modernization emerges when the return to the past deploys the future.

"If you have time to read only one book to learn about the intricacies of African philosophy, then read *Africa's Quest for a Philosophy of Decolonization*. The beauty of this volume is Kebede's clear presentation and thoughtful evaluation of each of the main schools in African Philosophy".
Joseph C. Kunkel
University of Dayton

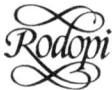

Rodopi

USA/Canada: One Rockefeller Plaza, Ste. 1420, New York, NY 10020,
Tel. (212) 265-6360, Call toll-free (U.S. only) 1-800-225-3998,
Fax (212) 265-6402
All other countries: Tijnmuiden 7, 1046 AK Amsterdam, The Netherlands.
Tel. ++ 31 (0)20 611 48 21, Fax ++ 31 (0)20 447 29 79
Orders-queries@rodopi.nl   **www.rodopi.nl**
Please note that the exchange rate is subject to fluctuations

African Diasporas in the New and Old Worlds:

Consciousness and Imagination.

Edited by Geneviève Fabre and Klaus Benesch.

Amsterdam/New York, NY 2004. XXI, 358 pp. (Cross/Cultures 69)
ISBN: 90-420-0880-6   Bound € 80,-/US$ 100.-
ISBN: 90-420-0870-9   Paper € 36,-/US$ 45.-

In the humanities, the term 'diaspora' recently emerged as a promising and powerful heuristic concept. It challenged traditional ways of thinking and invited reconsiderations of theoretical assumptions about the unfolding of cross-cultural and multi-ethnic societies, about power relations, frontiers and boundaries, about cultural transmission, communication and translation. The present collection of essays by renowned writers and scholars addresses these issues and helps to ground the ongoing debate about the African diaspora in a more solid theoretical framework. Part I is dedicated to a general discussion of the concept of African diaspora, its origins and historical development. Part II examines the complex cultural dimensions of African diasporas in relation to significant sites and figures, including the modes and modalities of creative expression from the perspective of both artists/writers and their audiences; finally, Part III focusses on the resources (collections and archives) and iconographies that are available today. As most authors argue, the African diaspora should not be seen merely as a historical phenomenon, but also as an idea or ideology and an object of representation. By exploring this new ground, the essays assembled here provide important new insights for scholars in American and African-American Studies, Cultural Studies, Ethnic Studies, and African Studies. The collection is rounded off by an annotated listing of black autobiographies.

USA/Canada: One Rockefeller Plaza, Ste. 1420, New York, NY 10020,
Tel. (212) 265-6360, Call toll-free (U.S. only) 1-800-225-3998,
Fax (212) 265-6402
All other countries: Tijnmuiden 7, 1046 AK Amsterdam, The Netherlands.
Tel. ++ 31 (0)20 611 48 21, Fax ++ 31 (0)20 447 29 79
Orders-queries@rodopi.nl   **www.rodopi.nl**
Please note that the exchange rate is subject to fluctuations

Rodopi

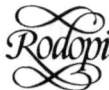